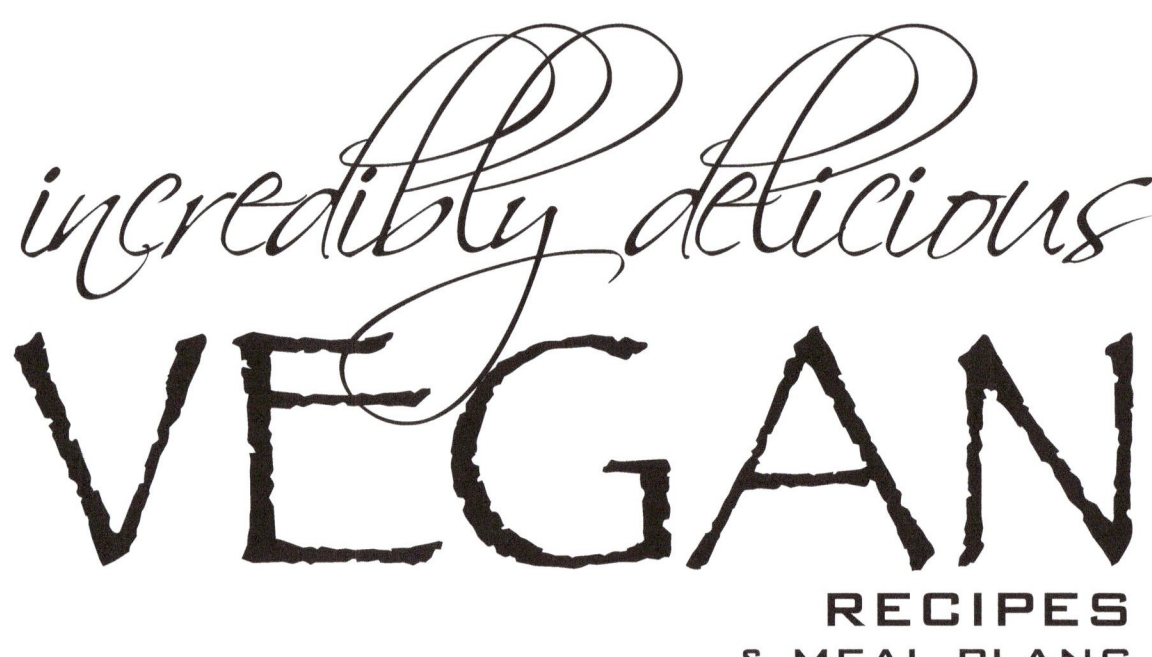

incredibly delicious VEGAN
RECIPES & MEAL PLANS

DR. DONA COOPER-DOCKERY
and Cooper Wellness Center

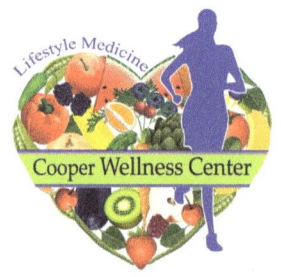

drdonacooper.com
cooperwellnesscenter.com
cooperinternalmedicine.com

$29.95 US

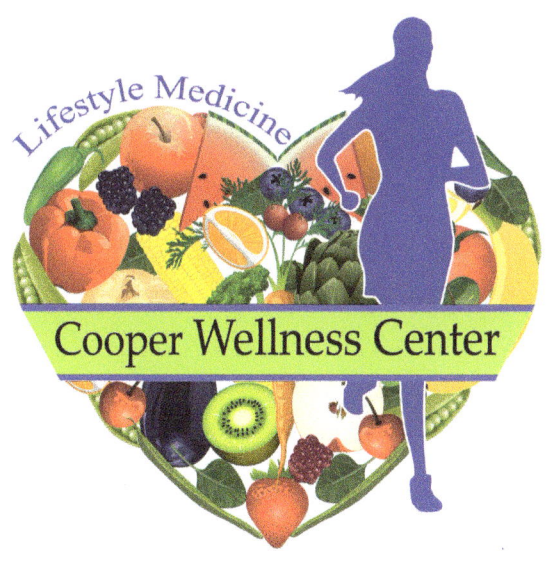

Get Healthy with Dr. Cooper™
3604 N. McColl Road
McAllen, TX 78501
www.drdonacooper.com
Copyright ©2019 by Dona Cooper-Dockery, M.D.

All rights reserved. No part of this book may be reproduced, stored in a retrieval system, or transmitted, in any form or by any means including electronic, mechanical, photocopying, recording or otherwise without prior written permission from the publisher and/or author.

Any Biblical quotations, unless otherwise noted, are taken from The Holy Bible, New King James Version (NKJV).

Copy edited by: Dahlia Burroughs
Cover design and interior design by: Debra Marcketti

ISBN: 978-1-7331654-1-9 (Print)
ISBN: 978-1-7331654-4-0 (eBook)

Printed in the U.S.A.

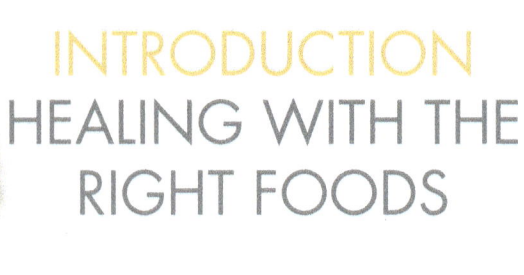

INTRODUCTION
HEALING WITH THE RIGHT FOODS

Most practicing physicians will confess that nutrition was not emphasized during their medical training. However, using food as medicine and focusing on a healthy lifestyle is now fast becoming the gold standard in managing patients with chronic diseases, such as diabetes, heart disease, hypertension, and even cancer.

If we were to review books throughout history, we would notice that the lack of consumption of certain foods led to a significant loss of lives. For instance, scurvy is now a rare disease, but in the 1600s and 1700s, it was a major medical concern. Soldiers were overcome with severe symptoms, such as loose teeth, loss of appetite, diarrhea, fever, numbness, skin lesions, internal hemorrhaging, and occasional paralysis. It was not uncommon for this disease to cause death. In fact, the history books tell us that Christopher Columbus lost many sailors as a result of scurvy. What was the cause of this dreadful disease? A lack of fresh fruits and vegetables! In 1747, while serving as a naval surgeon, Dr. James Lind carried out experiments and discovered the cause of scurvy and potential treatments. He discovered that the sailors who suffered from scurvy had their symptoms reversed when fed citrus fruits.[1]

Sailors were also afflicted with beriberi—a degenerative disease with symptoms such as weight loss, swelling extremities, body weakness and pain, brain damage, irregular heart rate, heart failure, and death, if left untreated. In the 1880s, beriberi reached epidemic proportions in the Dutch colonies. Toward the end of the 19th century, Christiaan Eijkman—a Dutch surgeon who was serving in the Dutch colonial army in exchange for his education as a physician—traced the cause of the disease to diets that included polished and processed white rice rather than unpolished brown rice.[2]

In 1906, the British biochemist Sir Frederick Gowland Hopkins demonstrated that food contained what he called accessory factors; but it wasn't until the chemist Casimir Funk found the vital substance that Eijkman called the anti-beriberi factor that the true

cure was identified. Funk gave it the name vitamine. He coined the word by combining vital and amine. This name later came to denote all vitamins and was accepted by the scientific community in 1912.[3]

What Does It All Mean?

Vitamins are nutrients which are present in food in small quantities, but in the 1800s this term was unheard of. According to the Centers for Disease Control and Prevention, (CDC) nearly two billion people are vitamin-deficient, with at least half of the children worldwide, ages 6 months to 5 years, suffering from one or more micronutrient deficiency.[4]

Let Food Be Thy Medicine and Medicine Be Thy Food.
~ Hippocrates

Micronutrients is the umbrella term for vitamins and minerals, called thus as you only need small (micro) quantities of them in order to stay healthy; if a person should fail to get the required amounts, disease and illness are virtually guaranteed. Micronutrients assist the body's development, function, ability to prevent disease, and overall well-being. Micronutrients must be derived from the food we consume. It is estimated that the average adult in developed countries eats approximately six hundred grams of food per day. Less than one gram of that food consists of vitamins.[5]

Nutrients

We have all heard the term nutrients, nutrition or some other variation of the word. Due to recent trends, people are becoming a lot more conscious of the kinds of foods they are eating. However, people are still becoming ill, and aging and dying prematurely. Cases of type 2 diabetes and obesity are still rising at an alarming rate—faster than they ever have before. How can this be? A lot of myths and false information surrounds this topic. In an effort to combat these issues, we are going to break down the subject into easy-to-digest sections….pun intended.

Nutrients are substances in foods that provide energy and materials for cell development, growth, and repair. There are six major types of nutrients in food:

- carbohydrates
- proteins
- lipids
- vitamins
- minerals
- water

Carbohydrates, proteins, vitamins, and fats are organic nutrients that can be broken down by heat, air, or acid. Unfortunately, their characteristics, cooking, storage, and even exposure to air, can inactivate these fragile compounds. Minerals and water, on the other hand, are inorganic and have a more robust chemical structure which can withstand more exposure.[7] It is also interesting to note that, unlike carbohydrates, proteins, vitamins, and fats which are made up of two or more molecules, minerals are stand-alone compounds that appear on the periodic table of elements. Nutritionists and other healthcare providers determine the recommended daily amount or RDA of a nutrient by how much the body needs of it to stay healthy. Nutrients can be obtained in a variety of ways, ranging from dietary choices to supplemental intake. A nutritional deficiency is when the body doesn't, or cannot, absorb the necessary amount of a nutrient.[8]

Carbohydrates

Although carbohydrates are not considered to be an essential nutrient, they are our body's main source of energy. They are comprised mostly of carbon (C), hydrogen (H), and oxygen (O) atoms. The body utilizes most carbohydrates to generate glucose, which serves as the basic functional particle of energy within the cells. Kilocalories (kcal) are the result, with an average of 4 kcal per gram (kcal/g) of carbohydrate. A kilocalorie is equivalent to one calorie on a nutritional label of a packaged food.[9] However, not all carbohydrates are the same. Simple sugars are the smallest carbohydrates and are made up of one or two sugar molecules. Polysaccharides are complex carbohydrates made up of many sugar molecules. Some examples of these forms of carbohydrates are potatoes, beans, and vegetables. Dietary fiber is another form of complex carbohydrates where the sugar molecules are linked together. However, the body cannot usually break these links apart and they pass through with minimal changes.

Proteins

I am sure that we have all heard of the importance of protein. The emphasis is not exaggerated at all. Every cell in our body contains protein. Proteins are essential for tissue growth and cellular repair. They are also the major component in the makeup of bone, muscle, and other tissues and fluids. They are created through the process of linking different combinations and large quantities of the twenty amino acids, or building blocks, found in our food. Our inherited genes typically dictate how the proteins are formed. When used as an energy source, protein supplies an average of 4 kilocalories per gram. In the American diet today, it is rare to come across a case of protein deficiency. Most Americans eat up to two times the required protein portion necessary to maintain adequate health.

Lipids

Lipids consist of fats and oils. Fat is basically concentrated energy that yields high volumes of energy-producing molecules. They are composed mostly of carbon (C), hydrogen (H) and oxygen (O). Lipids are an important part of our bodily functions. They assist in helping our bodies store fat-soluble vitamins and provide high levels of stored energy for when we need it. Fats, in the form of fat tissues, or adipose tissues, also cushion and protect our internal organs and skeletal infrastructure. A healthy diet should consist of no more than thirty percent fat. Unfortunately, we are seeing that fat consumption is rising above the recommended dosage in the average person's diets, leading to detrimental states of health, such as the obesity and diabetes crises. Studies show that four out of five people with type 2 diabetes are overweight or obese. Excess fat, especially abdominal fat, changes the way that the body responds to insulin, leading to a condition called insulin resistance. With this condition, the cells cannot use insulin to process blood sugar out of the blood, resulting in high blood sugar levels.

Vitamins

There are thirteen essential vitamins that are required for the human body to function properly. Four of these vitamins can be produced in the body naturally but usually in insufficient amounts and must be supplemented through dietary consumption. Otherwise, the body will experience the symptoms of deficiency for that particular nutrient. Vitamins are divided into two categories: water-soluble and fat-soluble. Vitamins A, D, E, and K are the four fat-soluble vitamins. The eight B vitamins and vitamin C make up the other nine water-soluble vitamins. Of the eight B vitamins, two are made in our intestines. Each vitamin contributes its own characteristics in the role of human and even animal health.

Contrary to popular belief, avoiding fats completely can be harmful to the body. Fats play an important role in fat-soluble vitamins' ability to be absorbed by the body, once stored in the body's fatty tissue. It is because of the presence of dietary fat that these nutrients can be absorbed. Because much of your body consists of water, many of the water-soluble vitamins circulate easily throughout the body. The kidneys continuously regulate their levels by discharging excesses out of the body in urine. They are absorbed directly into the bloodstream as food is broken down in the digestion process. Normally, water-soluble vitamins do not remain in the body for very long. Vitamin B12 is the only water-soluble vitamin that can be stored in the liver for many years.

Minerals

Trace minerals are exactly what they sound like. They are minerals where only traces are found in the human body. They are distinctly inorganic compounds with usually nothing more than a molecule or two of an element. Although minerals do not contribute to energy production, they support other vital functions that we require to survive. They promote cellular reactions, help to balance the water levels in the body and support structural systems, such as the skeletal system.

Major minerals are more prevalent in the body; however, they are no more important to a person's health than trace minerals. Major minerals travel through and enrich our bodies in different ways. For example, potassium behaves much like water-soluble vitamins do. It is quickly absorbed into the bloodstream where it can circulate freely until it is excreted by the kidneys. In contrast, calcium requires a carrier for absorption and transport. Iron is an essential mineral critical for motor and cognitive development. When iron levels are low, a condition called anemia occurs. Iron deficiency is considered the most common and widespread nutritional disorder in the world according to the World Health Organization.[10] It is not only a significant crisis in developing countries, but developed and industrialized countries as well.[11]

Food for Thought

There is no super-food that contains the full range of essential vitamins and minerals that a human needs in order to survive. However, there are plant-based foods that contain many of them. For example, kale is known to be a nutrient powerhouse and scientists are discovering more and more health benefits that are derived from plants such as the moringa tree. The wonderful thing about a plant-based diet is the fact that they are known to prevent and even reverse the onset of chronic illnesses such as diabetes, cardiovascular disease, hypertension, and more. This diet also contains no cholesterol and usually fewer calories and less fat than animal product-rich diet. Many studies now report the potential health risk with diets high in red and processed meat, animal fats, processed foods, sugar, salts, and additives. Scientists have also confirmed that a diet high in fruits, vegetables, nuts, seeds and whole grains is essential to prevent and cure chronic diseases and some cancers.

Vegetables

The doctor of the future will give no medicine, but will interest her or his patients in the care of the human frame, in a proper diet .
~ Thomas Edison

Nutrient-dense vegetables—especially leafy greens, cruciferous vegetables, and other green vegetables—are important for good health and their regular intake cannot be overemphasized. Medical professionals typically recommend that a person eats five or more servings of vegetables per day. Higher green vegetable consumption is associated with a lower risk of developing type 2 diabetes, and among diabetics, higher green vegetable intake is associated with lower HbA1c levels. A recent meta-analysis found that greater leafy green intake was associated with a 14% decrease in risk of type 2 diabetes. One study reported that each daily serving of leafy greens produces a 9% decrease in risk of developing diabetes.

As mentioned previously, kale is a powerhouse, nutrient-rich food that is an excellent source of vitamins A, C, and K, as well as calcium, folate, and potassium. Other noteworthy greens include:

- Spinach
- Collard Greens
- Broccoli
- Romaine Lettuce

Non-starchy vegetables like mushrooms, onions, garlic, eggplant, and peppers are essential components of a chronic illness prevention (or reversal) diet. These foods have almost non-existent effects on blood glucose and are packed with fiber and phytochemicals.

Fruits

Most fruits are naturally low in fat, sodium, and calories and, as with vegetables, none of them contain cholesterol. They are good sources of many essential nutrients that are under-consumed in our society today, including:

- Potassium
- Dietary Fiber
- Vitamin C
- Folate (folic acid)

Research shows that healthy potassium consumption in a person's diet may help to maintain healthy blood pressure. Dietary fiber obtained from fruits helps to reduce blood cholesterol levels and may even lower a person's risk of heart disease. Fiber is important for proper bowel function. It helps reduce constipation and diverticulosis. Fiber-containing foods, such as fruits, help provide a feeling of fullness with fewer calories. However, it is important to note that although whole or cut-up fruits are great sources of dietary fiber, fruit juices may contain little or no fiber at all. Fruits are also great sources of vitamin C, which is important for growth and repair of all body tissues, helps heal cuts and wounds, and keeps teeth and gums healthy.

Folate (folic acid) helps the body form red blood cells. Women of childbearing age who may become pregnant should consume adequate folate from foods, and in addition 400 mcg of synthetic folic acid from fortified foods or supplements. This reduces the risk of neural tube defects, spina bifida, and anencephaly during fetal development.

Nuts & Seeds

Thou should eat to live; not live to eat.
~ Socrates

Nuts and seeds are natural hunger-busters, not only because of their fat content but also because of their protein and fiber content. All nuts contain fiber, which helps lower cholesterol while anchoring a person's blood sugar. Most nuts, especially peanuts, contain other slimming nutrients. Peanuts could be considered the unsung heroes when it comes to building lean muscle mass because they contain the non-essential amino acid L-arginine. L-arginine is being studied for its ability to lessen body fat while helping to build lean muscle mass at the same time. Nuts also contain a wide array of antioxidants and vital minerals that most people lack, such as:

- Manganese
- Calcium
- Iron
- Chromium
- Zinc
- Selenium which is important for many physiological and metabolic functions.

If you're looking to lose fat, eating healthy fats for weight loss is important! It might seem counter-intuitive, but not getting enough good quality fats along with other vital nutrients in your diet can sabotage your weight loss efforts.

Grains

Healthcare practitioners recommend that people eat at least three or more servings of whole grains each day. Processed grains such as polished rice and white flour are stripped of their nutritional values and need to be artificially fortified with the necessary vitamins and minerals that the human body requires for good health. Whole grains, on the other hand, are packed with essential vitamins and minerals and are a great source of nutrients such as fiber, calcium, and others. Examples include:

- Brown rice
- Barley
- Rye
- Quinoa
- Bulgar wheat
- Whole wheat bread and pasta

Moreover, grains are essential because they offer great sources of good carbohydrates which the body uses as energy.

Beans, Lentils, and other legumes

Beans, lentils, and other legumes are the ideal carbohydrate source. Beans are low in glycemic load, due to their moderate protein, abundant fiber and resistant starch content. Beans contain carbohydrates that are not broken down in the small intestine. This reduces the amount of calories that can be absorbed from beans. Additionally, resistant starch is fermented by bacteria in the colon, forming products that protect against colon cancer. Accordingly, bean and legume consumption is associated with reduced risk of both diabetes and colon cancer.

Beans are very high in fiber and low on the glycemic index. They give you about 1/3 of your daily fiber requirements in just a 1/2 cup (at around 190 calories) and are also good sources of magnesium (important for heart health) and potassium (crucial for muscle function and hydration). Like berries and greens, beans are in the running for the top anti-oxidant rich foods, this is a little-known fact. Kidney and red beans rank highest, then black beans following close behind. Black beans are especially good for digestive tract health and have been studied in the context of colon cancer. If you have trouble digesting beans, here are two easy tips:

- Start by eating small portions, say 2 heaping tablespoons, to help your digestion become used to them until they cause less discomfort.
- If you don't mind cooking your beans from scratch, soaking dried beans helps remove some of the flatulence-causing substances.

As with everything in life, it is important to remember the rule of moderation. Portion size is a substantial aspect of healthy eating habits. Unrealistic portion sizes are one of the top causes of overeating. Today, modern packaging does not exemplify correct portion sizes for a healthy diet. A good example of an appropriate portion size is an amount equal to the size of a person's fist for most foods.

In Summary

By not fueling our bodies with foods that provide us with the nutrition we need, we are creating hazardous conditions inside of ourselves. Fueling our bodies and making sure that we have all the nutrients that we need, simply cannot be neglected if we want to maximize our health and our quality of life.

Just about 99% of human body mass is made up of six collective elements. They are oxygen, carbon, hydrogen, nitrogen, calcium, and phosphorus. Another five elements, potassium, sulfur, sodium, chlorine, and magnesium make up the other 0.85%. Every one of these elements is vital to life and we need to ensure that we do our part by giving our bodies what they need through healthy nutrition.

Heathy Swaps

As you transition to a healthier diet there are certain substitutions that might be challenging. Therefore, I decided to add this section in this book just to allow you to continue to enjoy the recipes that probably have been in your family for years.

Egg Replacements:

APPLESAUCE
Use 1/4 cup of unsweetened applesauce in place of one egg in most baking recipes. Some sources say to mix it with 1/2 teaspoon of baking powder. If all you have is sweetened applesauce, then simply reduce the amount of sugar in the recipe. Applesauce is also a popular healthy replacement for oil in many baked goods.

BANANA
Use 1/4 cup of mashed banana (about half a banana) instead of one egg when baking. Note that this may impart a mild banana flavor to whatever you are cooking, which could be a good thing.

FLAXSEEDS
Believe it or not, heart-healthy flaxseeds can be used as an egg substitute. Simply mix 1 tablespoon of ground flaxseeds with 3 tablespoons of water until fully absorbed and viscous. Use in place of one egg. (You can use pre-ground flaxseeds or grind them yourself in a spice or coffee grinder.)

WATER, OIL AND BAKING POWDER
Whisk together 2 tablespoons of water, 1 teaspoon of oil, 2 teaspoons of baking powder, preferably aluminum-free baking powder, and ½ teaspoon of baking soda. Use this in place of one egg. When used in cookies and other baked goods, it works so well no one would ever know.

AQUAFABA
The hot new egg replacement is bean juice — specifically the liquid that comes in your can of chickpeas called aquafaba. It may not work for everything, but if your recipe calls for egg whites, whip up some aquafaba instead; about 3 tablespoons per replaced egg. For best results, use an unsalted variety.

After successfully using these food substitutions, you may employ them for more than emergency backup in the future. They are all vegan alternatives and, with the exception of the vegetable oil, are more heart-healthy than eggs. Using banana, applesauce or other puréed fruit in baked goods is a wonderful tactic to boost flavor and make them incredibly moist, while adding extra nutrition, especially fiber.

Natural Sugar Substitutes/Sweeteners

Agave
Agave has a lower glycemic index than most other sweeteners, which means that it is less likely to cause a sudden spike in the blood glucose level. Agave has a high fructose content which could have negative effects on liver health.

Maple syrup
Maple syrup, made from the sap of maple trees, is a good alternative and contains traces of minerals like iron. Beware of "maple-flavored syrup" which is a counterfeit to the pure maple syrup; it is made with unhealthy refined sugar to which maple flavor was added, as a cheaper alternative.

- Coconut sugar
  It is made from the sap of the coconut palm.
  It is generally on the pricier end like maple syrup.
- Molasses

After fresh and dried fruits, molasses is the second best sweetener option. Obtaining organic blackstrap molasses would be a smart option as regular molasses is often derived from GMO (genetically modified) crops and sweeteners labeled "molasses" are generally a not the pure blackstrap molasses.[12]

Stevia

The sweetener stevia is extracted from the leaves of the plant Stevia rebaudiana. It appears however that its active ingredient, steviosides, is transformed by gut bacteria into a toxic substance, steviol, which has the potential of mutating DNA if taken in large amounts. The World Health Organization recommends limiting the intake of stevia to 4mg per kilogram of body weight, which is roughly 1.8 mg per pound of body weight.[13]

Honey

Honey is a sweetener that has been used for thousands of years. The Bible speaks well of it, in moderation (see Proverbs 24:13 and Proverbs 25:16). Honey has antibacterial properties and may help boost the immune system. When it comes to antioxidant levels, honey scores higher than maple syrup.[14]

Dates and other dried fruits (raisins, apple sauce, banana)

Outside of fresh fruits, dried fruits like dates or raisins, and date sugar (pulverized/ ground up dates), being whole foods, have the highest level of antioxidants and constitute the healthiest sweetener one can use.

Butter Substitutes

Coconut cream or oil

Coconut oil can be substituted for butter at a 1:1 ratio. A pinch of Himalayan salt or sea salt may be added to it for a buttery flavor.

Olive oil

Half a cup of butter (4 ounces) may be substituted with 3 ounces of olive oil (which is a quarter cup plus 2 tablespoons or 6 tablespoons of olive oil)

Applesauce or Pumpkin puree

Three-fourths of a cup may be used for 1 cup of butter.

Banana-mashed

Same principle as for apple sauce. Keep in mind this may add a slight banana flavor to your dish.

Proverbs 25:16 (NKJV)
Have you found honey? Eat only as much as you need,
Lest you be filled with it and vomit.

Salt Substitute

Celery or celery juice

Chopped celery or celery juice have a natural savory/ salty flavor that makes it a good salt substitute. Celery also has the advantage of helping control hypertension with long-term use. Dry celery seeds could also be used as a salt substitute.

Herbs and spices

Herbs and spices add much flavor to all sorts of dishes and thereby decrease the need for much added salt.

Lemon juice

Lemon juice enhances the flavor of dishes, especially meat substitutes.

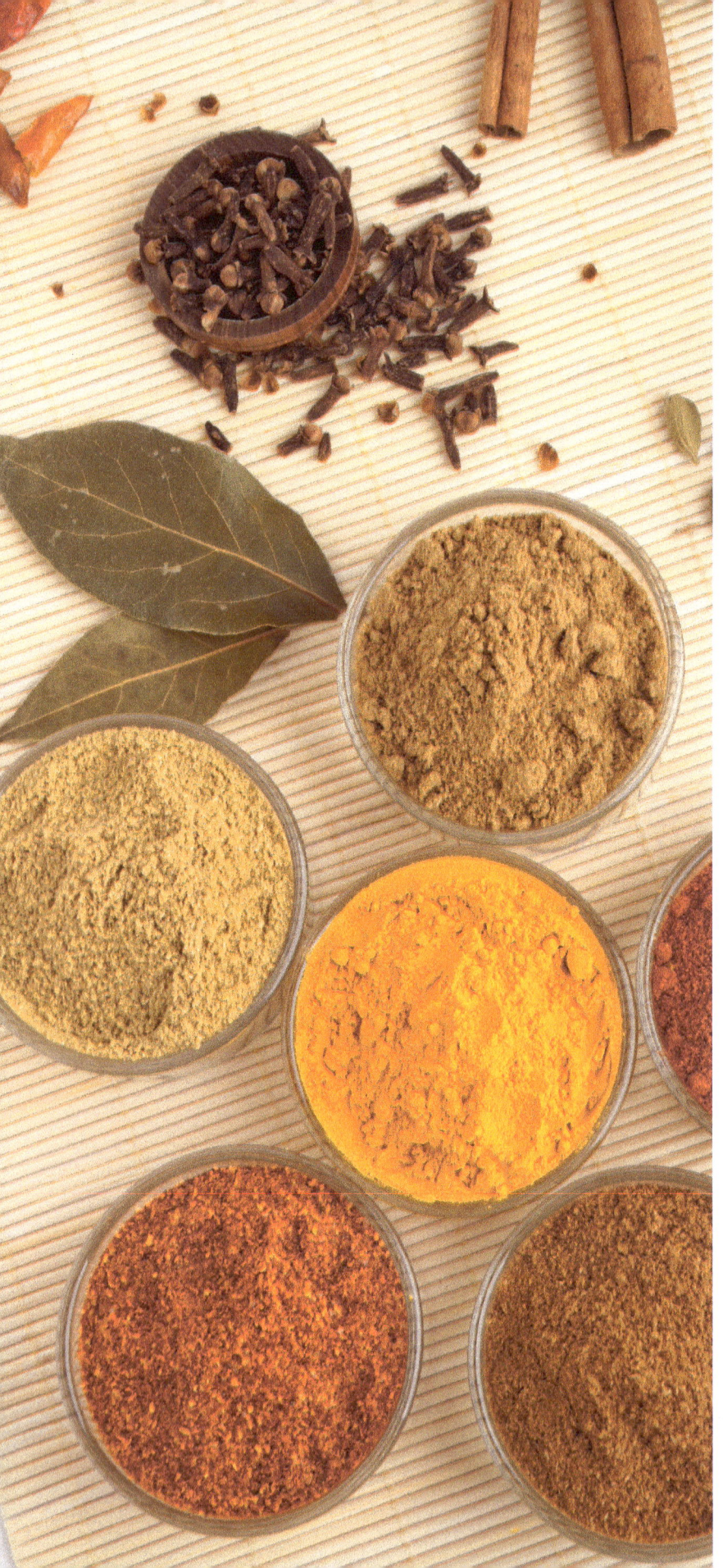

Seaweeds

Seaweeds, such as kelp or dulse, are good substitutes. They also contain trace minerals, like iodine.

Amino brags or Soy Sauce

There are some concerns about hydrolyzed proteins, like Bragg's Amino Acids or soy sauce, and their content of MSG. While Bragg's is non-GMO and lower in sodium than regular soy sauce the MSG concern is still something to consider.

Meats

- Tofu
- Mushroom
- Eggplant
- Beans
- Nuts and seeds
- Seitan (wheat gluten)
- Tempeh
- "Cauliflower meat" to replace ground meat
- "Bulgur meat" to replace ground meat
- Oat-burgers and other plant-based burgers

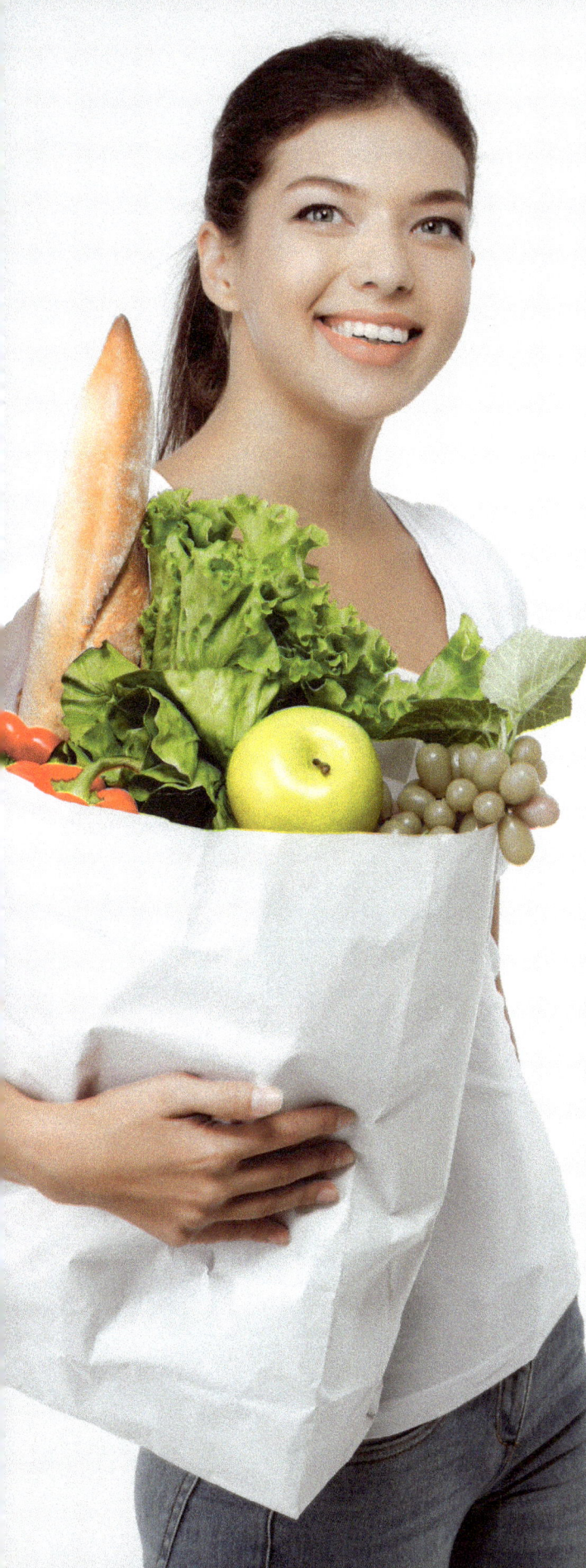

HOW TO CREATE A BALANCED PLATE

Breakfast is the most important meal. It fuels the body for the day ahead. Ideally, the last meal would have been consumed no later than 6 pm the day before, and the digestive system would have rested well throughout the night and would be ready to "break the fast" (a 12-hour or longer fast) in the morning.

For every meal, it is optimal to have at least half of that meal consist of fresh, raw fruits or vegetables. The other half should contain something cooked or steamed such as grains (millet pudding, oatmeal, etc.) to go with the fruits for breakfast or legumes and steamed vegetables for lunch. A handful of raw nuts or seeds may be added to either lunch or breakfast. It would be best to avoid drinks (whether water or juices) during meal times as liquid consumption during a meal will slow down digestion. An ideal time to drink water is between meals.

At any given meal, it would be best to limit the variety of dishes to no more than four different dishes at a time to ensure more optimal digestion. For instance, for lunch one may have a raw salad (with leafy greens, other raw veggies, and a healthy dressing), some black beans, and baked sweet potatoes. This would be three dishes.

Leave something on your plate.... Better to go to waste than to waist.
~ Micheal Pollan

Supper, if taken, should be light and 4-5 hours before bedtime so that the digestive organs have an opportunity to rest while sleeping instead of having to work overtime. Suppers should consist of foods that are easily digested like fresh fruits and smoothies; a slice of toast may be added, or healthy crackers, or some oil-free, organic popcorn. It is best to avoid nuts and other rich dishes at supper time; they are more suitable for breakfast and lunch.

A final tip to consider when eating a balanced diet is to avoid snacks, even when this snack is something generally considered healthy like an apple or celery sticks. Eating in between meals hinders the digestion of the meal taken before the snack, may encourage acid reflux, and may lead to weight gain in some cases. For optimal digestion and optimal health, it is best to leave about 5 hours between meals. If one is used to grazing throughout the day, in the beginning it may be challenging to not eat between meals. But after sticking to this practice for a couple of days, it gets easier and eventually becomes a habit. Those times in between meals are great to drink plenty of pure water and stay well hydrated! (For further reading on balanced meals, Counsels on Diet and Foods by Ellen G. White is a resourceful book).

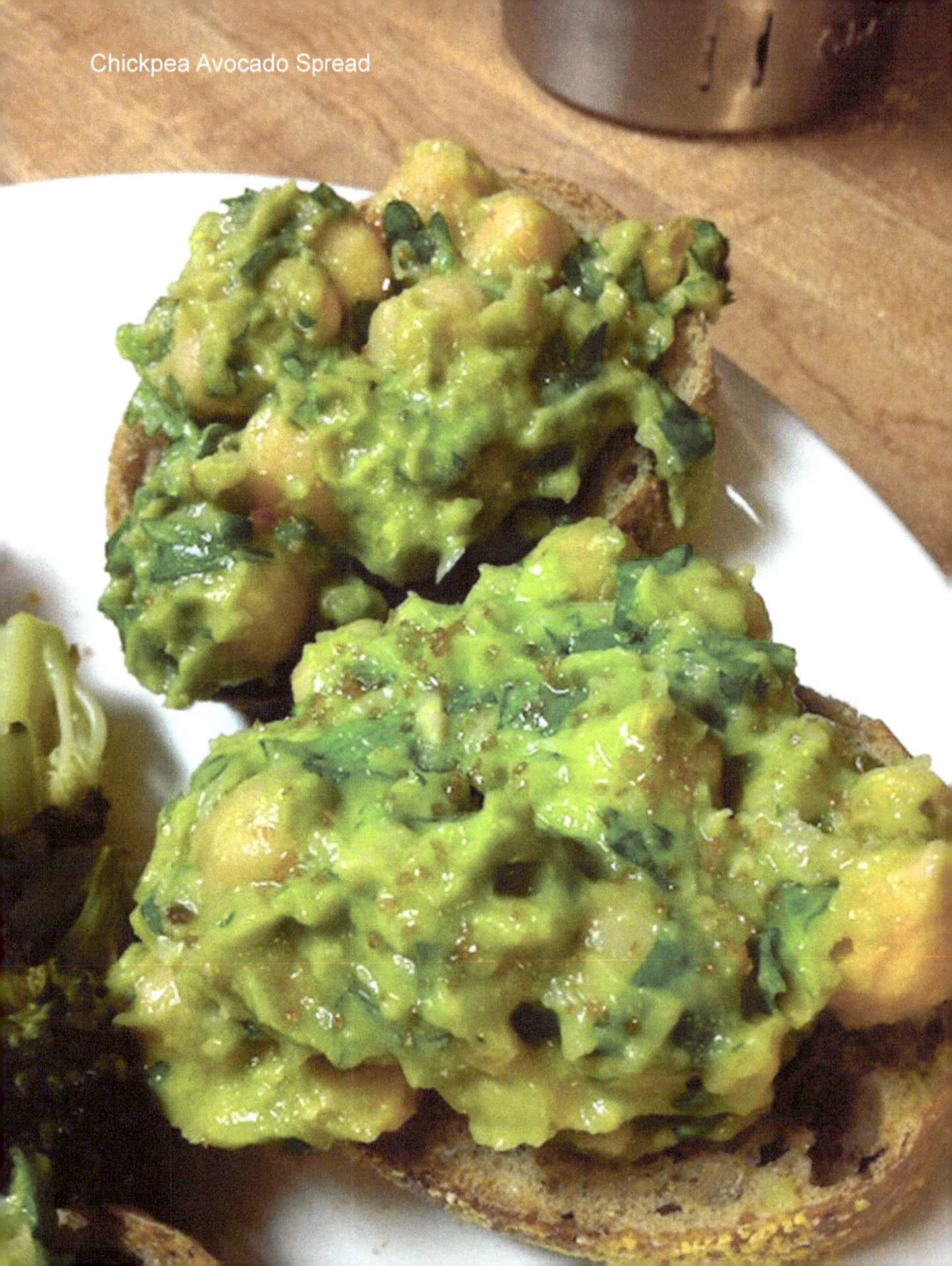
Chickpea Avocado Spread

CONTENTS

Healing Foods

Healing Foods for Specific Diseases 16-33

Meal Plans

Vegan 28 Day Meal Plan 34-35

Breakfast

Scrambled Tofu with Kale 38
Banana Whole-Wheat Muffins 39
Bean Burrito 40
Traditional Tofu Scramble 41
Oven Roasted Potatoes 42
Whole-Wheat Pancakes 43
Cashew-Oat Waffles 44
Strawberry Peach Smoothie 45
Mushroom and Kale Frittata 47
Baked Oats 48
Banana Berry Smoothie 49
Blueberry-Oatmeal Pancakes 50
French Toast 51
Huevos Rancheros 53
Jamaican Cornmeal Porridge 54
Hot Bulgur Wheat Cereal 55
Toast and Gravy 56
Steamed Spinach 57
Granola 58
Multigrain Waffles 59
Corn Bread 60
Detox Green Smoothie 61
Dr. Cooper's Oats-on-the-Go 62
Avocado Toast 63

Main Entrées

Heart-Healthy Bean Chili 67
Hummus and Veggie Wrap 68
Black Bean Burger 69
Tofu Thai Curry 71
Caribbean Curried Tofu 72
Baked Falafel 74
Tofu "Egg" Salad 75
Curried Bean Sandwich Spread 76
Coconut Chickpea Curry 77
Coconut Curry Eggplant 78
Seasoned Oven Fries 79
Roasted Vegetable Delight 80
Oats Walnut Balls 81
Chiles Rellenos 83
Dr. Cooper's Rosemary-Lemon Tofu Kabobs 85
Cashew Brown Rice Loaf 86
Oat-Nut Burgers 87
Spicy Tofu Burgers 88
5-Grain Brown Rice Pilaf 89
Eggplant Zucchini Bake 90
Mashed Cauliflower and White Beans 91
Eggplant Roll-Ups 93
Seasoned Vegetable Rice 94
Wild Rice and Mushroom Pilaf 95
Indian Rice 96
Seasoned Black Bean Brown Rice 97
Chickpea Avocado Spread 98
Lentil Walnut "Meatballs" 99
Pasta Primavera 101
Pasta with Vegetables 102
Veggie Wrap with Guacamole 103
Chickpea Curry 104
Lentil Patties 105
Walnut Balls 106
Sun-Dried Tomato, Black Bean and Rice Salad 107
Chinese Stir-Fry Vegetables 109
Mock Tuna Salad 110
Black Bean, Corn and Quinoa Salad 111
Quinoa Salad 112
Baked Mac & Cheese 113
Spicy Mexican Beans 114
Jamaican Stewed Peas 115

Soups

Corn and Potato Chowder 118
Quinoa Lentil Soup 119
Thai Coconut Curry Soup 120
Creamy Potato Broccoli Soup 121
Kale and White Bean Soup 122
Italian White Bean Soup 123
Zucchini and Califlower Soup 124
Split Pea Soup 125
Italian Minestrone Soup 126
Lentil Soup with Vegetables 128
Indian Lentil Soup 129
Jamaican Kidney Bean Soup 130
Spinach Kale Soup 131
Cream of Pumpkin Soup 132
Lentil Stew 133
Easy Green Pea Soup 134
Summer Soup 135
Cream of Broccoli Soup 136

Sauces, Gravies and Dips

"Meatball" Tomato Sauce 140
Alfredo Sauce 141
Lima Bean Cheese Sauce 142
Tofu Cheese Sauce 143
Vegan Cheese Sauce 144
Cashew Cheese Sauce 145
Hummus 146
Mango Avocado Salsa 147
Guacamole 148
Chickpea Spread or Dip 149
Mushroom Gravy 150
Country-Style Brown Gravy 151

Salad Dressings

Cucumber Salad Dressing 154
Avocado Salad Dressing 155
Caesar Salad Dressing 156
Strawberry Dressing 157
Orange Ginger Dressing 158

Desserts

Vegan Gluten-Free Black Bean Brownies 161
Banana Peanut Butter Ice Cream 162
Banana Coconut Ice Cream 163
Papaya Banana Ice Cream 164
Strawberry Banana Sorbet 165
Berry Sorbet 166
Carrot Cake 167

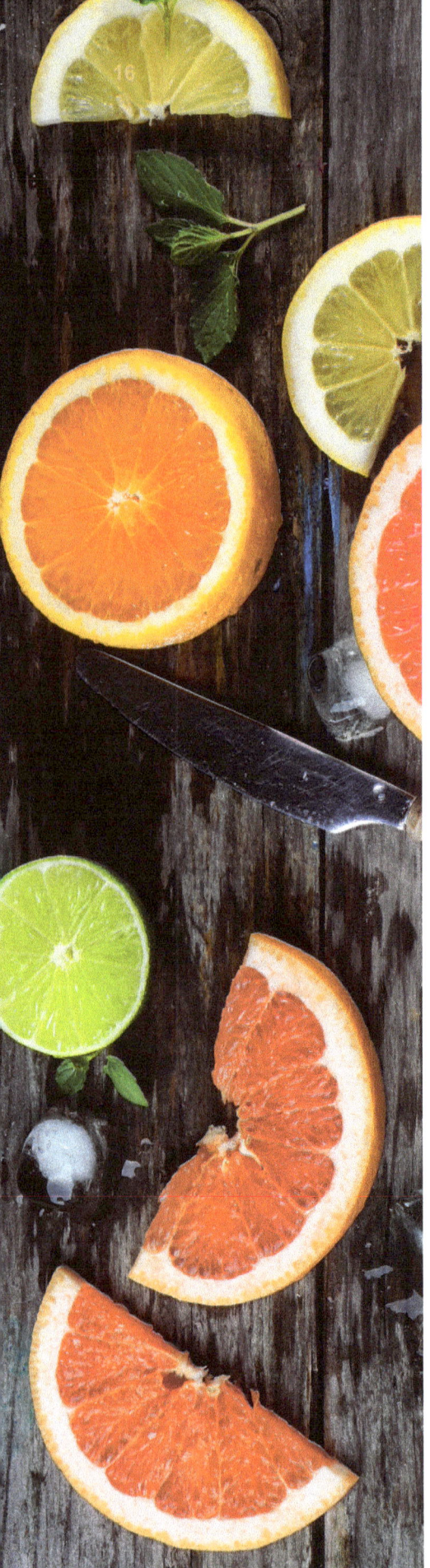

Incredibly Delicious VEGAN

HEALING FOODS

ANEMIA

LEGUMES
Rich source of Iron, folate, and protein which are used for blood production.

SOY
Soybeans are very rich in iron and contain all the essential amino acids. Soy is the most iron-rich legume. It is best to use whole soybeans and avoid processed soy products, such as soy protein or TVP. It is also important to select organic soy products (whether whole soybeans, soymilk, tempeh or tofu) as much of the soy crop is genetically modified. Selecting organic soy helps prevent or at least minimize the consumption of GMOs.

FRUIT
Fruits, especially citrus fruits, help facilitate the absorption of iron. Examples are oranges, lemons, limes, etc.

GREEN LEAFY VEGETABLES
Green leafy vegetables like spinach, romaine lettuce and kale, are a rich source of iron, magnesium and copper, all of which play a role in blood production. Some of these green leafy vegetables will be discussed individually below.

ALFALFA

It contains about the same amount of iron as beef. It also contains vitamin C which facilitates absorption of iron. One can easily grow alfalfa sprouts at home.

WATERCRESS

It contains iron, some vitamins and minerals used in blood production.

RED BEETS

They contain iron and vitamin C and help stimulate blood production in the bone marrow.

SPINACH

Contains iron, but slow to absorb. It also contains various vitamins and trace elements for blood production.

AVOCADOS

They are rich in iron and also contain vitamin C.

SUNFLOWER SEEDS

They are rich in iron, vitamins B and E. It is recommended to consume them unsalted. They are also more healthly when raw or soaked.

PISTACHIOS

Rich in iron and copper. Copper facilitates the absorption of iron.

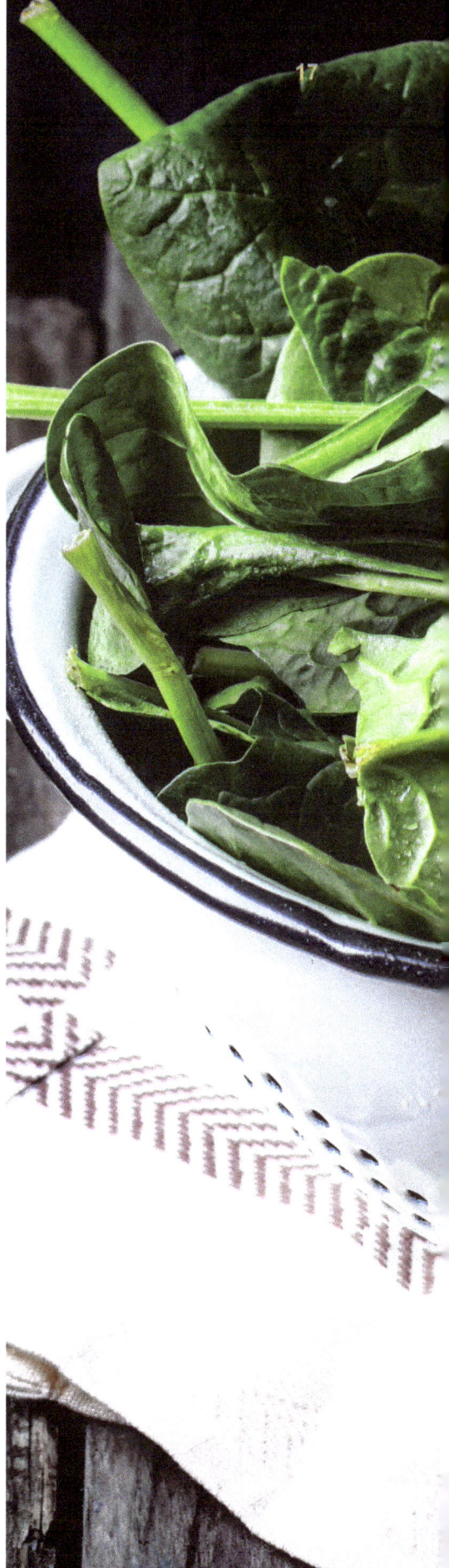

GRAPES
Grapes are rich in iron and also contain copper.

PASSIONFRUIT
It contains iron and vitamin C.

APRICOTS
They have anti-anemic effects despite the fact that they are not very rich in iron.

LEMON
Lemon facilitates the absorption of iron found in other fruits, grains and vegetables due to its vitamin C and organic acid content.

SPIRULINA
This is a blue-green bacterium which was previously considered an alga until recently, and contains high amounts of iron and vitamin B12, although some scientist state that the vitamin B12 is slightly different than true vitamin B12, hence making it difficult to absorb.

MOLASSES
It is a rich source of iron and other needed minerals. It is an excellent replacement for sugar.

VITAMIN B12

Vitamin B12 deficiency causes megaloblastic (large red blood cells) anemia. Strict vegetarians with a poorly managed diet are at risk of vitamin B12 deficiency. Vegans would do well to check their B12 regularly and take a vegan B12 supplement as needed. A methylcobalamin supplement is more effective than its cyanocobalamin counterpart; a sublingual l B12 is also more readily absorbed than a capsule or tablet. We must also add that interestingly many meat eaters have a B12 deficiency, despite the consumption of animal products. In these individuals, the cause is typically a lack of an intrinsic factor in their body. B12 deficiency is thus not an issue that affects only vegans.

FOLATE

Essential in the production of red blood cells. Folate deficiency reduces the number of cells and increases the size of cells. They can be found in legumes and leafy green vegetables, especially lentils, pinto beans, garbanzos, spinach, collard and turnip greens.

B GROUP VITAMINS

Vitamins B1, B2 and B6 contribute to blood production.
or soaked.

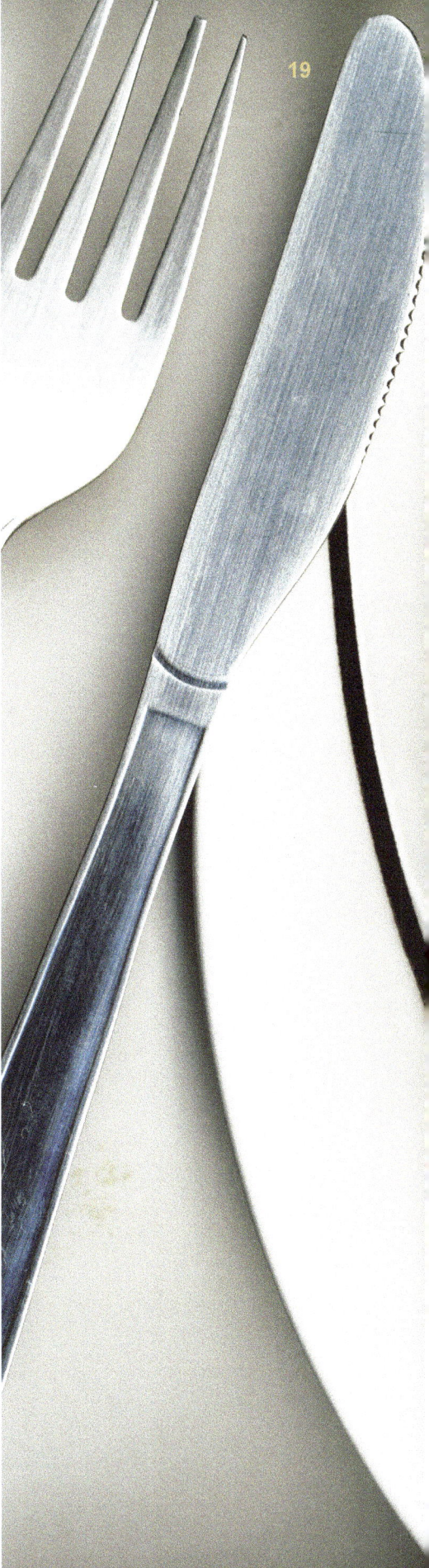

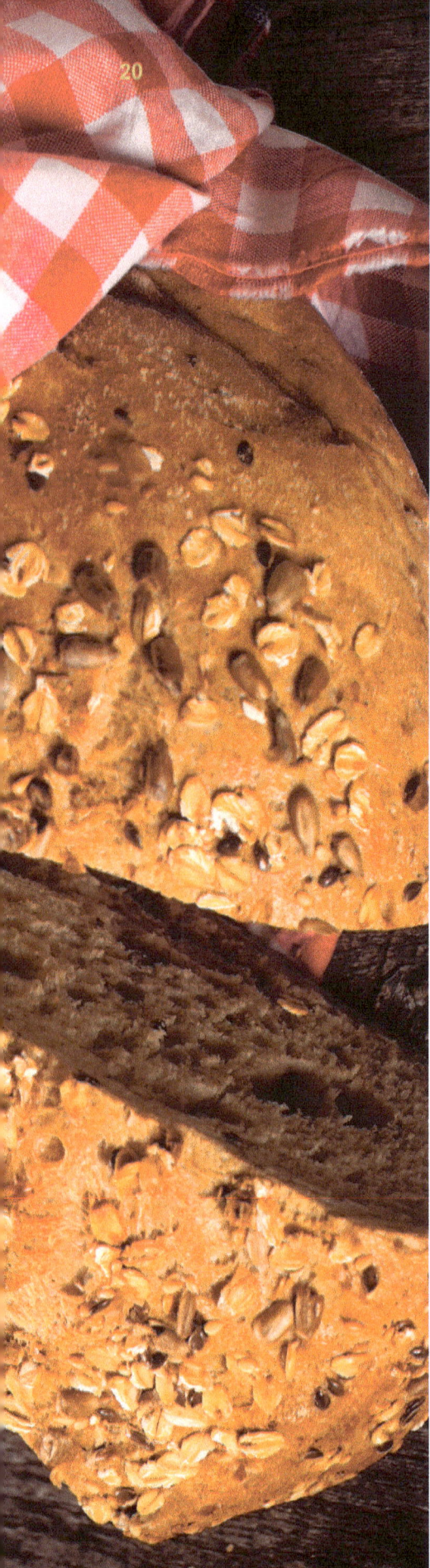

VITAMIN E

Its deficiency leads to the production of fragile red blood cells that are easily destroyed. Nuts and seeds are good sources (especially sunflower seeds and almonds), as well as avocados, red bell peppers, mangoes, raw turnip greens, and kiwi fruit.

VITAMIN C

It increases the measure of absorption of iron by double. Best sources, better than supplements, are citrus fruits, berries, and tomatoes.

DIABETES

LEGUMES

Well tolerated by diabetics because it has high fiber content which helps regulate glucose in the blood.

VEGETABLES

All vegetables are well tolerated by diabetics because of their low-calorie content, which makes them excellent for the prevention and treatment of obesity.

WHOLE GRAINS

Whole grains are well tolerated and can be consumed freely as they help prevent diabetes.

FRUIT

Fruits are necessary in diabetic diets because of their antioxidant properties that protect against cardiovascular disease. Caution on the quantity of fruits used. Diabetics would do well to avoid dried fruits, though these are healthy for individuals who do not have issues with carbohydrate metabolism.

NUTS

They are poor in carbohydrates and high in easily assimilated fatty acids and vitamins B that provide energy.

ARTICHOKE

Its active ingredient, Cynarin, has mild hypoglycemic properties. It also contains ulin, a beneficial carbohydrate in diabetics.

CELERY

It helps regulate blood sugar levels, decreases cholesterol, and neutralizes acids.

AVOCADO

It helps regulate blood sugar, decreases cholesterol and also regulates fat composition in blood.

ONION

Onions help reduce blood sugar. They alkalize the blood and protect against arteriosclerosis.

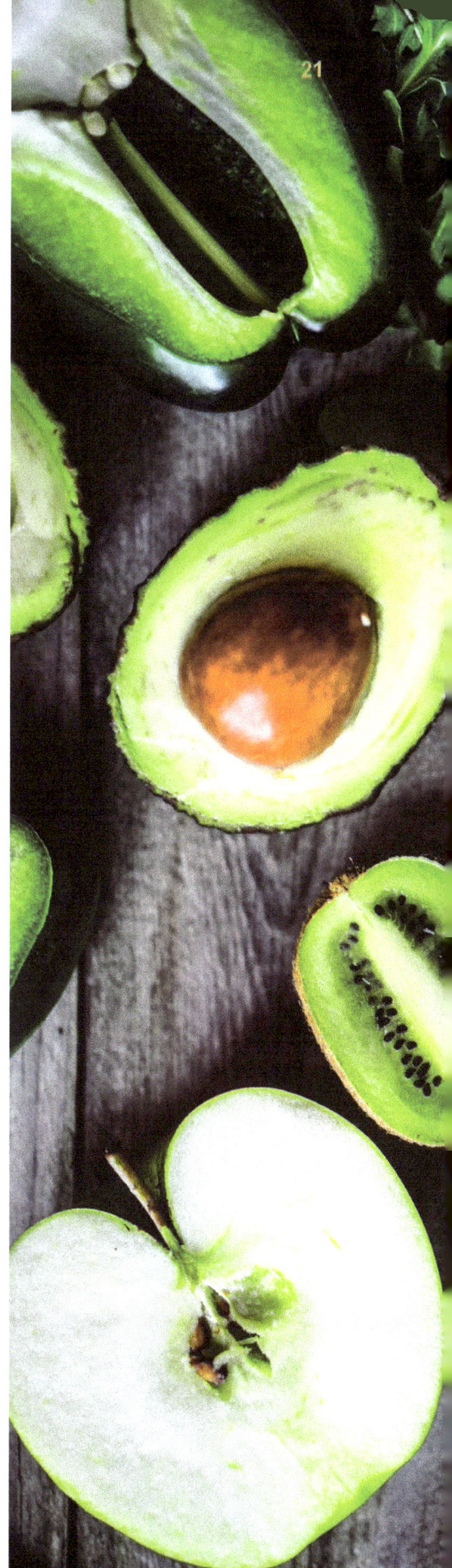

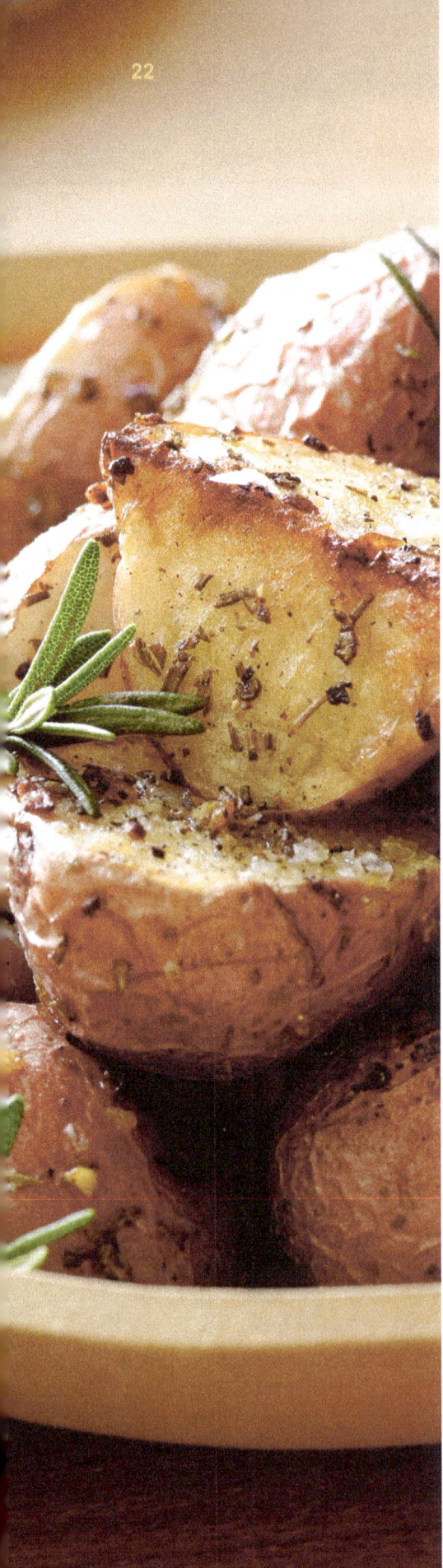

MUSHROOM

Studies have shown that mushrooms produce improvement in the disease course, and also contain proteins and group B vitamins. They reduce the need for insulin.

NOPAL

Some studies in Mexico show a drop in blood sugar levels in non-insulin dependent individuals after the consumption of Nopal leaves.

POTATO

They are rich in complex carbohydrates and fiber, which releases glucose slowly during digestion. Caution on the amount of regular potatoes used by diabetics. Sweet potatoes have a lower glycemic index and thus are better for diabetics.

WHEAT GERM

It contains vitamins B1 and E that have anti-diabetic effects. 4-5 spoons can reduce glucose level and need for insulin.

GUAR

It slows the absorption of glucose from other foods, hence preventing its level from increasing in the blood.

ANTIOXIDANTS

Protects cells from harm caused by excess sugar. Provitamin A, vitamins C and E and flavonoids are natural antioxidants.

B GROUP VITAMINS

Vitamins B1, B2 and B6 are essential in glucose metabolism and transforming it to energy.

MAGNESIUM

Diabetics run the risk of lacking this mineral involved in insulin production. Wheat germ, legumes, and nuts are rich sources.

TRACE ELEMENTS

Minerals involved in insulin production are copper, chromium and manganese. Chromium is found in fresh fruits and vegetables (especially broccoli and green beans), barley, and wheat germ.

HYPERTENSION

DIURETIC FOODS

In some cases, they are as effective as medications. They increase urine production, and decrease blood volume, thus reducing blood pressure. They are rich in potassium, fiber and antioxidants. Some examples include celery, dandelion, parsley, garlic, asparagus, pears, watermelon, and cucumber.

FRUIT

Eating a lot of fruits protects against hypertension. People suffering from hypertension should consume lots of fruits.

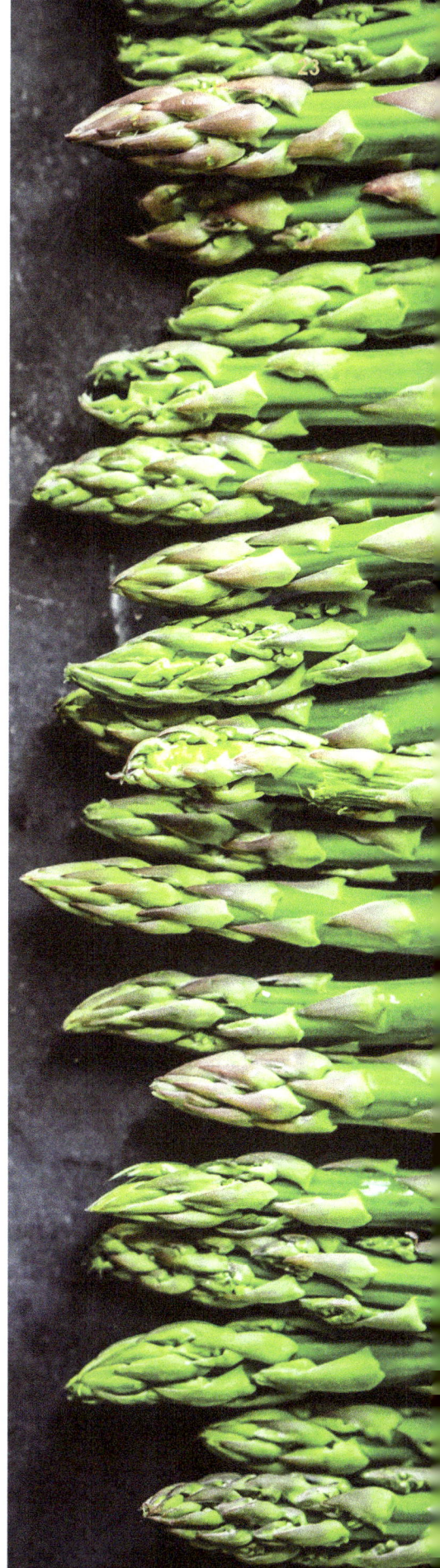

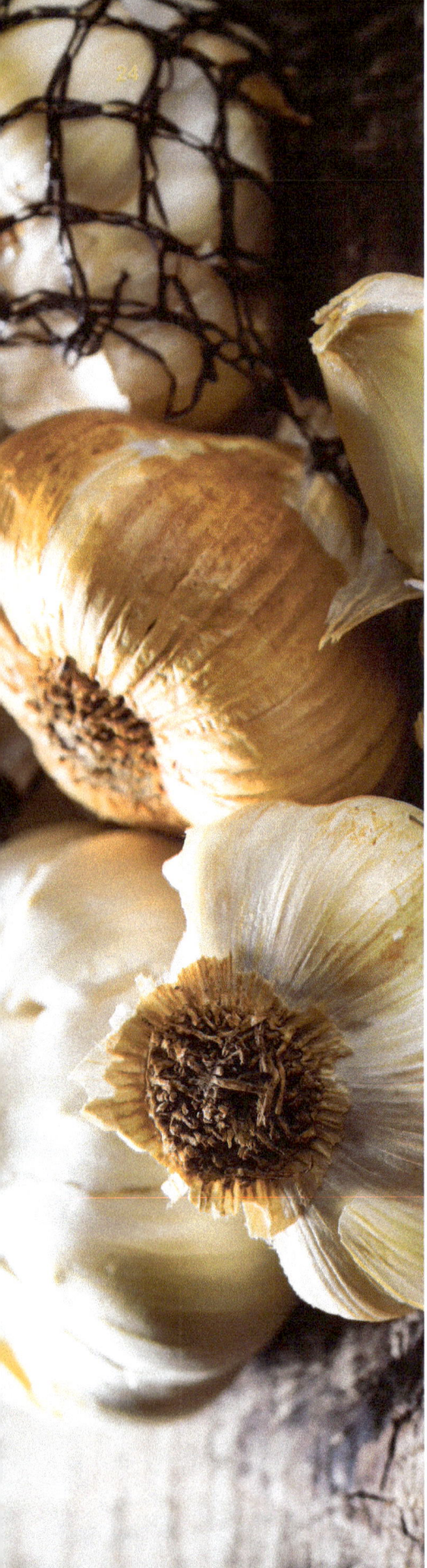

GREEN LEAFY VEGETABLES

They are rich sources of potassium, magnesium and nitrates which help lower blood pressure. A vegetarian diet lowers blood pressure.

DEPURANT BROTH

Broth made with onion and celery that detoxifies blood waste and helps prevent hypertension. A half to one liter of this broth is consumed a day instead of water.

LEGUMES

Contain potassium, magnesium and calcium which help control blood pressure. They are low in sodium and high in fiber.

CELERY

Celery contains a compound called 3-n-butyl phthalide which has been shown to lower blood pressure. It functions as a vasodilator and diuretic, thus helps with hypertension.

SQUASH

Rich in potassium and low in sodium.

GARLIC

It has nitrates which potentiate nitric oxide production. Nitric oxide has vasodilatation and hypotension properties. Need to consume an average of 8 cloves of slightly steamed garlic a day to achieve this effect.

GUAVA
Eat guava every day to reduce blood pressure.

PEARS
They have diuretic properties and are rich in potassium.

GRAPEFRUIT
Protects the arteries and has diuretic properties.

FIBER
More fiber in the diet lowers the risk of hypertension. Animal products do not contain fiber while plant foods, especially unrefined plant foods (such as whole fruits, vegetables and whole grains) are rich in fiber.

POTASSIUM
A potassium-rich diet protects against hypertension. Foods rich in potassium include chia seeds, green leafy vegetables, oranges, bananas, etc.

CALCIUM
Dairy products are a good source as well as legumes, broccoli, cabbage and nuts. Low calcium can lead to hypertension.

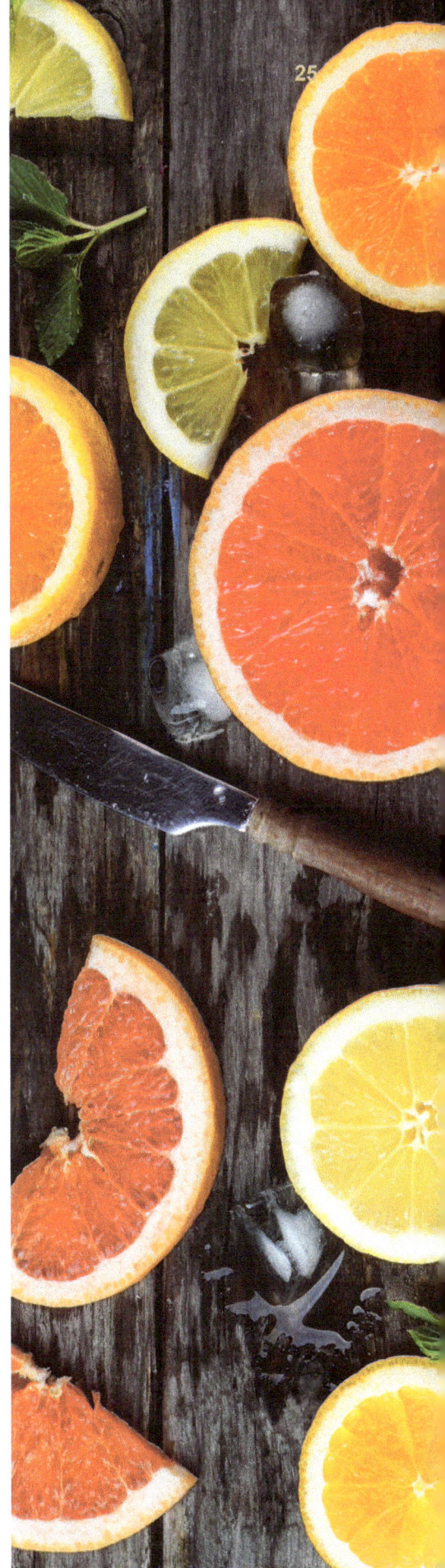

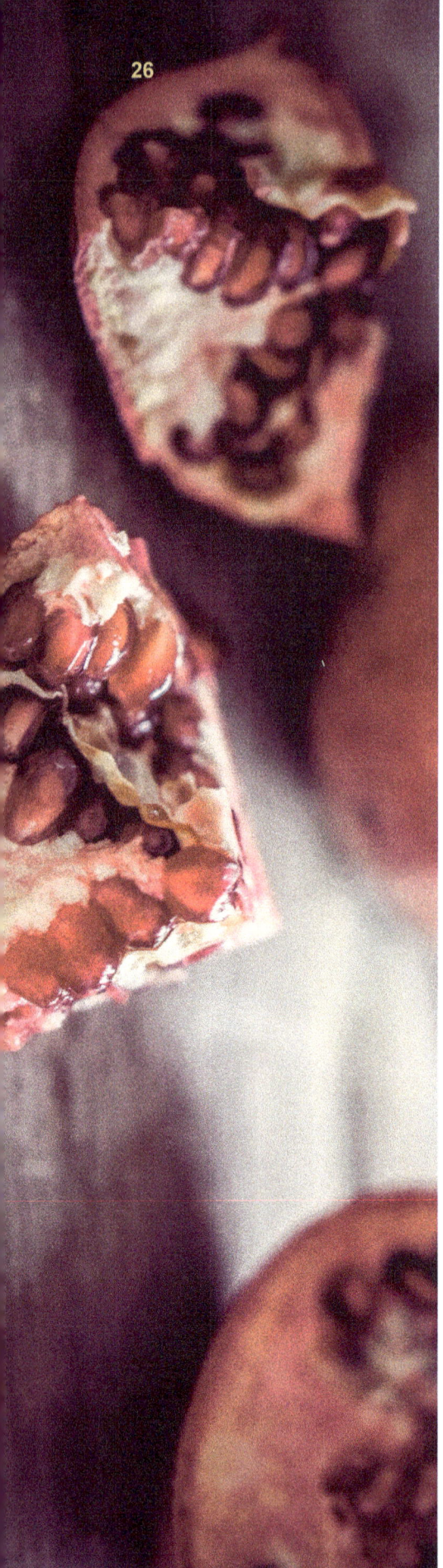

MAGNESIUM

A magnesium deficiency can lead to hypertension. Good sources are green leafy vegetables, fruits (especially figs, avocado, bananas, and raspberries).

BEETS

Rich in dietary nitrates which are converted to nitric oxide, which has vasodilatory and hypotensive properties.

HIBISCUS FLOWERS

Hibiscus tea has been shown to lower blood pressure in people with hypertension.

CURCUMIN

Turmeric is very rich in curcumin, which is shown to improve blood flow and decreases blood pressure especially in those with kidney disease.

POMEGRANATE

Pomegranate juice is a strong source of nitrates, which helps to keep blood vessels soft and elastic. The daily intake of 150ml (5oz) of pomegranate for 2 weeks can markedly lower blood pressure.

OBESITY

DIURETIC FOODS
Their effect helps with the elimination of fluid and sodium and helps with weight loss.

PINEAPPLE
Eaten before a meal helps curb appetite. Also has diuretic properties.

SWEET POTATO
Good source of complex and easily digestible carbohydrate. It produces satiety, and relieves hunger for several hours.

CHERRIES
Do not contain fat or sodium, have diuretic and depurant properties. Should be eaten slowly.

CABBAGE
Provides a feeling of satiety due to its high fiber. It also has a low-calorie content which can help create a caloric deficit and thus promote weight loss.

CALCIUM
Provides feeling of satiety due to its high fiber. It also has a low calorie content which can help create a caloric deficit and thus promote weight loss.

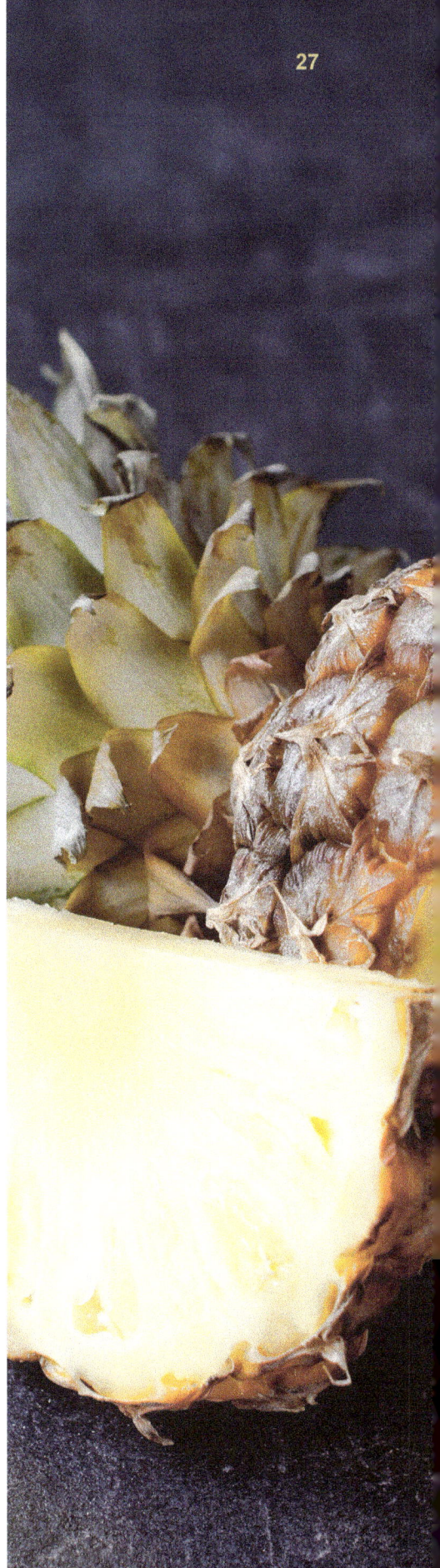

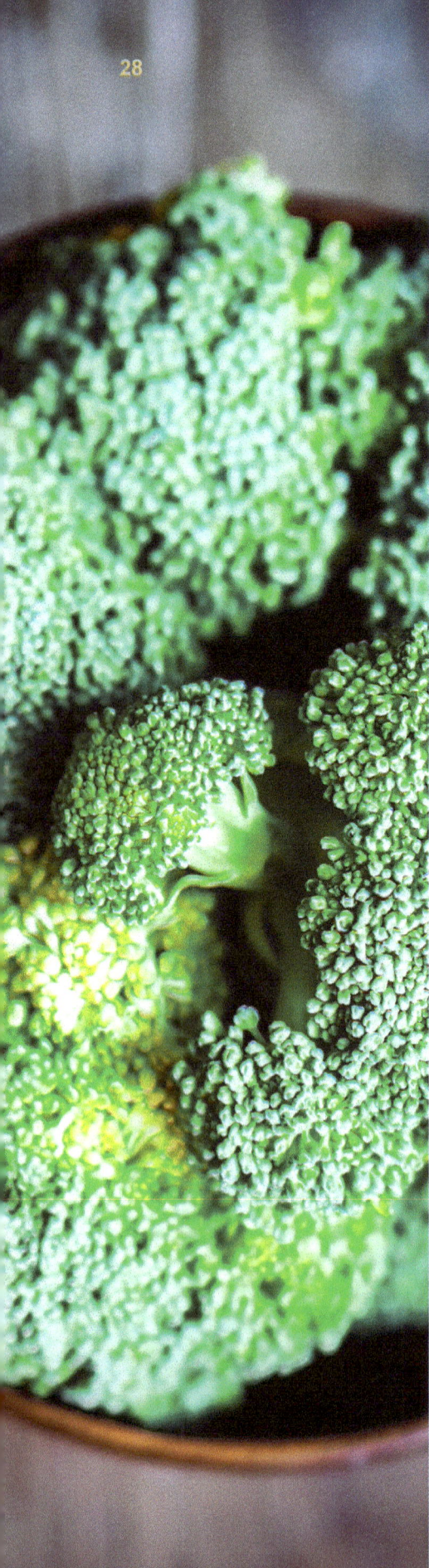

BROCCOLI

It is low in calories and sugars. Provides a source of vitamins A and C making suitable for weight loss.

SEAWEED

It functions by retaining water in the stomach due to is mucilage structure, hence stretches the stomach and give the feeling of satiety.

ZUCCHINI

It has diuretic properties and also has a smoothing effect on the digestive tract, making it suitable for weight loss.

ASPARAGUS

It nourishes without weight gain due to its high protein and low-calorie content. It is also rich in fiber.

GARCINIA

Derived from a Southeast Asian fruit, it acts as an appetite reducer.

SPIRULINA

Used as a dietary supplement in weight loss. It is rich in proteins vitamins and iron, but extremely low in calories.

LETTUCE

Good source of vitamins and minerals but few calories. Produces feelings of satiety.

CUCUMBER
Rich in mineral, low in fat and calories.

PEACH
Contains low calories, helps with the elimination of acidic wastes. Good source of vitamins A and C. Provides satiety.

GRAPEFRUIT
Functions as a depurant. Contains vitamins A, B1 and C and other minerals and fiber.

MUSHROOM
Contains low calories and produces a satiety effect.

CHERIMOYAS
Have a high carbohydrate content and produce satiety.

BELL PEPPERS
Contain vitamins A and C but are low in calories and carbohydrates.

TURNIPS
They have a low-fat content, few calories and are easily digested.

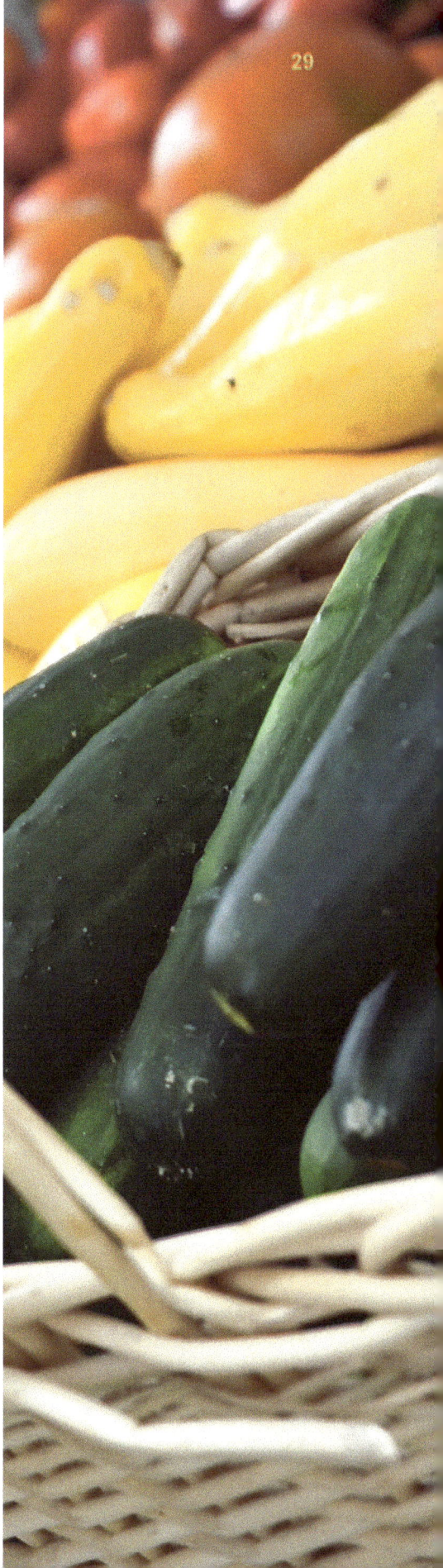

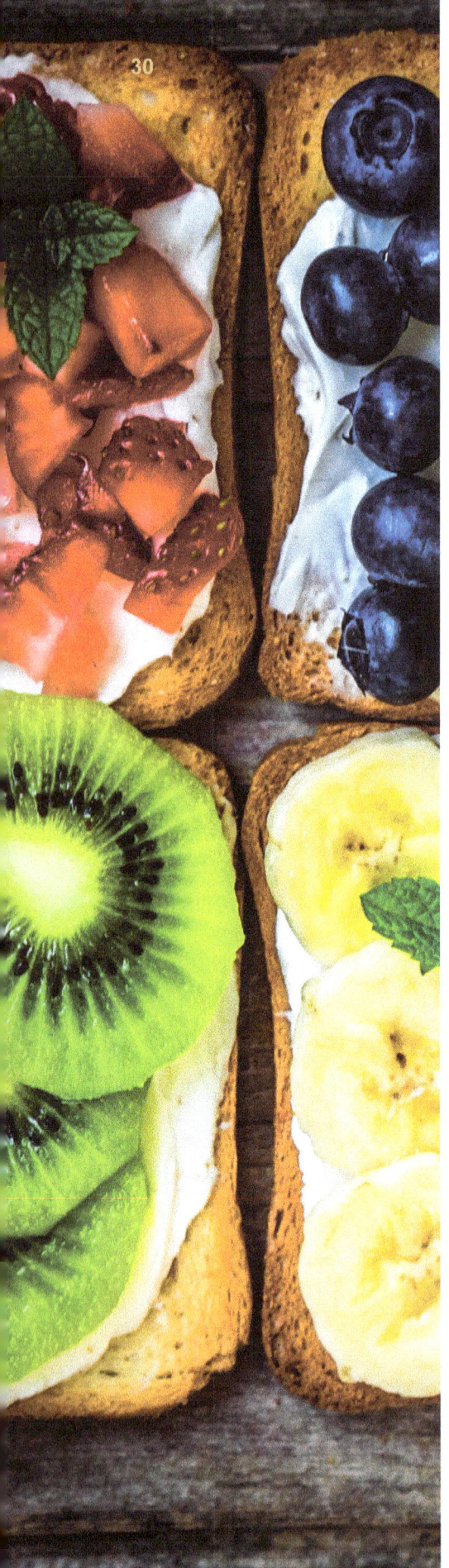

CANCER

FRUITS

(oranges, lemons, grapefruit, pineapples, plums, berries, guavas, kiwis, acerolas, mangoes, and apple)

They are rich in antioxidant vitamins, fiber and phytochemicals that help prevent the development of cancers.

According to the current scientific data, lemons and cranberries are among the most effective fruits in decreasing the proliferation of cancer cells, followed by apples, berries, and grapes, then grapefruits and bananas.

Bear in mind that most commercial dried cranberries are sweetened with table sugar and therefore are not as healthy as fresh cranberries or unsweetened dried cranberries.[16]

VEGETABLES
(red beet, carrots, tomatoes, sweet peppers, eggplant, onion, garlic, cabbage, cauliflower, radishes, and spinach)

They contain provitamin A, vitamin C, and antioxidant phytochemicals that protect against cancer development and growth. Cruciferous vegetables (kale, cabbage, Brussels spouts, and broccoli sprouts) contain chemical components such as sulphoraphane and Indol-3-carbinol which have anti-carcinogenic properties.

WHOLE GRAINS
(rye, wheat germ)

They contain phytates that have anti-cancer properties. High fiber content promotes intestinal motility. Also helps retain harmful substances in the gut and excreted with feces.

OLIVE OIL
Contains antioxidants and monounsaturated fatty acids. Studies have shown to reduce the risk of breast cancer.

LEGUMES
(soy and tofu)

They contain fiber and anti-carcinogenic phytochemicals that help prevent cancer.

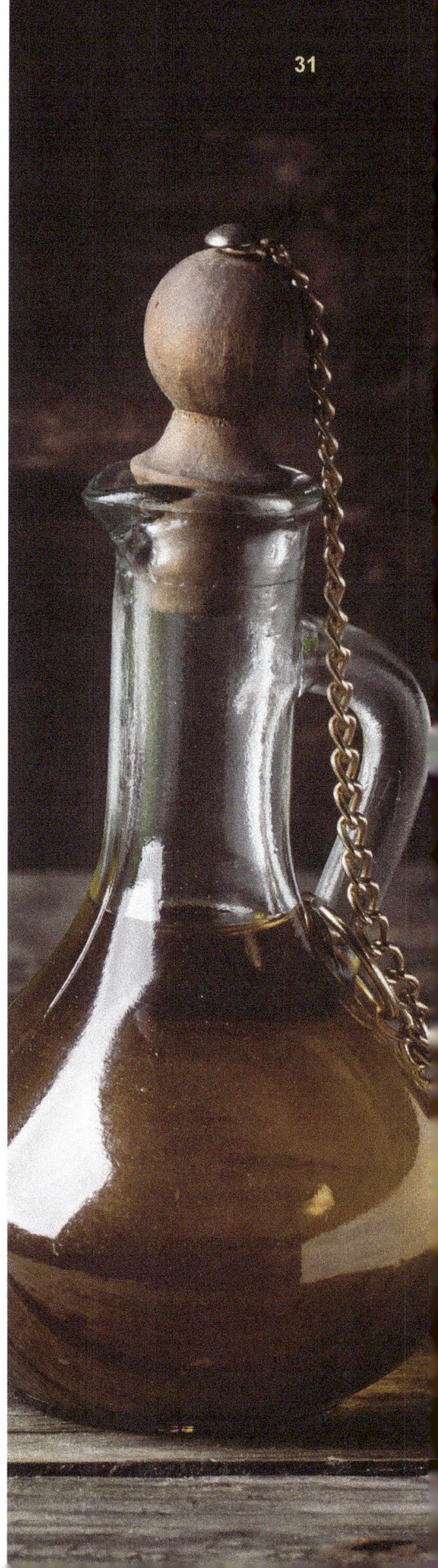

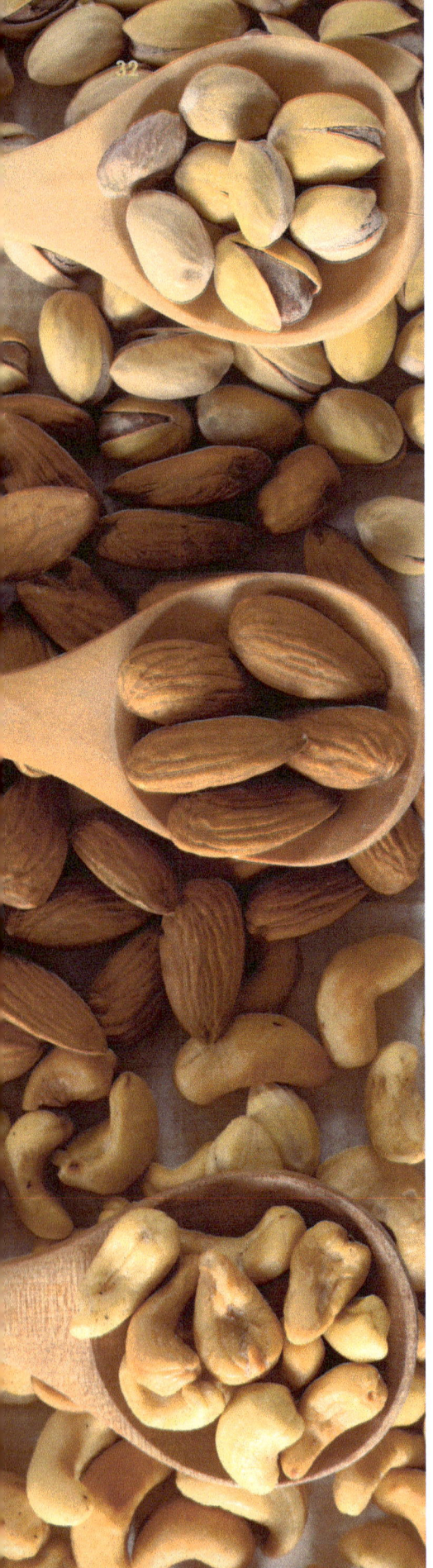

CORONARY ARTERY DISEASE/ARTERIOSCLEROSIS AND HYPERLIPIDEMIA

FRUITS

Consuming a lot of fruits is the best way to help prevent the development of arteriosclerosis. Fruits have anti-oxidative properties and are low in fat.

WHOLE GRAINS

High consumption of whole grains helps prevent formation of arteriosclerosis as opposed to consuming products of refined flour such as white bread, white pasta, white flour, or white rice.

LEGUMES

Are high in proteins and carbohydrates and in fat. Also provide phytoestrogen which protects the arteries.

VEGETABLES

They are rich in antioxidants and phytochemicals and low in fat and sodium.

NUTS

They are rich in unsaturated fatty acids that help reduce cholesterol. They also contain vitamin E which is an antioxidant and helps prevent arteriosclerosis.

FIBER

Found in whole grains, fruits, vegetables, and legumes. They reduce the risk of arteriosclerosis.

OILS

Vegetable oils contain unsaturated fatty acids that help lower cholesterol. They should be used instead of animal oils, such as butter. However, one must be cautious with their use of oils as they are very high in calories. Furthermore, cheap oils and GMO oils like canola oil, corn, soybean, and palm oil, promote inflammation in the body and are not healthy.

ANTIOXIDANTS

They prevent arteriosclerosis by preventing oxidation of lipoproteins. They include provitamin A, vitamins C and E, and flavonoids.

GARLIC

Functions as an antioxidant, preventing the oxidation of lipoprotein, hence reducing the risk of arteriosclerosis.

FOLATE

Together with vitamin B6, folate reduces homocysteine levels which have been shown to play a role in arteriosclerosis formation. Folates are found in legumes and green vegetables.

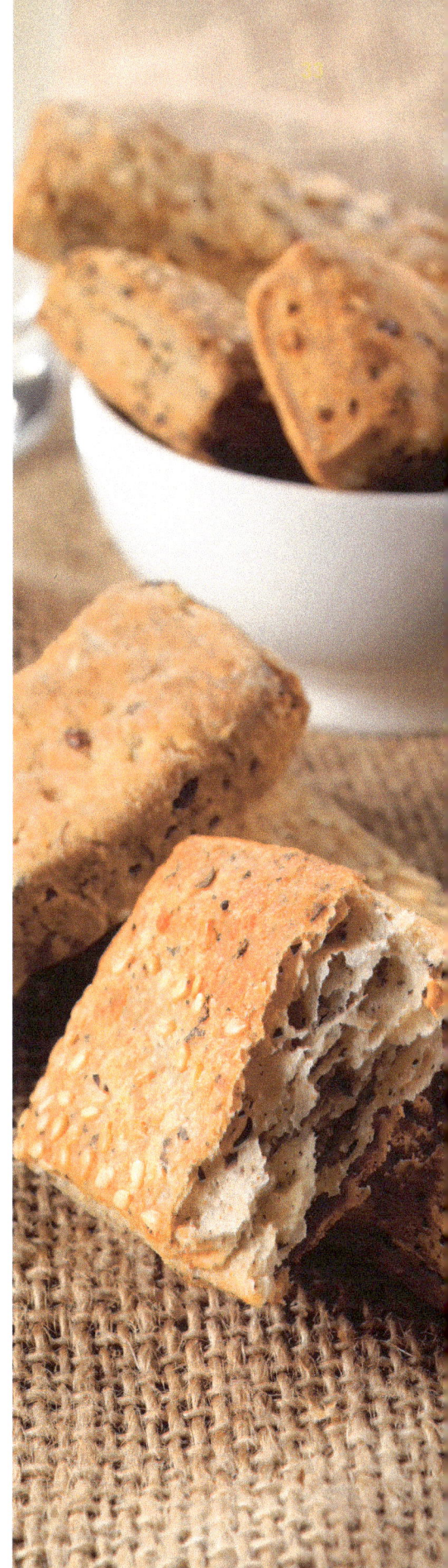

VEGAN 28 DAY MEAL PLAN
(Weeks 1 & 2)

Week 1	Sun.	Mon.	Tue.	Wed.	Thu.	Fri.	Sat.
Breakfast	1 Oven Roasted Potato 1 cup Scrambled Tofu 1 small apple	2 Banana Whole-Wheat Muffins 1 cup non-dairy milk 1 pea	1 Bean Burrito ½ grapefruit 1 oz walnuts	1 cup Scrambled Tofu with Kale 1 whole-wheat tortilla or 2 large lettuce leaves 1 cup cantaloupe 1 oz cashews	1 cup Scrambled Tofu 2 slices whole-wheat bread ½ cup mixed berries	1 Whole-Wheat Pancake 1 ripe banana sliced 1 oz walnuts or pecan nuts 1 cup non-dairy milk	1 Cashew Oat Waffle ½ cup fruit topping (banana or mixed berries) 1 cup non-dairy milk (optional)
Lunch	1 cup Heart-Healthy Bean Chili 1 medium baked sweet potato	1 Black Bean Burger 1 whole-wheat bun 1 slice tomato and lettuce	2 Baked Falafel 2 whole-wheat pita pockets 2 slices tomato and lettuce	1 cup Tofu "Egg" Salad 2 slices whole-wheat bread or 2 lettuce leaves 1 oz mixed nuts	¾ cup Coconut Chickpea Curry ½ cup brown rice or 1 cup steamed vegetables 1 cup raw vegetables	¾ cup Coconut Curry Eggplant 1 cup whole-wheat pasta 1 cup raw vegetables	1 cup Seasoned Oven Fries ¾ cup Heart-Healthy Bean Chili
Dinner	1 Hummus and Veggie Wrap 1 cup cantaloupe	½ cup Hummus 1 cup celery, carrot sticks and bell pepper slices	½ cup Jamaican Stewed Peas ½ cup rice (brown or wild) 1 cup fresh vegetable salad	¾ Mashed Cauliflower and White Beans 2 Baked Falafel	½ cup Chickpea Avocado Spread 2 slices whole-wheat bread 1 slice tomato ½ cup lettuce leave ½ cup alfalfa sprouts	1 cup Quinoa Lentil Soup 1 cup fresh vegetable salad	1 Veggie Wrap with Guacamole 1 apple

Week 2	Sun.	Mon.	Tue.	Wed.	Thu.	Fri.	Sat.
Breakfast	Mushroom and Kale Frittata (serving size: 2-5x5 inch squares) 1 cup mixed fruit 2 oz walnuts	Baked Oats (one serving) 1 cup Detox Green Smoothie 1 tablespoon Flax seed	8 oz Strawberry Field Smoothie 2 oz almond nuts	8 oz Banana Berry Smoothie 1 slice whole-wheat bread 1 tbsp nut butter	2 Blueberry-Oatmeal Pancakes 1 cup mixed fruits 1 tablespoon flax seed	1 slice French Toast 1 cup berries 1 cup nut milk	¾ Huevos Rancheros 2 corn tortillas ½ grapefruit
Lunch	1½ cups Roasted Vegetable Delight 2 cups raw green vegetables	1 Chile Relleno 1 apple	2-3 Oats Walnut Balls ½ cup cooked brown rice or whole wheat pasta 1 cup steamed broccoli	Dr. Cooper's Rosemary-Lemon Tofu Kabobs 1 cup cantaloupe	2 slices Cashew Brown Rice Loaf 1 cup steamed spinach or broccoli	1 Oat-Nut Burger 1 whole-wheat burger bun 1 slice tomato 2 lettuce leaves	1 Spicy Tofu Burger 2 slices whole-wheat bread 1 slice tomato 2 slices avocado
Dinner	1 cup Lentil Soup with Vegetables 2 oz nuts	1 cup Mock Tuna Salad 3 lettuce leaves 1 pear	1½ cups Black Bean, Corn and Quinoa Salad 1 oz cashew nuts	¾ Mashed Cauliflower and White Beans 2 Baked Falafel	1 cup Corn and Potato Chowder 2 cups mixed fresh vegetable salad	1 cup Thai Coconut Curry Soup 1 kiwi	1 cup Creamy Potato Broccoli Soup 2 oz mixed nuts

VEGAN 28 DAY MEAL PLAN
(Weeks 3 & 4)

Week 3	Sun.	Mon.	Tue.	Wed.	Thu.	Fri.	Sat.
Breakfast	1 cup Jamaican Cornmeal Porridge 1 slice whole-wheat bread with nut butter ½ grapefruit	1 cup Hot Bulgur Wheat Cereal 1 cup mixed fresh fruits	1 Toast and Gravy 1 cup cantaloupe	½ cup Steamed Spinach 1 whole-wheat tortilla 2 oz walnuts or roasted pumpkin seeds	¾ cup Granola 1 cup nut milk 1 medium pear	2 Multigrain Waffles ½ cup mixed berries	2 slices Corn Bread 1 cup steamed spinach 1 oz nuts or baked seeds
Lunch	1 cup Italian White Bean Soup 1 cup papaya	Eggplant Zucchini Bake ½ cup whole-wheat pasta	2-3 Lentil Walnut "Meatballs" ¾ cup whole wheat spaghetti 1 cup steamed mixed vegetables	1 cup Italian Minestrone Soup ¼ cup Hummus with vegetable sticks	½ cup Chickpea Curry ½ cup brown rice or 1 medium baked potato 2 cups fresh vegetable salad	2 Lentil Walnut Meatballs ¼ cup avocado, mashed ¼ cup vegetable sprouts 2 slices whole-wheat bread	1 ½ cups Sun-Dried Tomato, Black Bean and Rice Salad 1 cup papaya
Dinner	Eggplant Roll-Ups 2 cups fresh salad	1 cup Kale White Bean Soup 2 oz mixed nuts	1½ cups Pasta Primavera 1 apple	1 cup Split Pea Soup 2 cups Fresh Vegetable Salad	1 cup Indian Lentil Soup 1 apple	1 cup Jamaican Kidney Bean Soup 2 cups vegetable salad	Eggplant Roll-Ups 1 whole-wheat tortilla

Week 4	Sun.	Mon.	Tue.	Wed.	Thu.	Fri.	Sat.
Breakfast	1 cup Breakfast Quinoa Bowl 1 pear	1 slice Loaded Toast 1 cup non-diary milk	1 Breakfast Quesadilla 1 cup cantaloupe	Avocado Toast ½ grapefruit	8 oz Detox Green Smoothie 2 oz mixed nuts	1 cup Banana Berry Fruit Salad 1 Slice whole-wheat bread 1 tablespoon nut butter	8 oz Oatmeal/Fruit Smoothie 1 slice whole-wheat bread 1 tbsp nut butter
Lunch	1 Lentil Patty 1 whole-wheat burger bun 2 cups green vegetable salad	1 cup Chinese Stir-Fry Vegetables ½ cup steamed brown rice	½ cup Lentil Stew 1 baked sweet potato 1 cup steamed broccoli	½ cup 5-Grain Brown Rice ½ cup Coconut Chickpea Curry 4 steamed asparagus	½ cup Seasoned Vegetable Rice 2-3 Oats Walnut Balls	½ Wild Rice and Mushroom Pilaf 2 Lentil Patties 2 cups green vegetable salad	½ cup Lentil Stew ½ cup Indian Rice 1 cup steamed cauliflower
Dinner	1 cup Spinach Kale Soup 1 pear	1 cup Cream of Pumpkin Soup pita chips	1 cup Easy Green Pea Soup 2 cups green vegetable salad	1 cup Summer Soup Hummus and pita chips	1 cup Cream of Broccoli 1 slice whole-wheat bread with avocado spread	2-3 Walnut Balls 2 cups steamed spinach	1 cup Spicy Mexican Beans pita chips

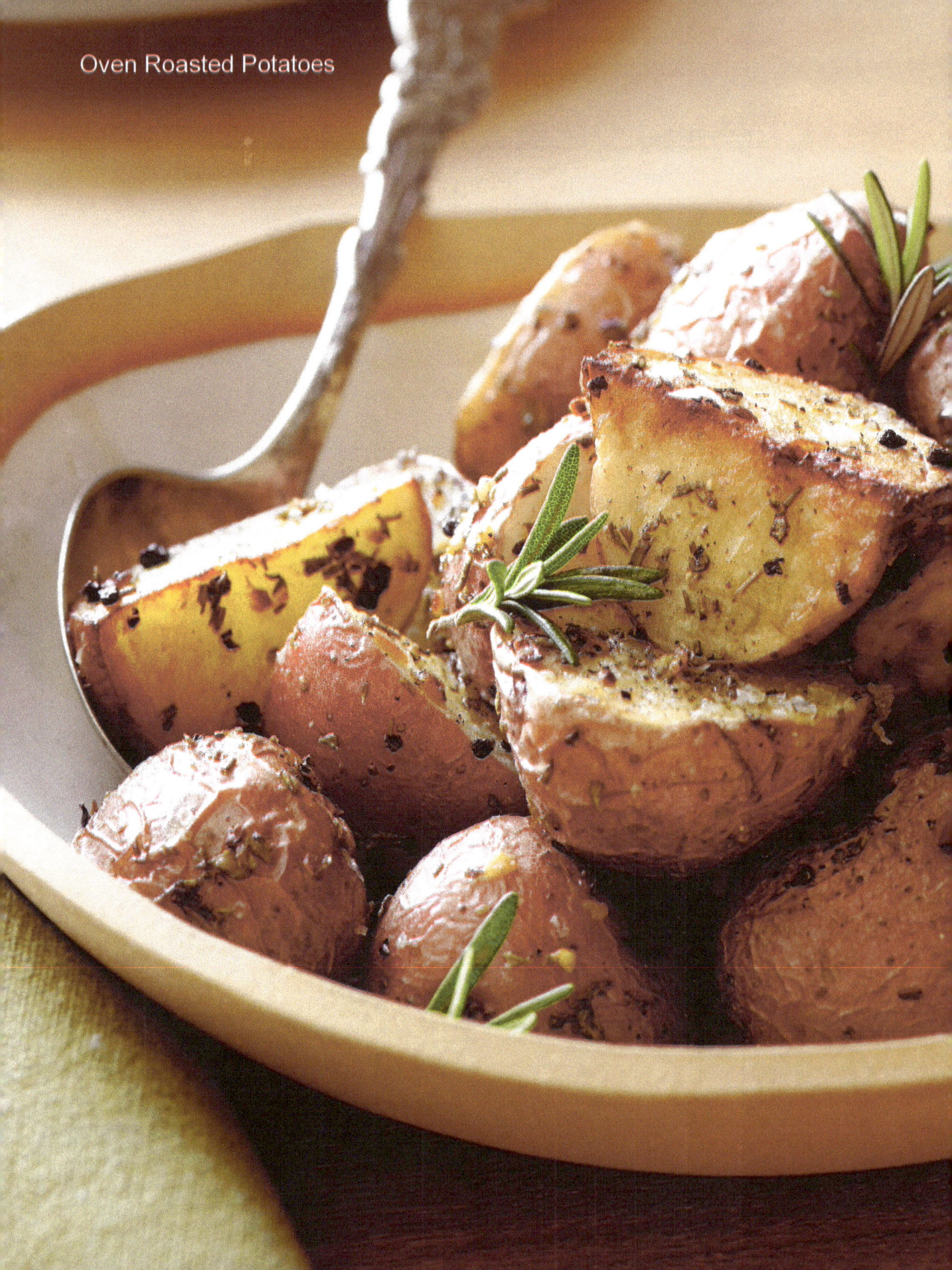

Oven Roasted Potatoes

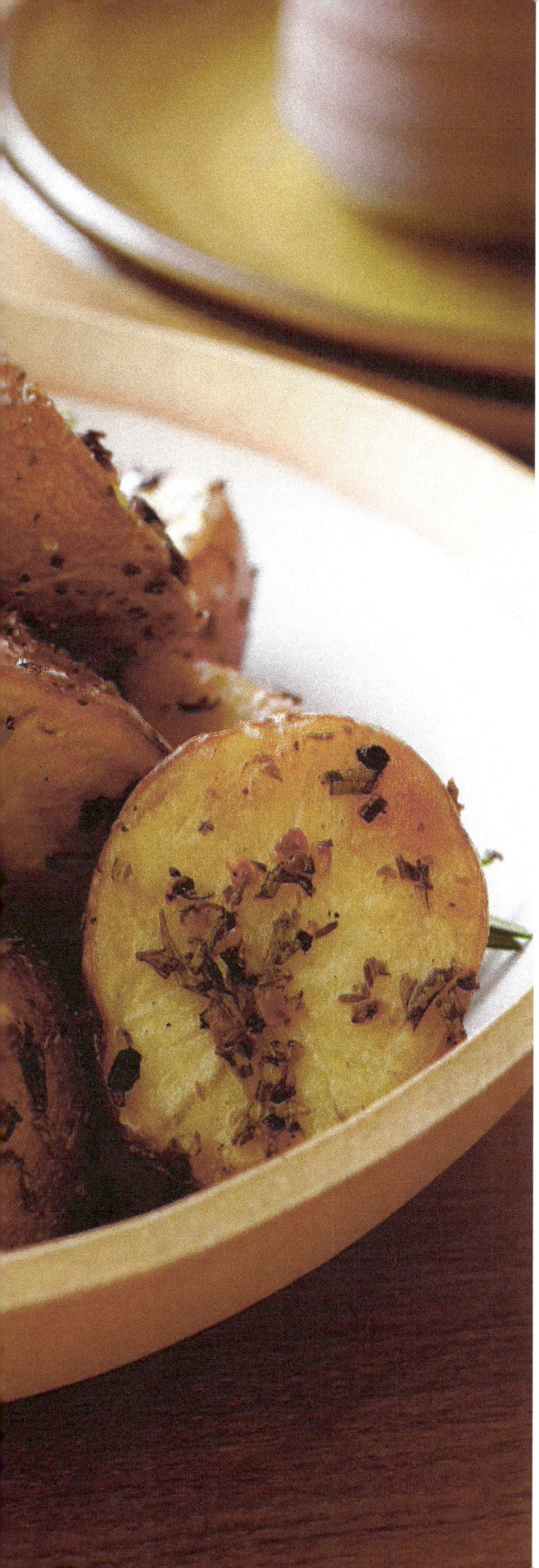

BREAKFAST

Scrambled Tofu with Kale
Banana Whole-Wheat Muffins
Bean Burrito
Traditional Tofu Scramble
Oven Roasted Potatoes
Whole-Wheat Pancakes
Cashew-Oat Waffles
Mushroom and Kale Frittata
Strawberry Fields Smoothie
Baked Oats
Banana Berry Smoothie
Blueberry-Oatmeal Pancakes
French Toast
Huevos Rancheros
Jamaican Cornmeal Porridge
Hot Bulgur Wheat Cereal
Toast and Gravy
Steamed Spinach
Granola
Multigrain Waffles
Corn Bread
Detox Green Smoothie
Dr. Cooper's Oats-on-the-Go
Avocado Toast

Scrambled Tofu with Kale

- 1 (16-ounce) water-packed package of extra-firm organic tofu
- 2 teaspoons vegetable oil
- ½ cup chopped onion
- ¼ cup bell peppers
- 2 teaspoons savory seasoning
- ½ teaspoon turmeric powder
- ½ teaspoon salt
- ½ teaspoon onion powder
- ½ teaspoon garlic powder
- ½ teaspoon thyme
- 2 teaspoons Mrs. Dash
- ½ cup tomatoes
- 4 cups kale, coarsely chopped

This great dish is filled with lots of vitamins, antioxidants, protein, fiber, and phytochemicals.

Remove the tofu from its package, rinse, drain, and set aside. In a large skillet or saucepan, sauté in hot oil the onion, peppers, and spices for 5 minutes. Scramble tofu in skillet and add remaining ingredients except kale. Allow to cook for 7 minutes on medium heat. Add kale. Stir occasionally. Cover until kale is wilted, about another 3 to 5 minutes. Serve with whole wheat bread or baked potatoes or over brown rice (main dish).

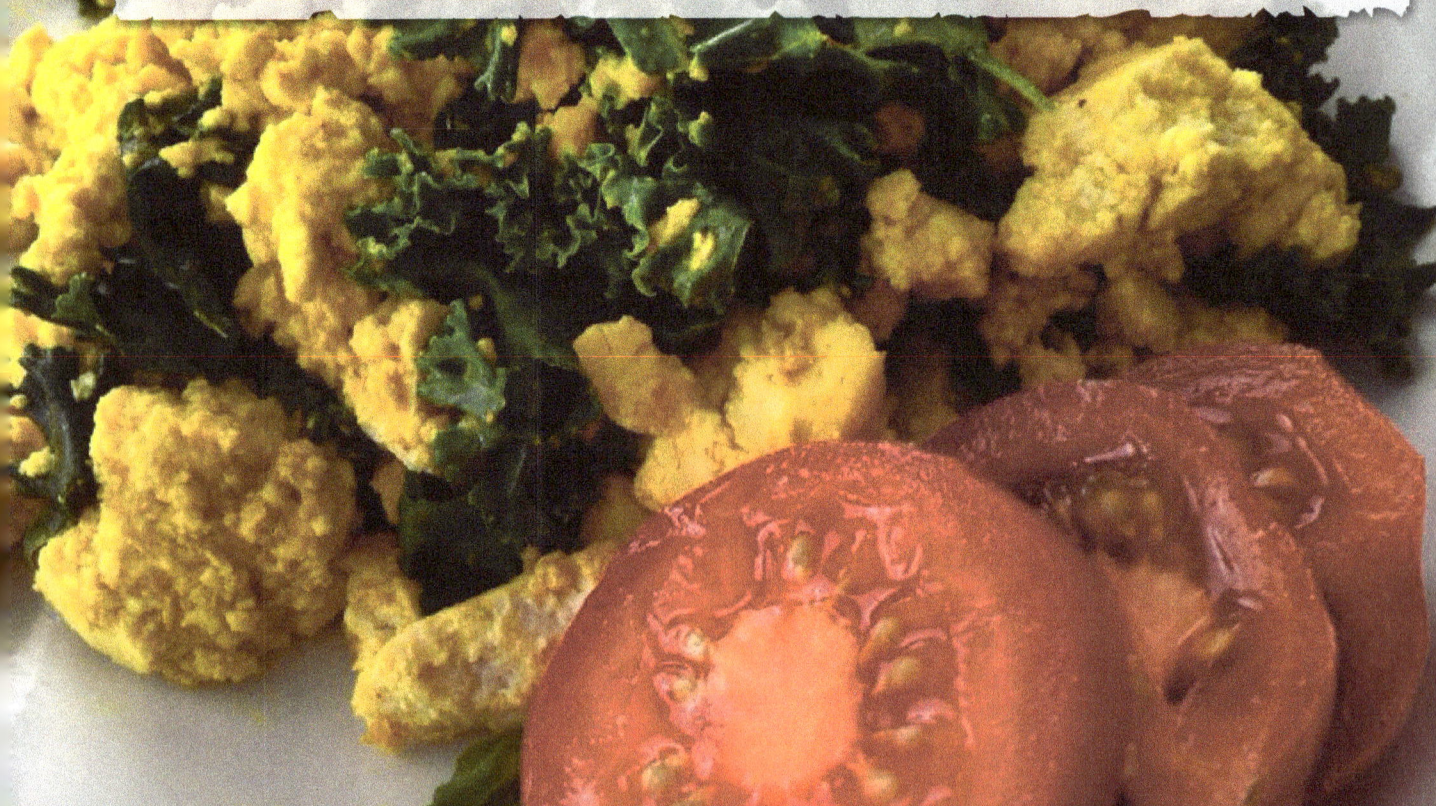

Banana Whole-Wheat Muffins

- 1 ¾ cups whole wheat flour
- 2 teaspoons baking powder
- ½ teaspoon baking soda
- ½ teaspoon salt
- ¼ teaspoon ground nutmeg
- 1 teaspoon cinnamon
- ⅔ cup crushed pineapple
- ⅔ cup coconut cream
- 1 cup mashed, very ripe banana
- 1 teaspoon vanilla
- ½ cup raisins
- ¼ cup chopped pecans

This is a great breakfast option but eat with moderation if you are diabetic.

Preheat oven to 375 degrees Fahrenheit. Line 12 standard muffin cups with paper baking cups or grease bottoms. Stir together whole wheat flour, baking soda, salt, and nutmeg in a medium-sized bowl. Mix crushed pineapple, milk, banana and vanilla in a large bowl. Stir in the flour mixture just until just moistened (batter will be lumpy). Fold in raisins and pecans. Divide batter evenly among muffin cups. Bake 18 to 20 minutes or until golden brown and a toothpick inserted into the center comes out clean. Remove from pan to wire rack. Serve warm.

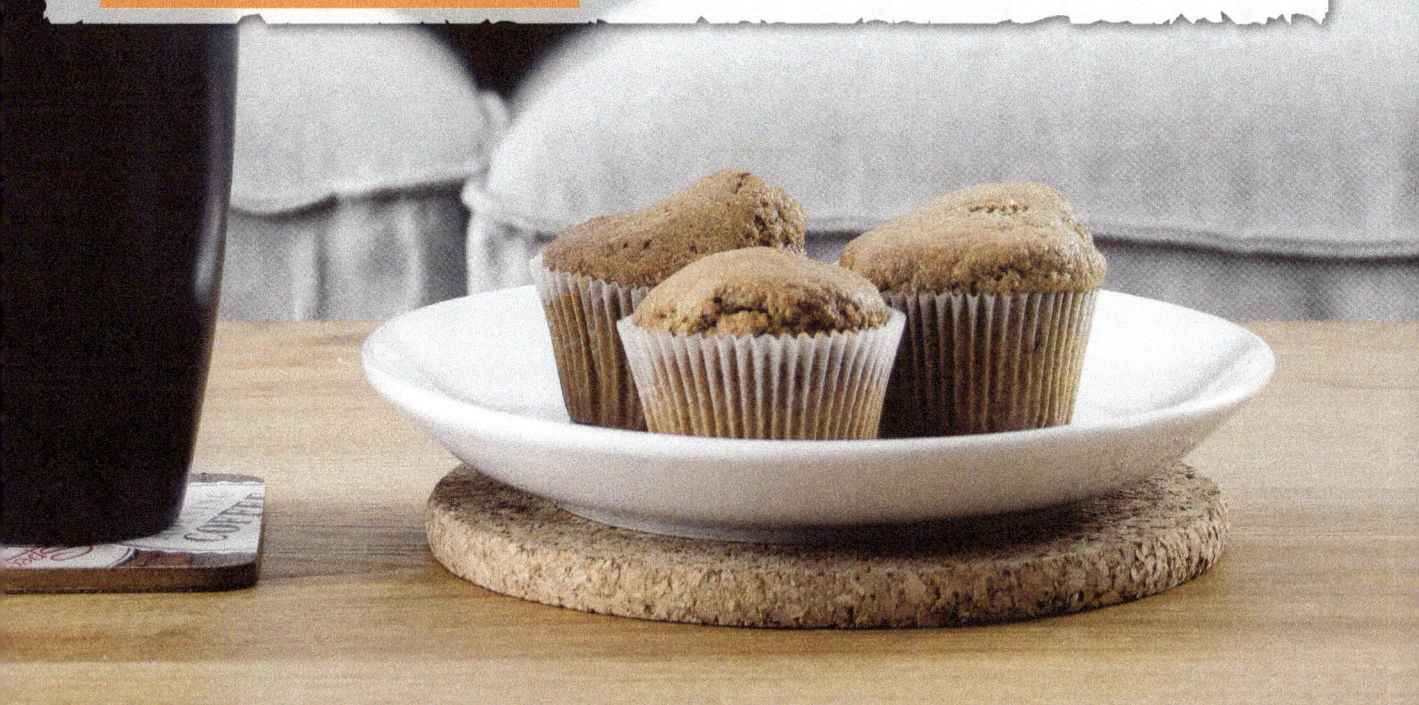

Bean Burrito

- 1 whole-wheat tortilla
- ¼ cup spicy Mexican beans (mashed)
- Desired amount of:
- Chopped lettuce
- Chopped tomatoes
- Diced onions
- Olives
- Avocado
- Salsa
- Soy sour cream (non-dairy)

This is a well-known and easy to prepare Mexican dish. These can be served at any time of the day.

Warm tortillas and spread the beans over the tortillas. Fold like an envelope. Serve with lettuce, tomato, onions, olives, and avocado and top with salsa and soy sour cream.

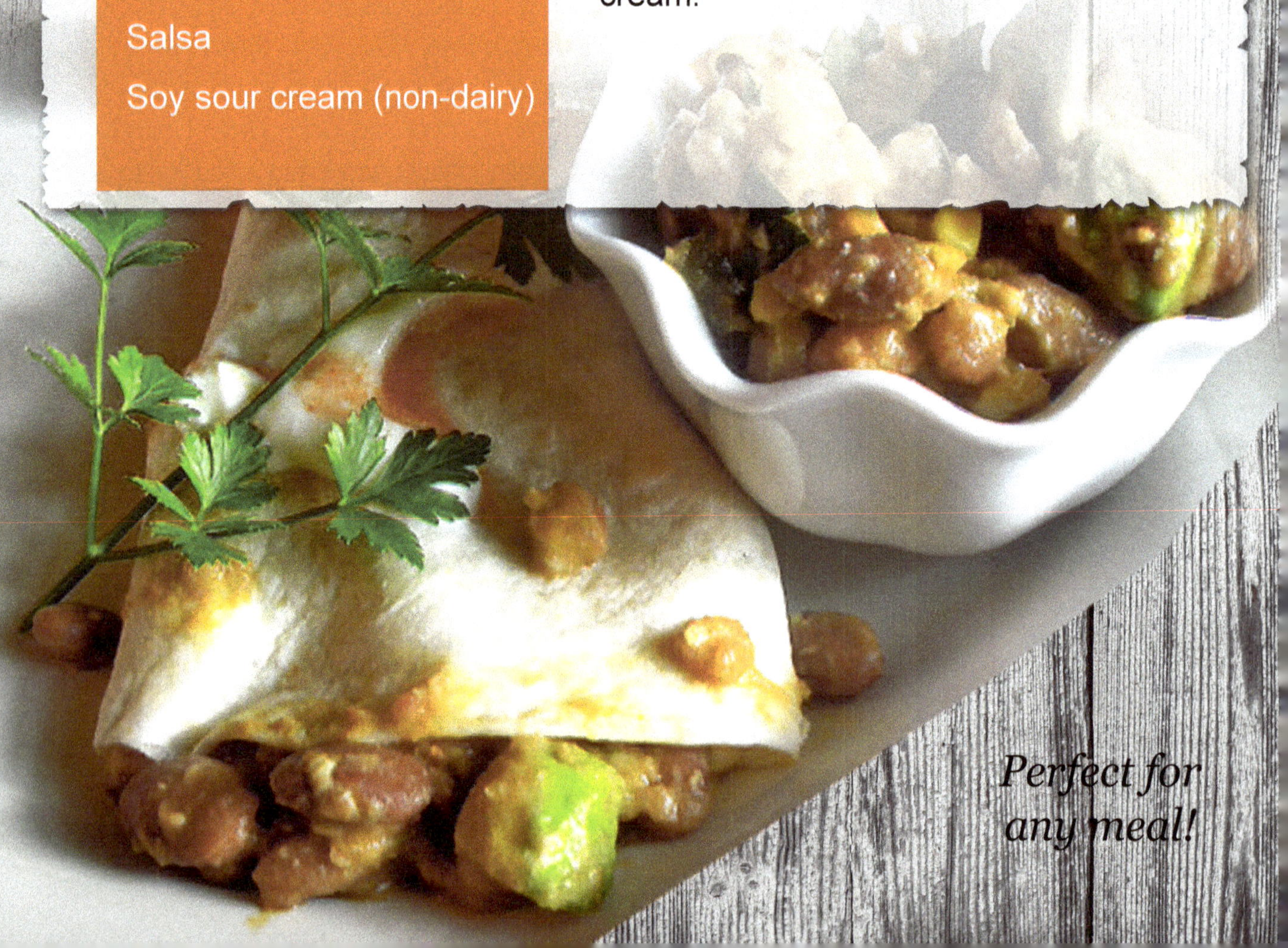

Perfect for any meal!

Traditional Tofu Scramble

1 (16-ounce) water-packed package of extra-firm organic tofu
2 teaspoons vegetable oil
½ cup chopped onion
¼ cup bell peppers
2 teaspoons McKay's savory seasoning
½ teaspoon turmeric powder
½ teaspoon salt
½ teaspoon onion powder
½ teaspoon garlic powder
½ teaspoon thyme
1 teaspoon Mrs. Dash
½ cup tomatoes

This dish looks and taste like eggs but without the cholesterol. It is even more delicious when left overnight in the refrigerator.

Remove the tofu from its package, rinse, and drain. Use fork to mash tofu into small pieces and set aside. In large skillet/saucepan sauté in hot oil the onion, peppers, and spices for 5 minutes. Add tofu to the skillet with oil and vegetables, add the remaining ingredients. Cover and allow to cook for another 10 minutes. Serve as filling for tacos or with whole wheat bread.

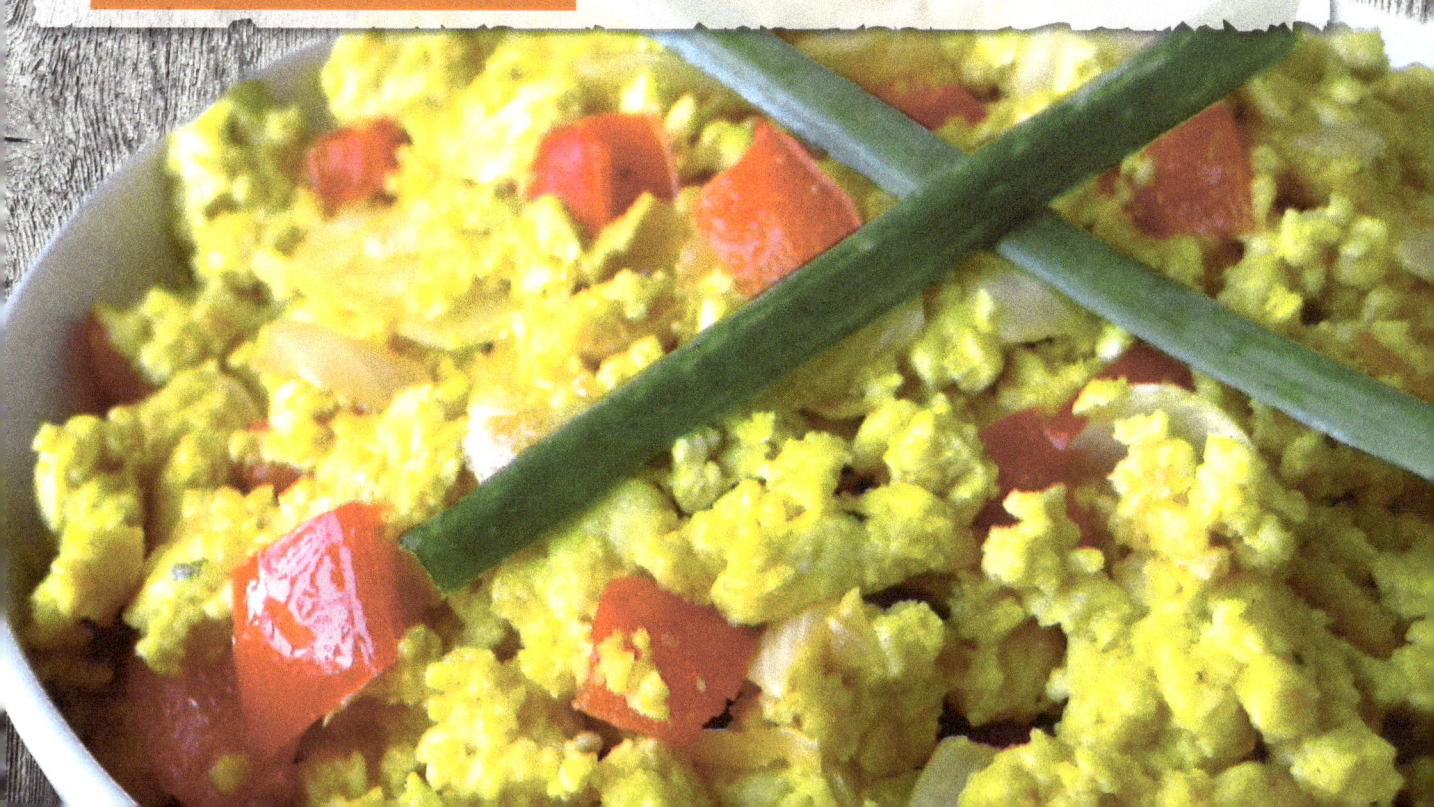

Oven Roasted Potatoes

- 4 pounds small red potatoes, halved
- 1 ½ tablespoon olive oil
- 4 teaspoons fresh rosemary, chopped
- 2 teaspoons Mrs. Dash seasoning
- 1 medium onion, chopped
- 2 tablespoons savory seasoning
- 1 teaspoon salt, to taste

This is a great side dish you can enjoy any time of the day. You could also add firm tofu (cubes) and bake. Makes a great main dish.

Preheat oven to 400 degrees Fahrenheit. Place potatoes in a single-layer baking sheet and sprinkle oil over potatoes. Then evenly mix in all the other ingredients. Cover with foil and bake for 12 to 15 minutes. Remove foil and continue to bake for an additional 15 minutes or until golden brown.

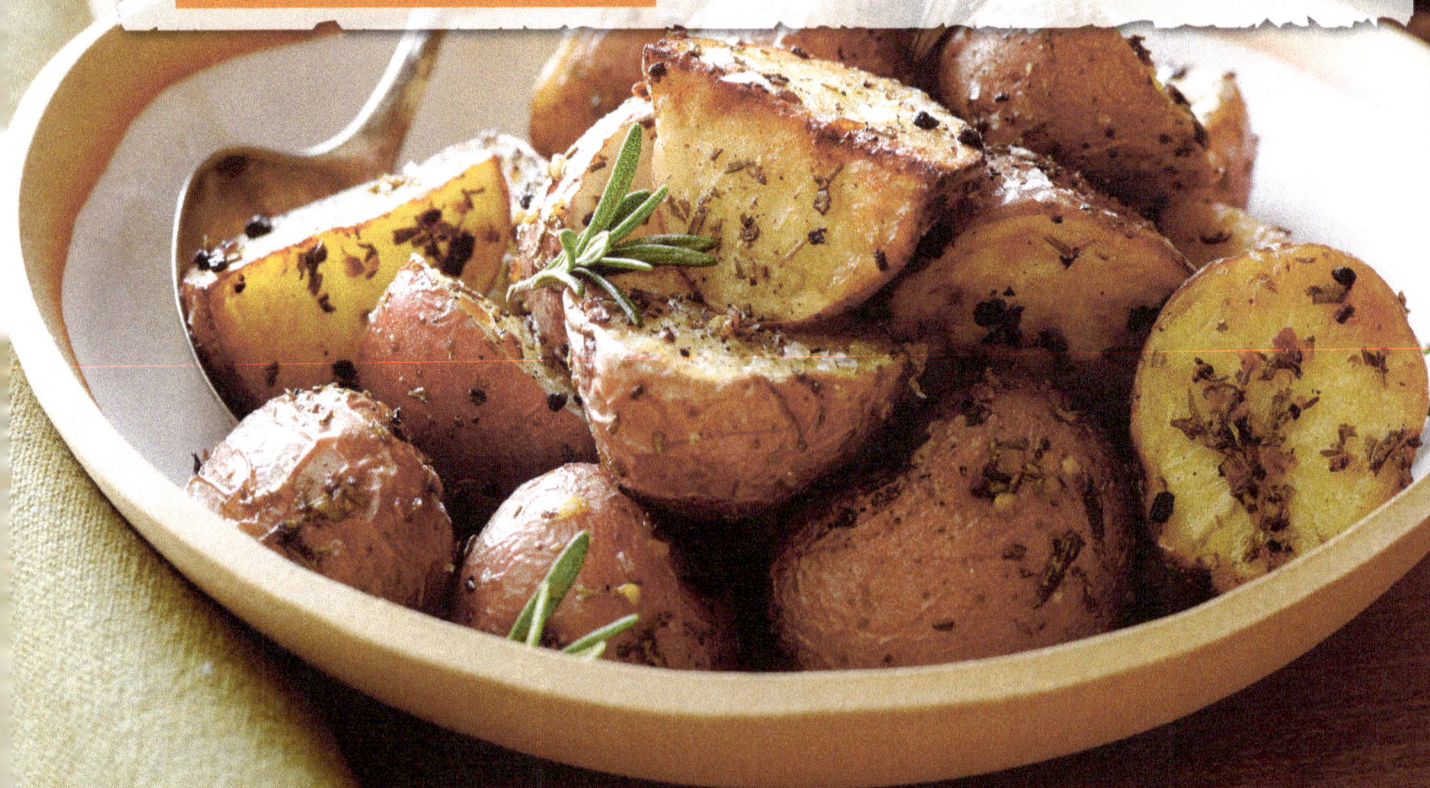

Whole-Wheat Pancakes

- 3 cups whole wheat flour
- 2 ½ teaspoons baking powder
- ½ teaspoon salt
- 2 cups soy milk
- 3 tablespoons applesauce

These delicious pancakes will not raise your cholesterol.

Mix dry ingredients together. Add remaining ingredients and mix well gently. Drop mixture by spoonful on a hot, nonstick griddle. Fry until golden brown. Flip pancake and repeat for the other side. Serve with fruit topping.

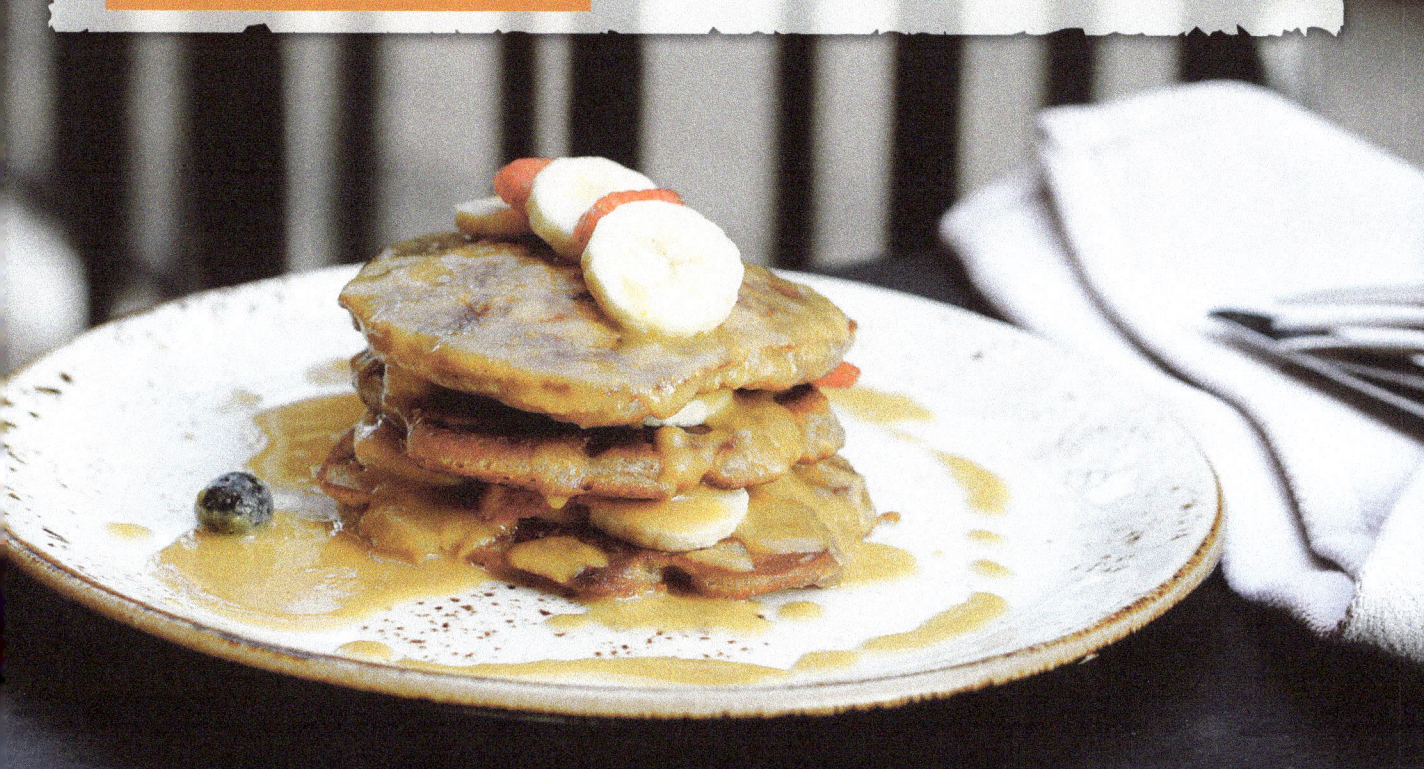

Cashew-Oat Waffles

- ⅓ cup raw cashews
- 2 cups water or 1 cup soy milk
- 1 teaspoon vanilla extract
- 2 cups old-fashioned oats
- ½ teaspoon salt

These waffles are filling and great for people with heart disease, diabetes and high cholesterol. A diet high in fiber will promote better glucose and cholesterol levels. Serves 2 to 3.

Blend cashews in water or soy milk until smooth. Add remaining ingredients, and then blend together. Let mixture stand 5 minutes to thicken. Cook approximately 7 minutes in the waffle iron until golden brown. Serve hot with your favorite fruit topping. Waffles freeze well and can be easily reheated in a toaster or microwave.

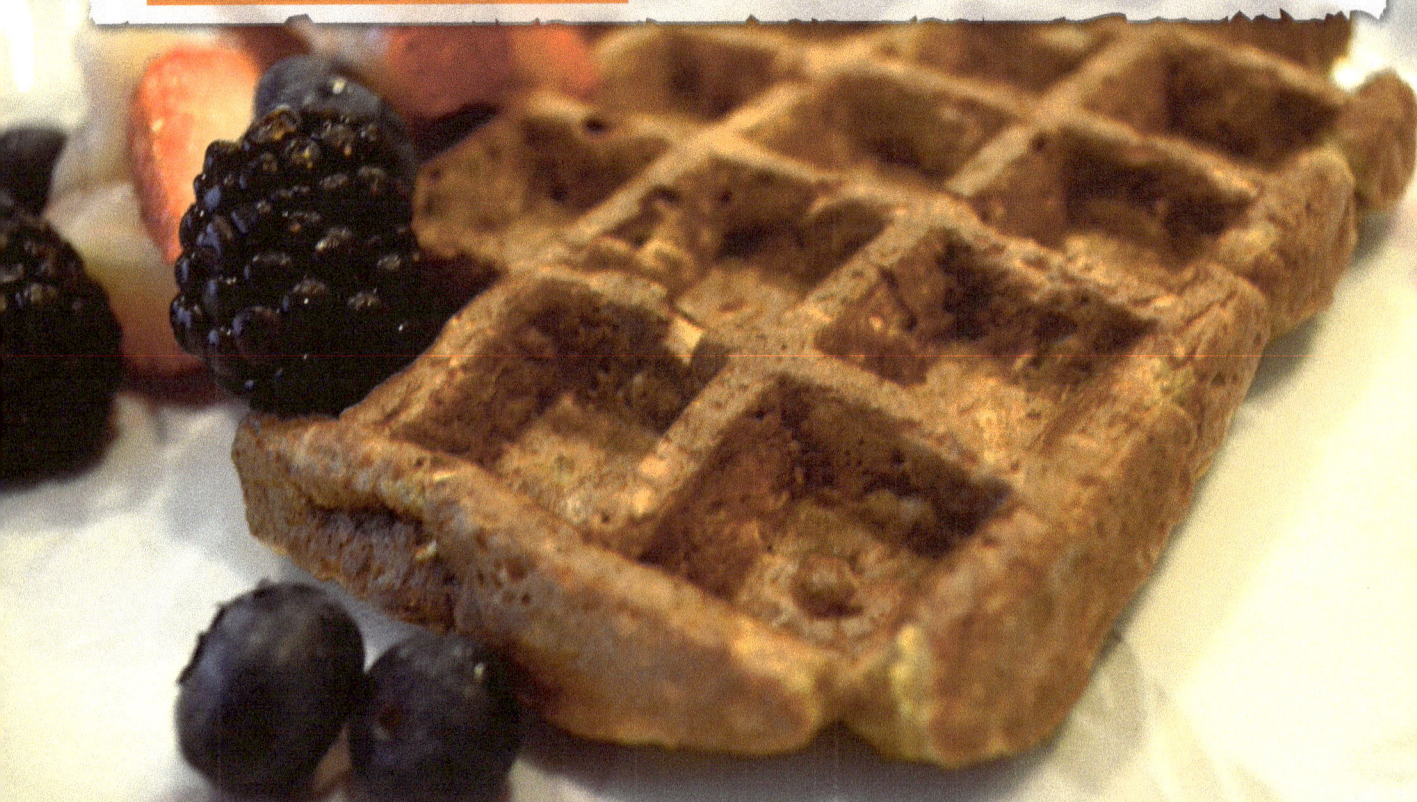

Strawberry Peach Smoothie

- 4 cups strawberries, frozen
- 4 cups peaches, frozen
- 2 tablespoons flax seeds
- 1 cup vanilla almond milk

Smoothies are quick and easy to make. Keep small bags of frozen fruits and vegetables handy.

Place everything in a high-speed blender and blend until smooth.

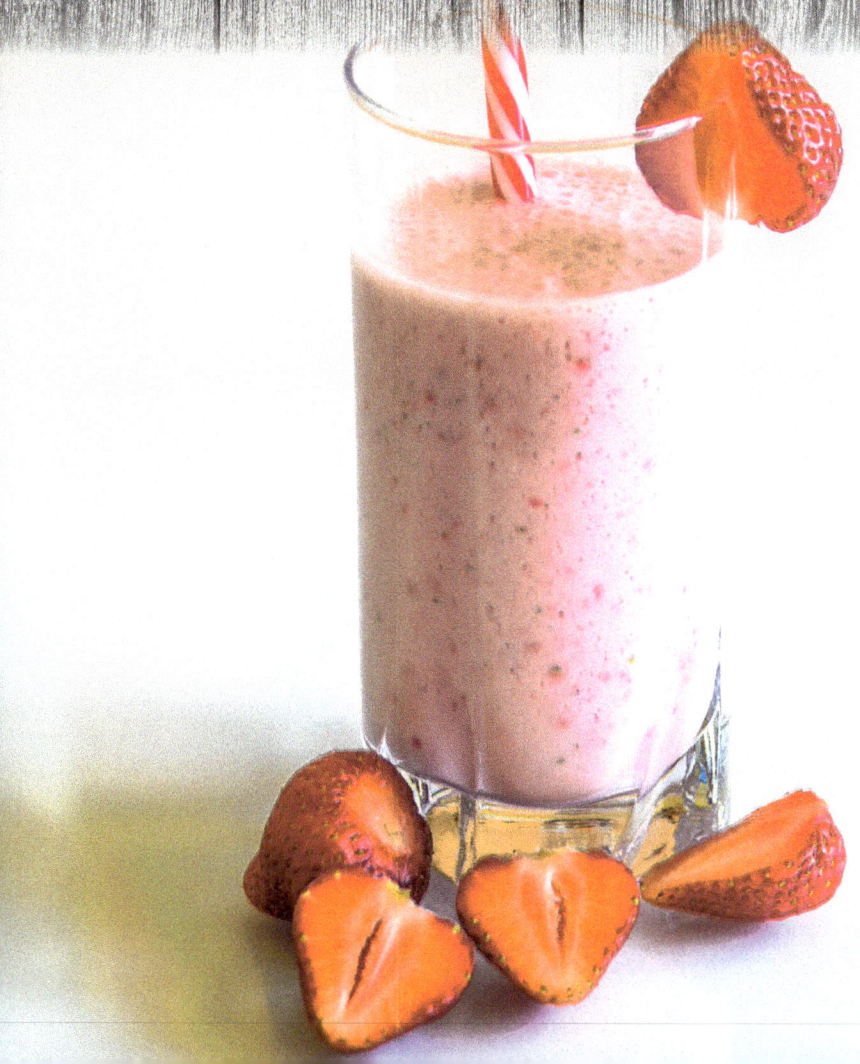

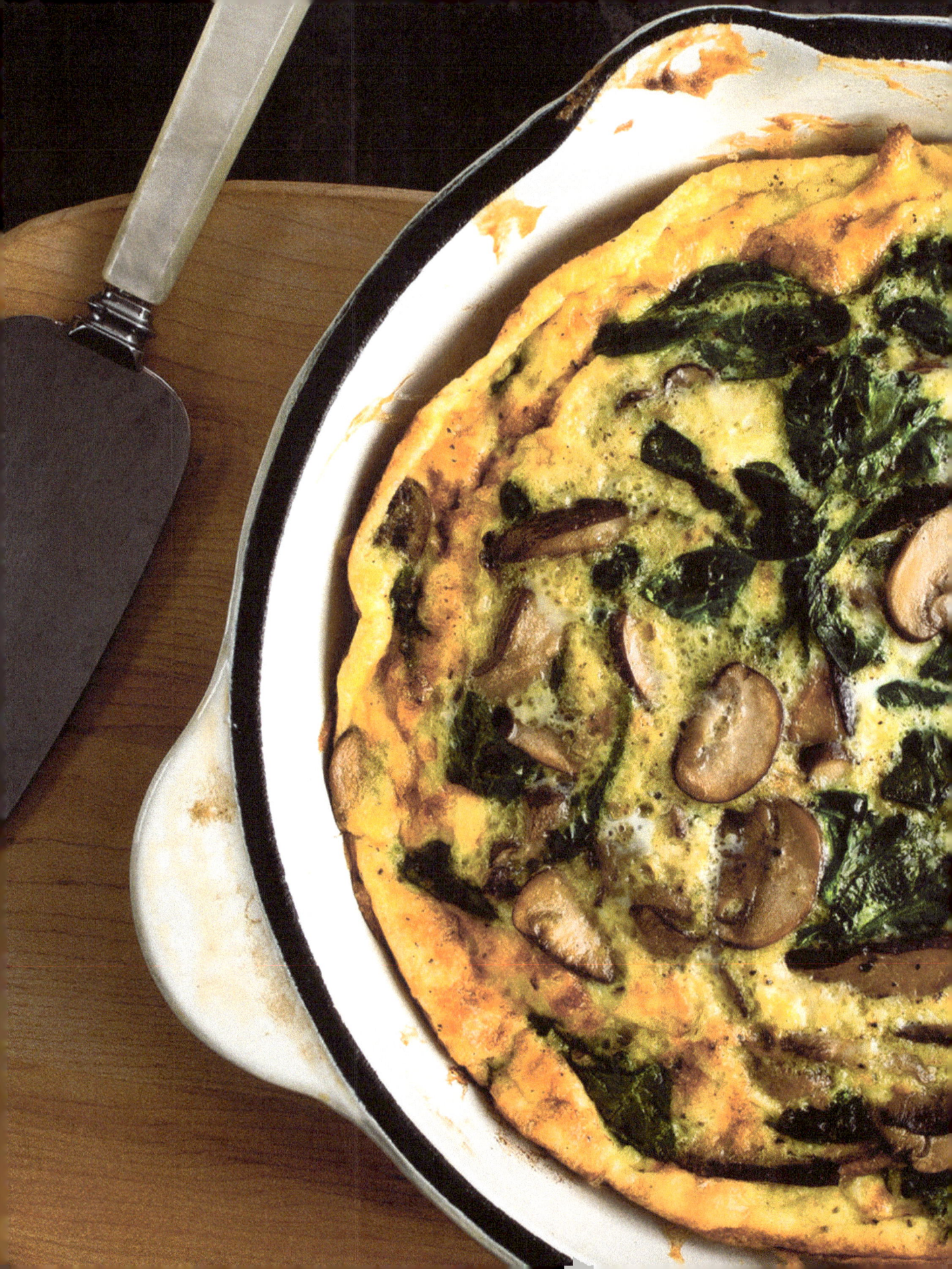

Mushroom and Kale Frittata

1 cup rolled oats

½ cup whole wheat flour

½ teaspoon baking soda

¼ teaspoon salt

1 cup soy milk

2 tablespoon olive oil

1 small onion, chopped

2 cups mushrooms

2 cups scrambled tofu (refer to recipe on page 41)

4 cups coarsely chopped kale leaves

2 cloves garlic, mashed and minced

This simple dish is good for breakfast but could be eaten at any time of the day. Store leftovers in the refrigerator and re-warm in the oven. Makes 6 servings.

Blend oats; add wheat flour, baking soda, and salt. In a separate bowl, mix milk and oil. Then combine both and set aside. Spray large ovenproof skillet with nonstick cooking spray, and heat over medium heat. Add onion and mushrooms, cook and stir 6 to 8 minutes or until onion is light golden. Add kale and garlic, cook 3 to 5 minutes or until kale is wilted. Evenly spread mixture to cover the bottom of the skillet. Pour scrambled tofu over the kale mixture. Cover and cook 6 to 7 minutes or until almost set. Poor batter mixture over sautéed vegetable tofu and slightly mix, then allow to cook on low-medium heat for 5-7 minutes or until dough is cooked. Or may place mixture in an oiled baking dish and baked at 375 degree Fahrenheit for 7-10 minutes or until dough is baked. Let stand 5 minutes before cutting into 6 wedges.

Baked Oats

- 2 cups rolled oats
- ¼ cup raisins
- ¼ cup dates, chopped
- 1 teaspoon ground cinnamon
- 1 ½ teaspoon baking powder
- 1 cup soy or almond milk
- ½ cup blended apple
- 1 teaspoon vanilla extract
- ½ cup almond slivers

This is an excellent breakfast dish and is filled with fiber and good fat, which are very filling and will eliminate the urge to snack.

Mix all dry ingredients in a bowl, and then add the wet ingredients and mix well. Preheat oven to 350 degrees Fahrenheit. Place mixture in a lightly oiled baking dish, spread evenly, and cover and bake for 25 to 30 minutes. Serve warm or cold.

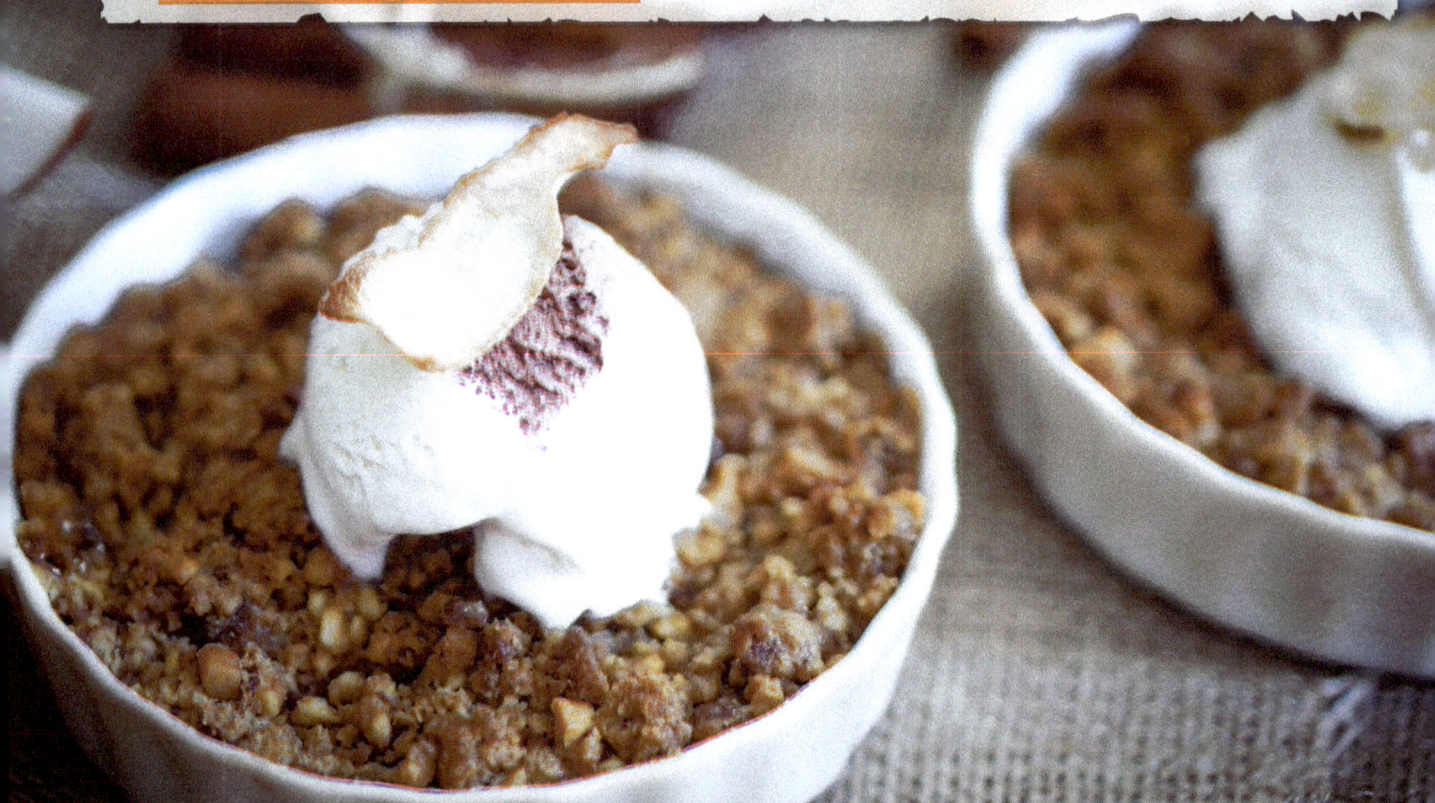

Banana Berry Smoothie

- 4 cups strawberries, frozen
- 3 ripe bananas, frozen
- 3 cups soy or almond milk
- ½ cup rolled oats

Smoothies are quick and easy to make. Keep small bags of frozen fruits and vegetables handy.

Place everything in a high-speed blender and blend until smooth.

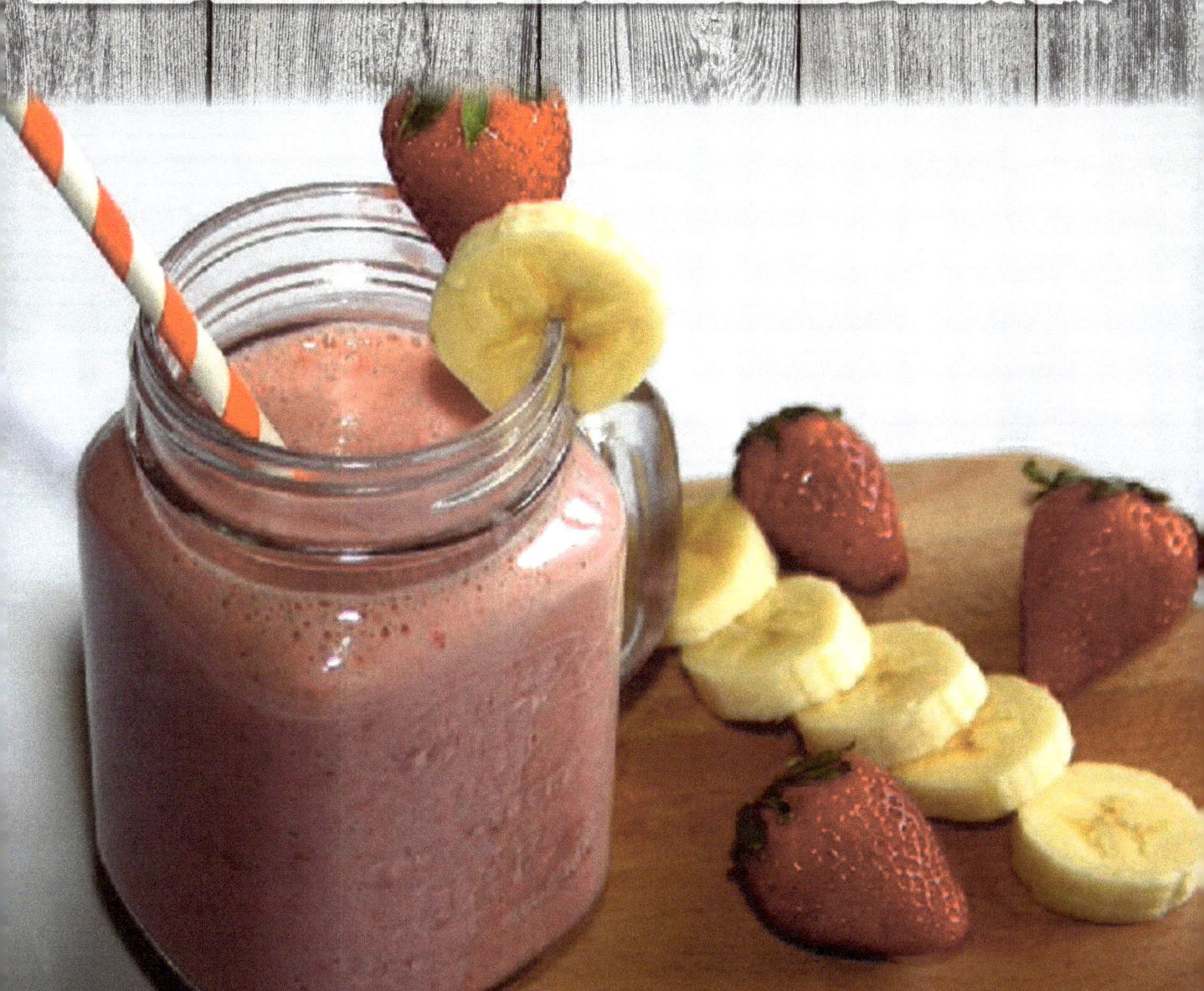

Blueberry-Oatmeal Pancakes

- 2 flax eggs (2 tablespoons ground flaxseed + 6 tablespoons water)
- 1 cup rolled oats
- 1 ½ cup unsweetened soy or almond milk
- ¼ cup walnuts
- ½ cup whole wheat flour
- ½ teaspoon baking soda
- ½ teaspoon baking powder
- 6 dates, pitted
- ½ teaspoon salt
- 1 cup fresh or frozen blueberries

These pancakes are a little denser, heartier, and more filling than the regular pancakes.

Mix ground flax with 6 tablespoons of water and let the mix stand for 10 minutes. The consistency should be that of an egg. Place oats, nuts, and milk in a blender and blend until smooth. Place mixture in bowl, and then fold in other ingredients. Add more milk if necessary for the desired consistency. Lightly grease the hot skillet or pan with additional oil. Pour ½ cup pancake rounds on the skillet and cook until bubbles form on the surface. Carefully drop 6 to 8 (optional) blueberries onto one side of each pancake, and then flip and cook on the other side until golden brown.

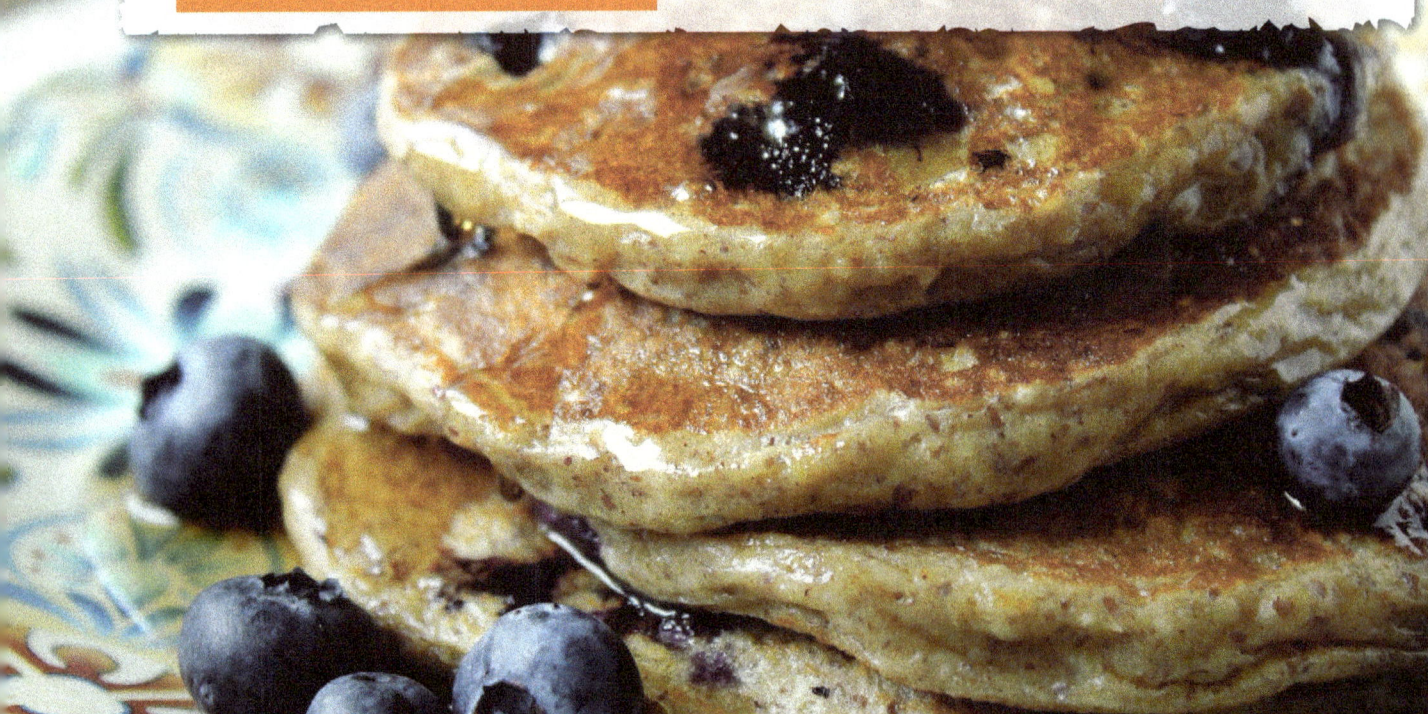

French Toast

- 1 ripe banana
- 1 cup unsweetened soy or almond milk
- 2 tablespoons cornstarch
- ½ teaspoon pure vanilla extract
- ½ teaspoon nutmeg
- Tiny pinch of salt
- 6 slices whole wheat bread

This is a healthier and delicious spin on the traditional fat-laden French toast.

Mash banana in a wide, shallow bowl. Mix in other ingredients, except the bread. Soak bread in the liquid mixture. Heat nonstick pan or griddle on medium heat and lightly spray with vegetable oil. Transfer the soaked bread to a heated surface and cook until both sides are golden brown. Serve with fruit sauce or berries.

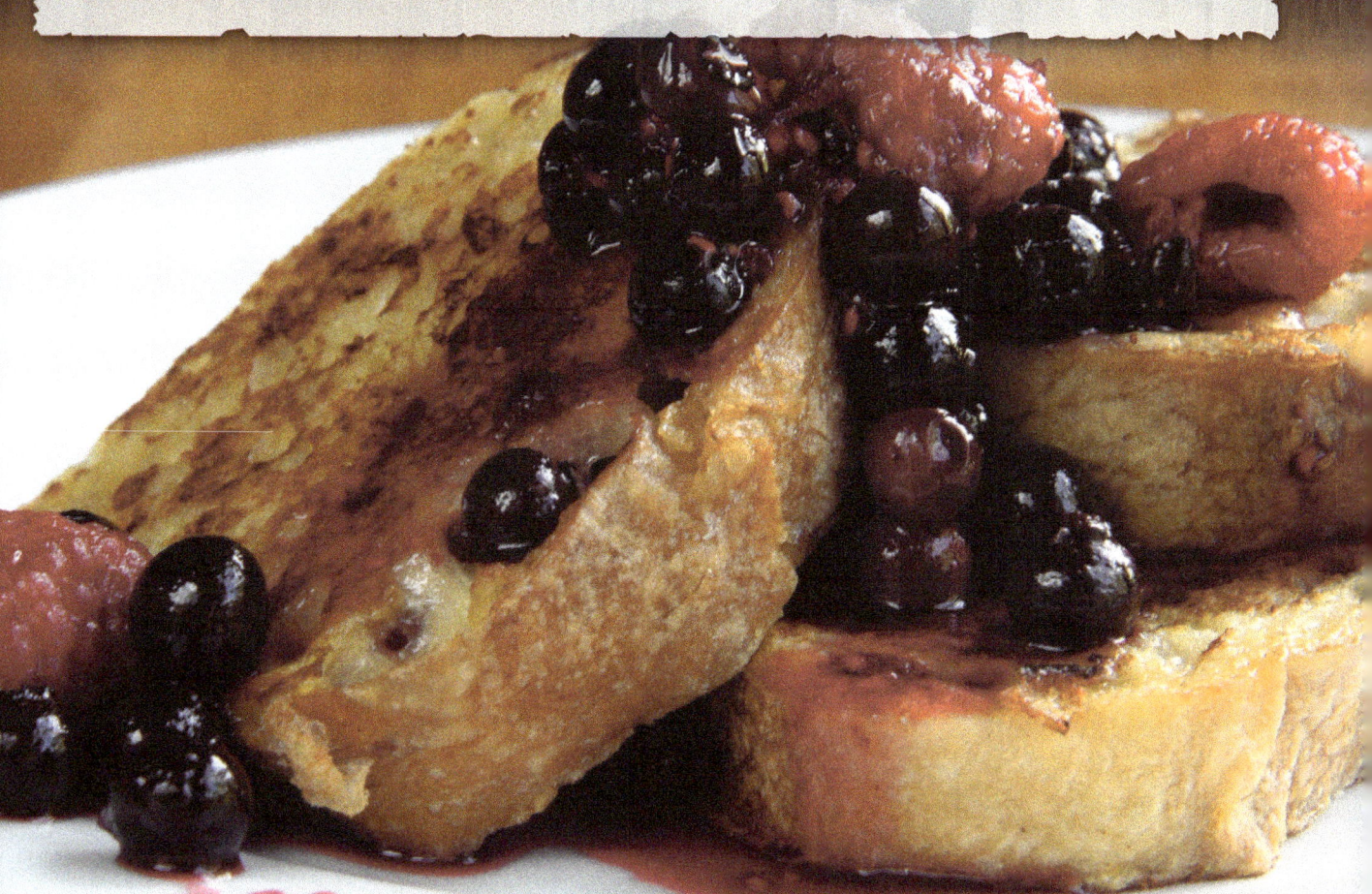

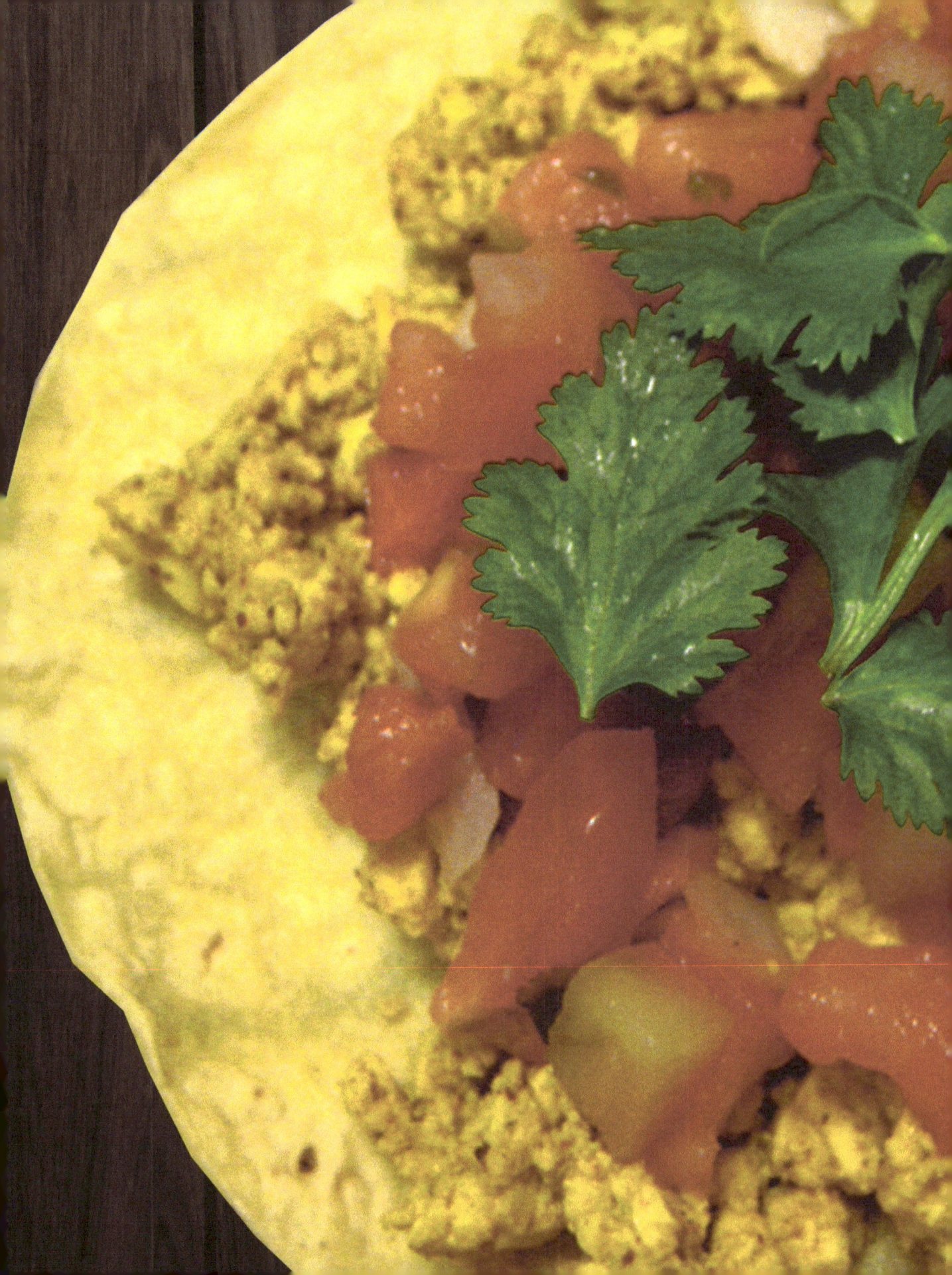

Huevos Rancheros

1 ½ teaspoon olive oil
1 (14- to 16-ounce package) firm tofu, drained and mashed with fork
1 medium onion, chopped
1 large clove garlic (mashed and minced)
1 medium green bell pepper, chopped
1 cup prepared medium or mild salsa, plus more for serving
2 medium tomatoes, diced (1 cup)
1–2 small fresh jalapeño chilies, seeded and minced
2 tablespoons nutritional yeast
2 teaspoons ground cumin
½ teaspoon ground turmeric
1 teaspoon Savory Seasoning powder
1 cup cilantro leaves, chopped
8 corn tortillas, warmed

This great breakfast option is high in protein content and goes well with smashed cooked kidney beans.

Heat oil in large skillet over medium heat. Add onion and garlic and sauté 5 minutes or until translucent. Add bell pepper, crumbling each as it goes in. Stir in salsa, tomatoes, and chilies, followed by nutritional yeast (if using), cumin, savory seasoning, and turmeric. Cook 5 to 8 minutes or until tomatoes have softened and ingredients are melded. Stir in cilantro. Taste and add salt, if desired. Divide tofu mixture among tortillas, and serve with salsa.

Jamaican Cornmeal Porridge

- 1 cup yellow cornmeal
- 4 cups water
- 2 cinnamon sticks
- ½ teaspoon salt
- ½ teaspoon nutmeg
- 1 cup soy or almond milk

This classical warm breakfast cereal is widely served in Jamaica. May add coconut cream for a creamier taste.

Mix cornmeal in 1 cup water and set aside. Place 3 cups of water and cinnamon sticks in a deep, medium-sized pot. Bring water to a boil and then pour the cornmeal mixture into the boiling water. Turn heat down to low and stir continuously until thickened and smooth. Cover pot and allow to cook for 20 minutes. Add milk, salt, and nutmeg, and allow to cook for 10 minutes more. Sweeten to taste with natural sweetener, such as agave. Serve hot in a bowl.

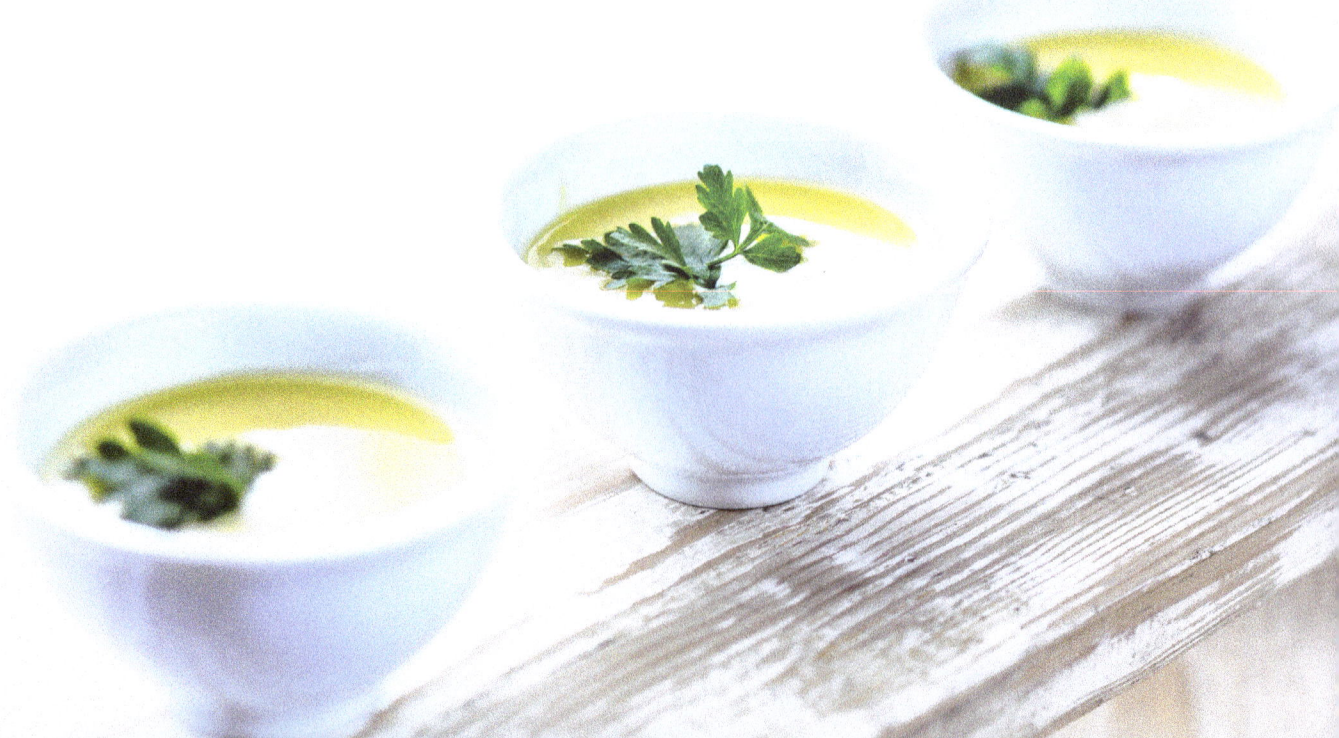

Hot Bulgur Wheat Cereal

- 2 cups bulgur wheat
- 4 cups almond or soy milk
- 2 cinnamon sticks
- 2 tablespoons whole wheat flour
- ½ teaspoon nutmeg
- ½ teaspoon salt (optional)
- ½ cup raisins
- ¼ cup walnuts, chopped
- 1 ripe banana

Delicious hearty breakfast ideal for diabetics because of the high fiber content but great for everyone.

Place bulgur wheat, cinnamon sticks, and milk in a deep, small- to medium-sized pot and allow to cook on low to medium heat for 25 minutes. Mix whole wheat flour in a small amount of water and then pour this mixture into the pot. Stir and allow to cook for another 7 to 10 minutes more. Add nutmeg to mixture just before removing pot from heat. Serve hot in a bowl topped with raisins, walnuts, and ripe banana to sweeten.

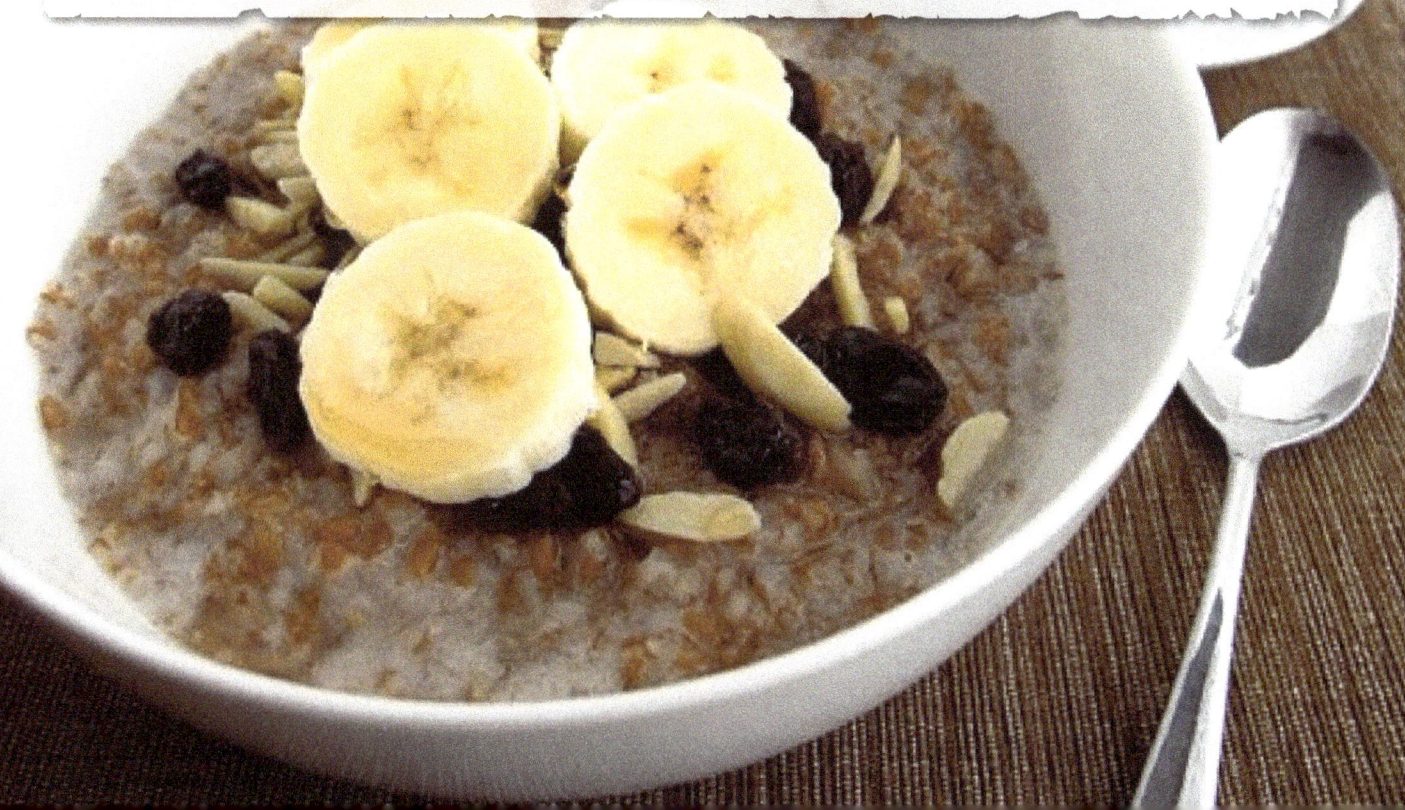

Toast and Gravy

- ½ cup almonds
- 2 cups water
- 2 tablespoons McKay's chicken-style seasoning
- 2 tablespoon Bragg's Amino Acids
- 1 tablespoon nutritional yeast
- ½ teaspoon garlic powder
- ½ teaspoon onion powder
- 1 small onion
- ½ teaspoon dry basil
- 2 tablespoons cornstarch

If you are a lover of biscuits and gravy, then this breakfast option is for you. It is fast and easy to prepare, and, most important, it is healthy with good fats.

Place all ingredients except cornstarch in a high-speed blender with 1½ cup of water. Blend until smooth. Place mixture in a saucepan. Allow to simmer on medium heat. Mix cornstarch in remaining water and incorporate to boiling mixture. Stir frequently until smooth. Place toast bread on plate. Pour gravy over toast and enjoy!

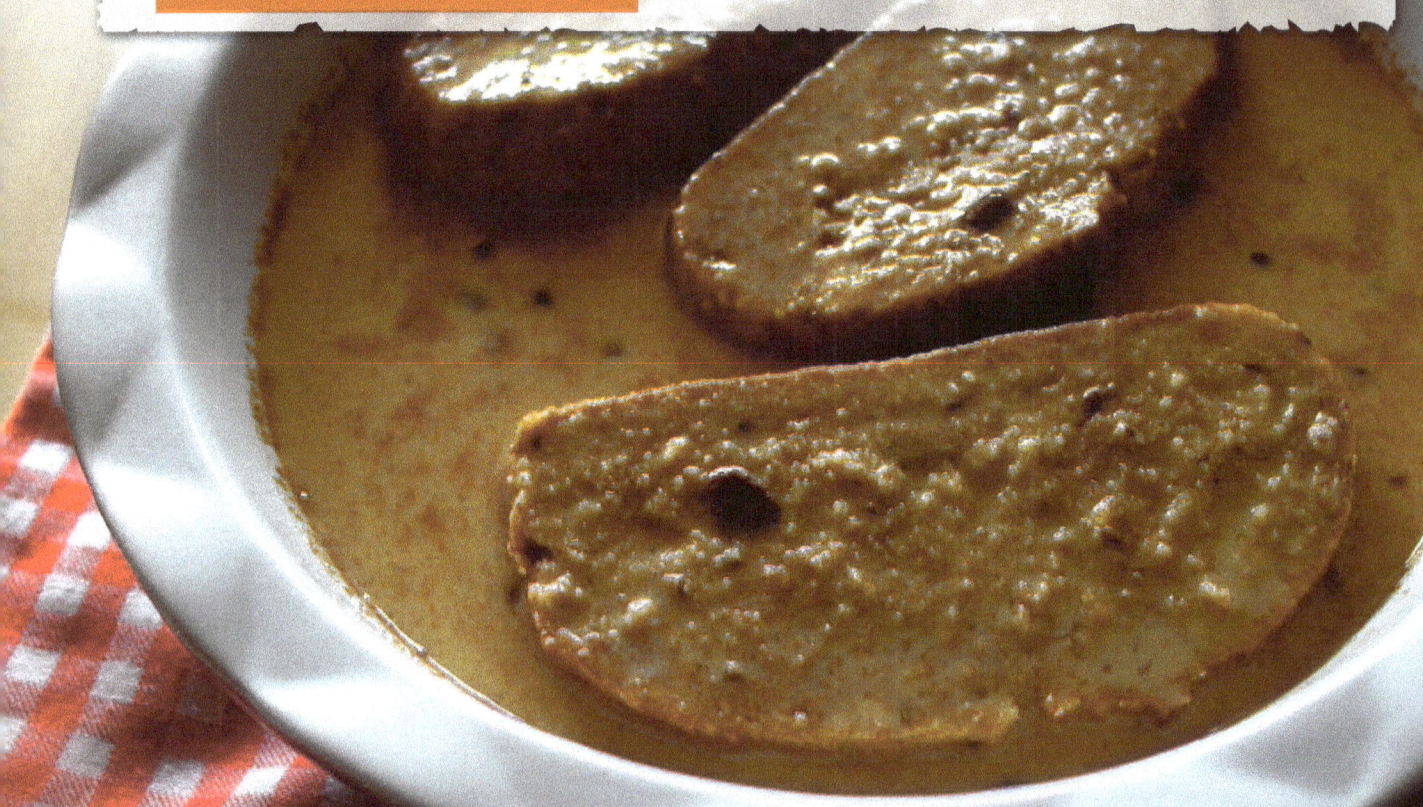

Steamed Spinach

- 1 tablespoon olive oil
- ½ medium onion, chopped
- 1 small tomato, chopped
- ½ medium green bell pepper, chopped
- 2 (10-ounce) packages frozen spinach
- 2 sprigs fresh thyme
- 1 teaspoon McKay's chicken-style seasoning

This dish is filled with vitamins, minerals, and antioxidants. You may use kale instead of spinach. Remember not to cook your vegetables, as this will destroy vital nutrients.

Place oil in saucepan on low-medium heat. Sauté onion, bell pepper, and tomato for 3 to 5 minutes. Remove water from spinach and then add to saucepan. Add remaining ingredients. Allow to simmer for another 7 to 10 minutes. Taste and add extra seasoning or salt if desired. Serve with oven-roasted potatoes.

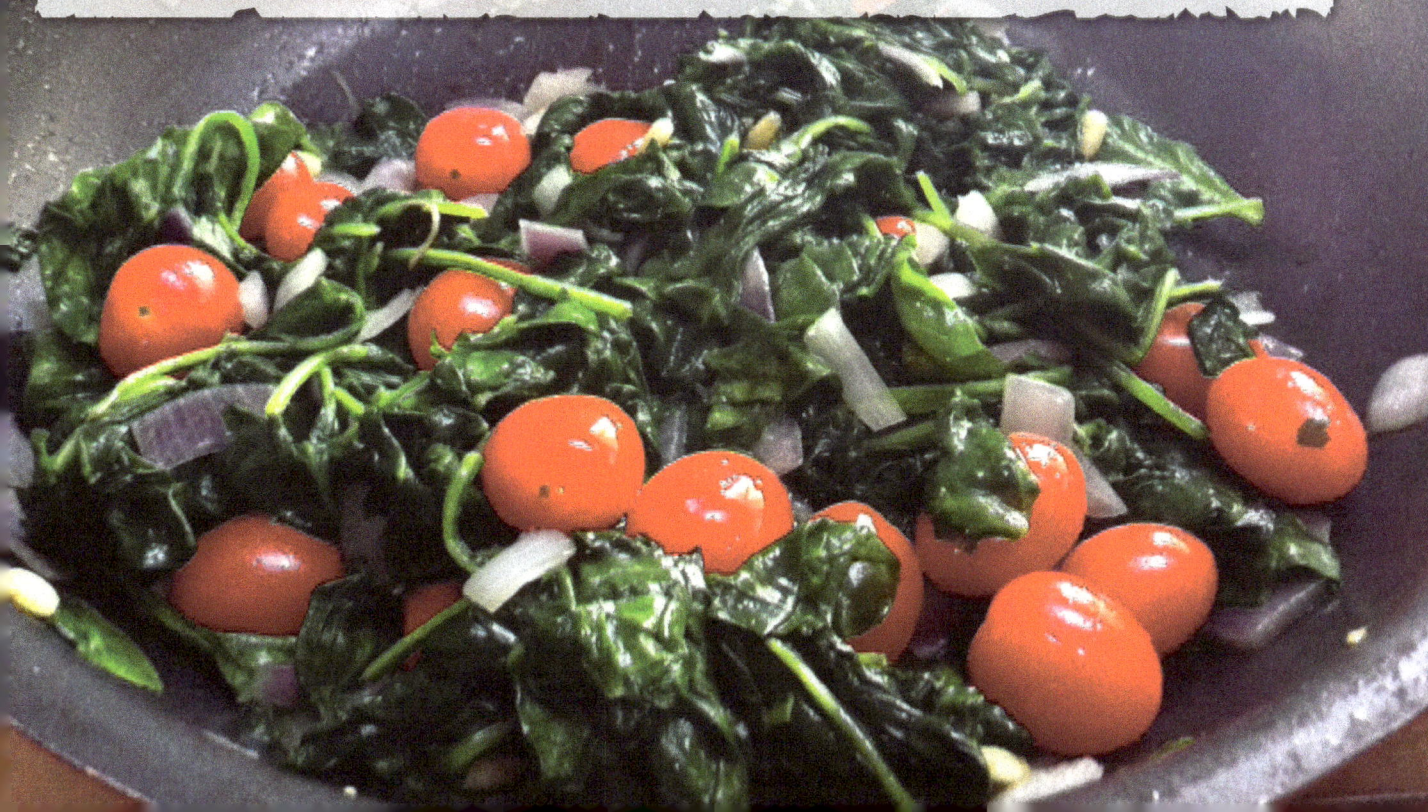

Granola

- 3 cups whole rolled oats
- ½ cup unsweetened coconut, shredded
- ½ cup almond slivers
- ½ cup wheat germ
- 1 cup raw sunflower seeds
- ½ cup sesame seeds, unsalted
- 3 cups banana, mashed
- ½ cup raisins
- ½ teaspoon salt

This recipe can be prepared on the weekend and then stored. You may serve with nondairy milk or consume dry as a snack. You could also add your favorite seeds and dried fruits. For diabetics, remember that dried fruits could raise your blood sugar, so limit your portion.

In a large bowl, mix together dry ingredients, except raisins, and then add the banana. Lightly oil-spray three baking sheets and then divide granola between the baking sheets and spread out evenly. Bake at 350 degrees Fahrenheit until golden brown. Stir every 5 minutes. Remove granola from oven and cool. Mix in raisins. Later, store granola in an airtight container to retain freshness.

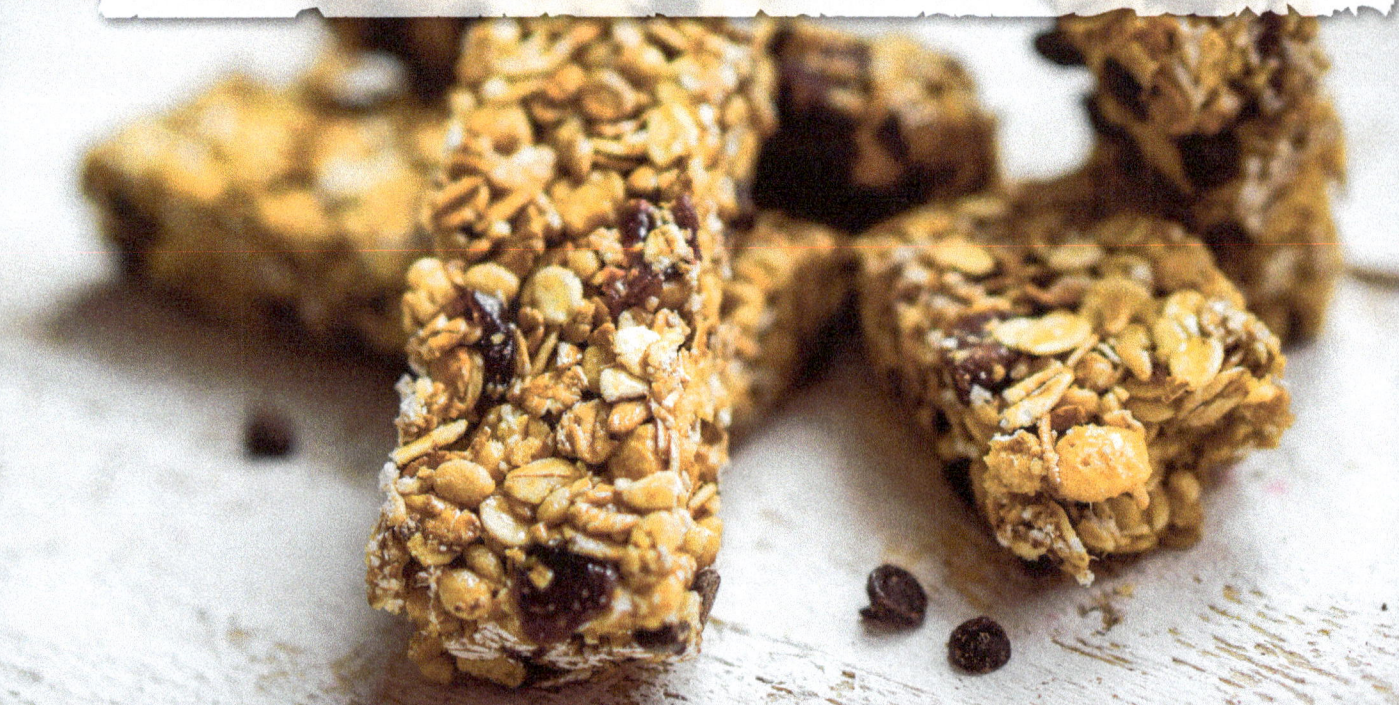

Multigrain Waffles

- ½ cup rolled oats
- ½ cup rye flour
- ½ cup whole wheat flour
- ½ cup soy flour
- 2 ¼ cups water or almond milk
- ½ teaspoon nutmeg
- 1 teaspoon cinnamon
- 2 tablespoons dates, chopped
- ½ teaspoon salt

Delicious and filling! These waffles can be made ahead, stored in the freezer, and warmed in a toaster when needed.

Blend all ingredients until smooth. Let batter stand for 5 minutes to thicken. Blend again, and then pour onto a hot, slightly oiled waffle iron. Bake for 10 minutes. Serve hot with fruit topping.

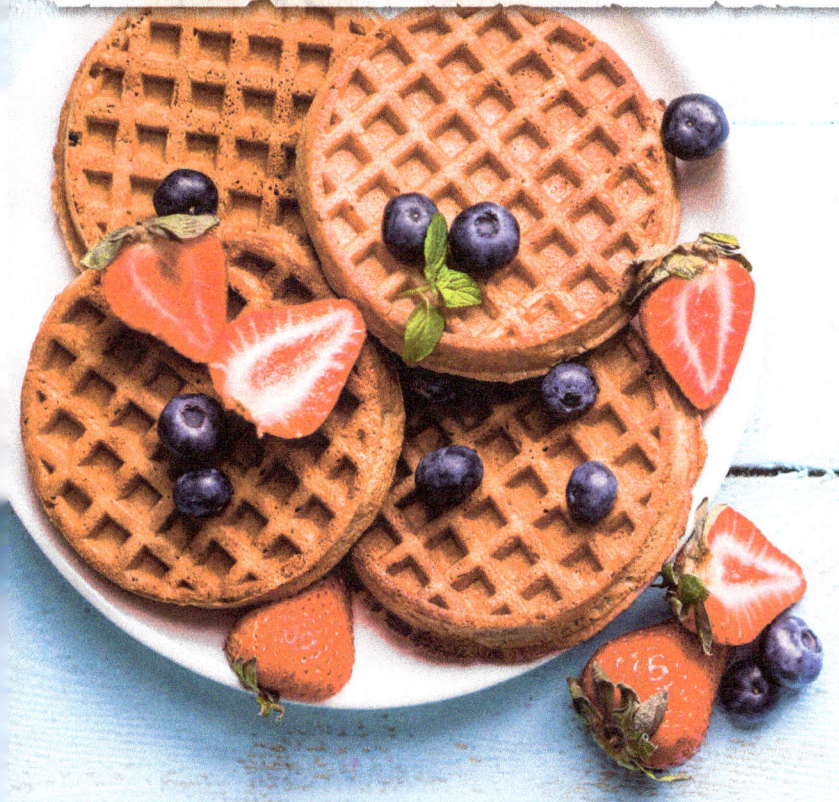

Corn Bread

- 1 ¼ cups flour
- 1 cup cornmeal
- ½ cup pureed corn
- ¾ cup pureed sweet potato
- 4 teaspoon baking powder
- 1 teaspoon baking soda
- ½ teaspoon salt
- ½ cup coconut cream
- ½ cup nut milk
- 2 tablespoon olive oil
- 2 tablespoon maple syrup

This is a tasty cornbread without the cholesterol from eggs or batter. Makes a great side dish.

Place milk, oil, pureed corn and potato, then add other liquid ingredients in a bowl, then add all the other ingredients and continue mixing until smooth. Pour batter into a slightly oil-sprayed 9-x-9-inch baking pan. Bake at 400 degrees Fahrenheit for 25 minutes or until golden brown. Allow to stand for a few minutes before serving.

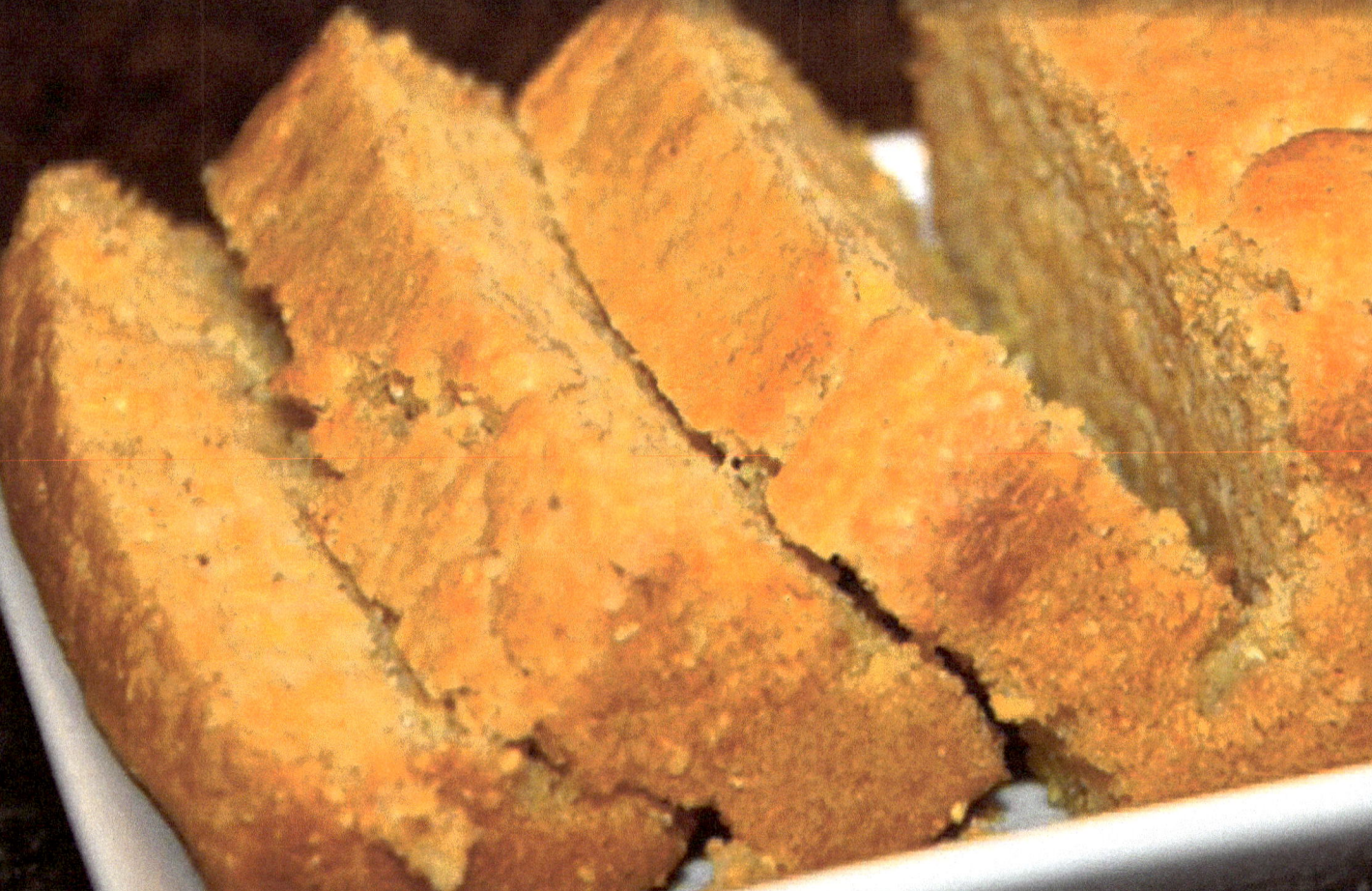

Detox Green Smoothie

2 cups kale
2 cups romaine lettuce
2 cups spinach
1 green apple
1 cup water

Place all the ingredients in a high-speed blender and blend until smooth.

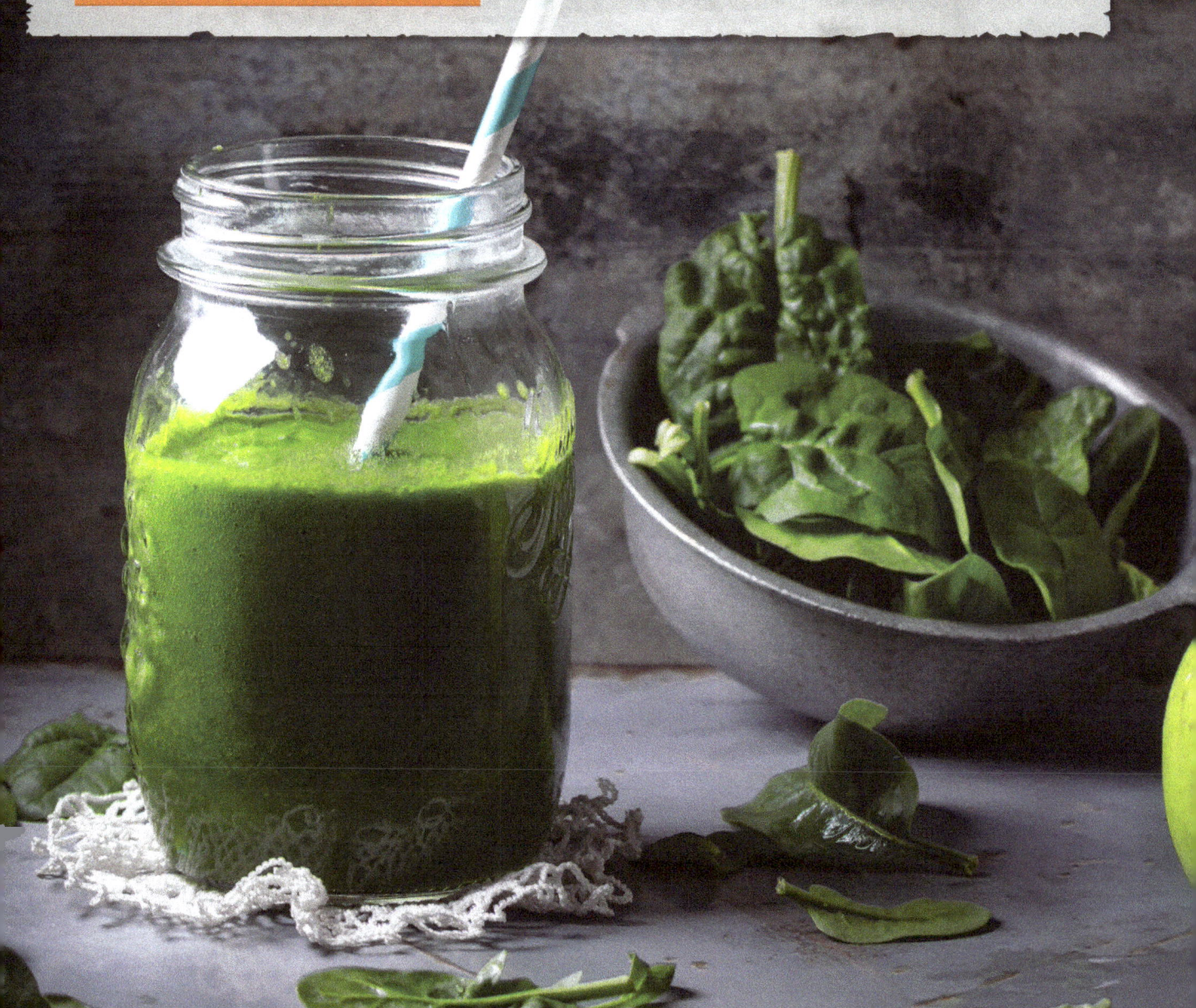

Dr. Cooper's Oats-on-the-Go

- ½ cup old-fashioned oats
- ¾ to 1 cup non-diary milk
- 1 ounce walnuts
- 1 ripe banana or ½ cup berries
- ¼ teaspoon cinnamon

This breakfast is quick and easy to prepare. It is filled with fiber to keep you satisfied all morning. It is also packed with protein, vitamins, and good fats.

Place oats and milk in a microwavable bowl and microwave for 3 to 4 minutes. Carefully remove and top with banana slices or berries, nuts, and cinnamon. Enjoy!

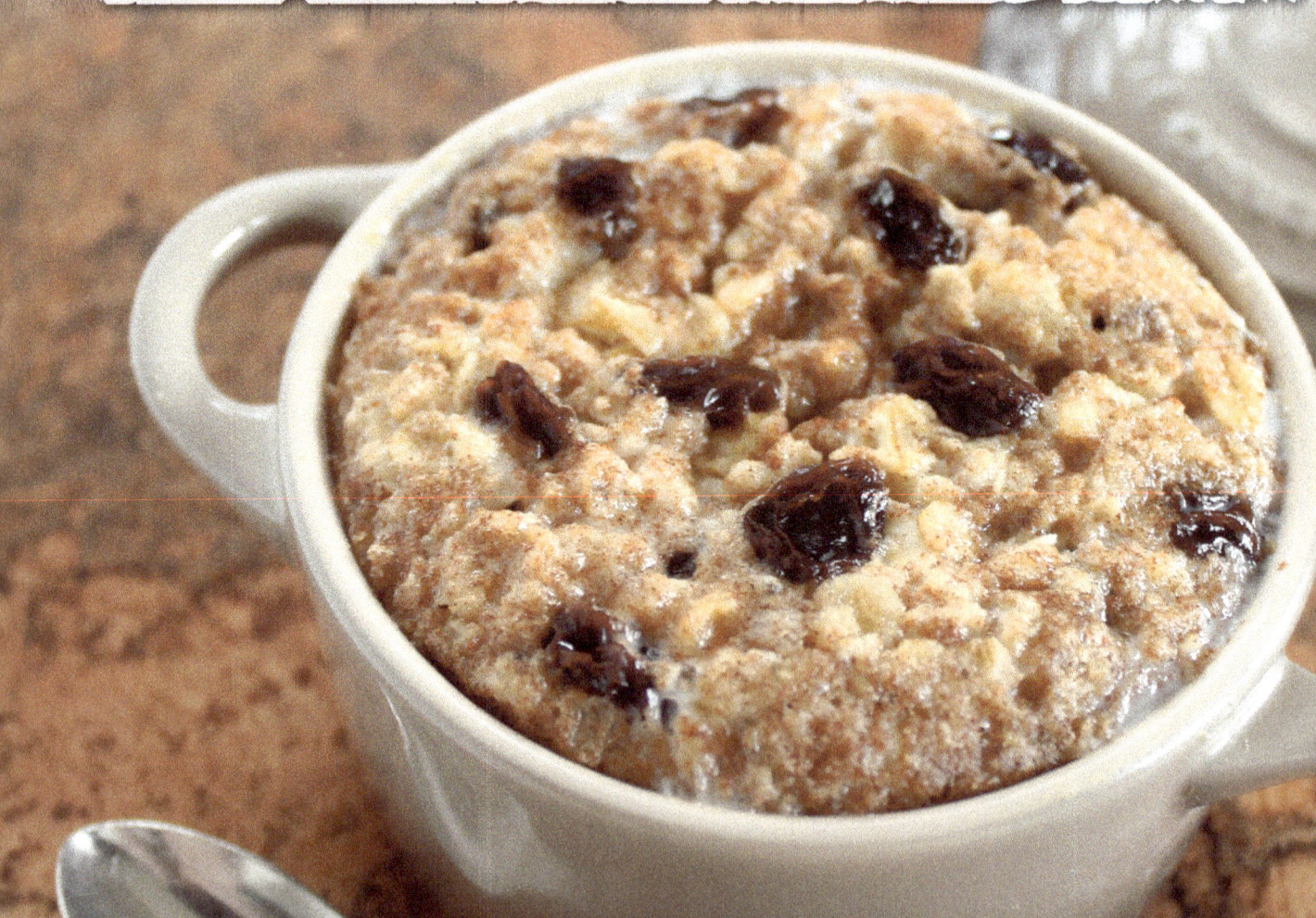

Avocado Toast

- 4 thick slices of multigrain bread
- 1 ripe avocado
- ¼ cup lime juice + pinch of salt
- 1 large sliced tomato
- ½ cup black beans (warmed)
- ½ small red onion, chopped

Mash avocado with a fork until smooth, sprinkle salt, add onion and lime juice. Toast bread, then spread the avocado and add sliced tomato and spoonful of black beans for added protein.

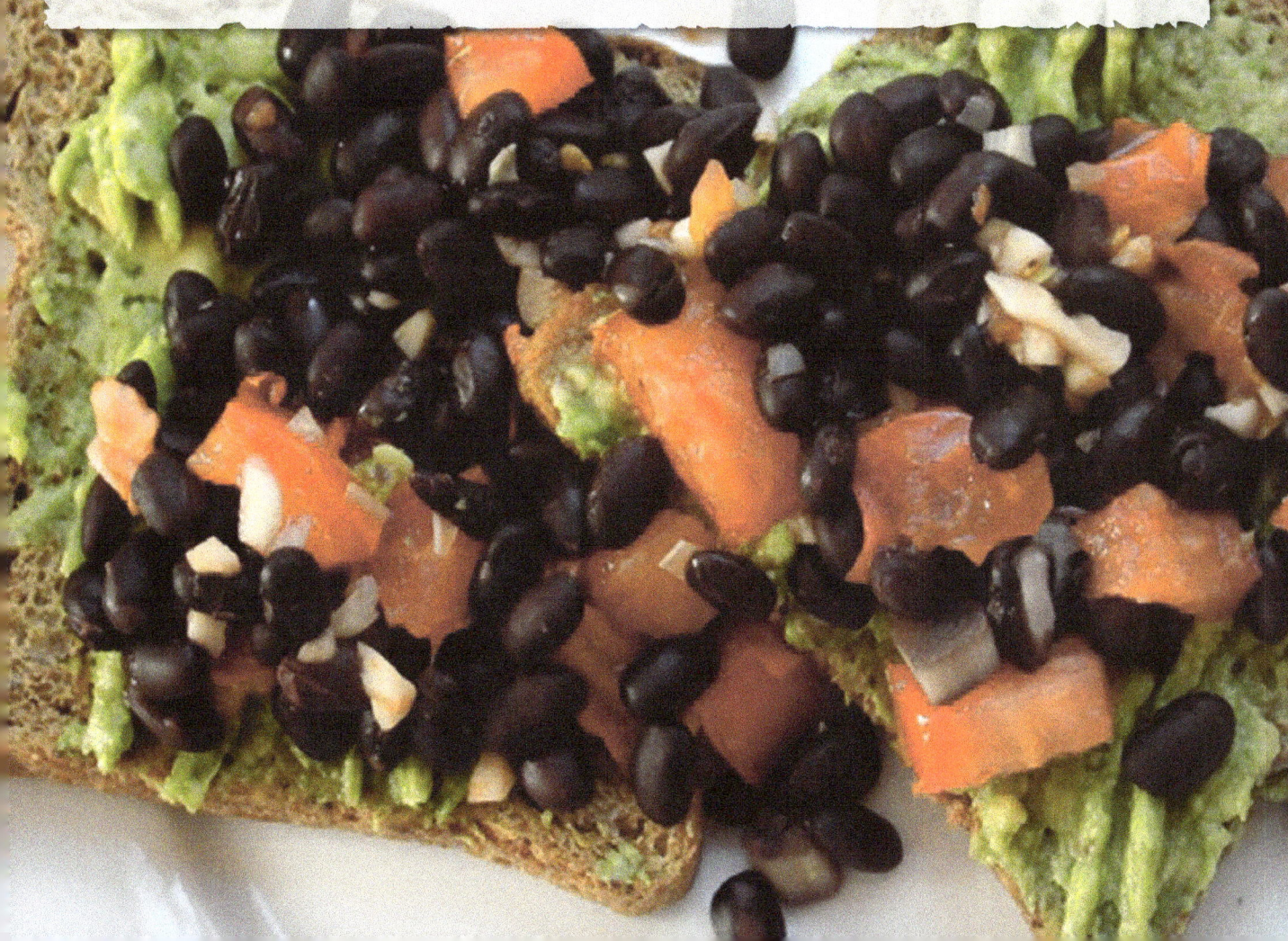

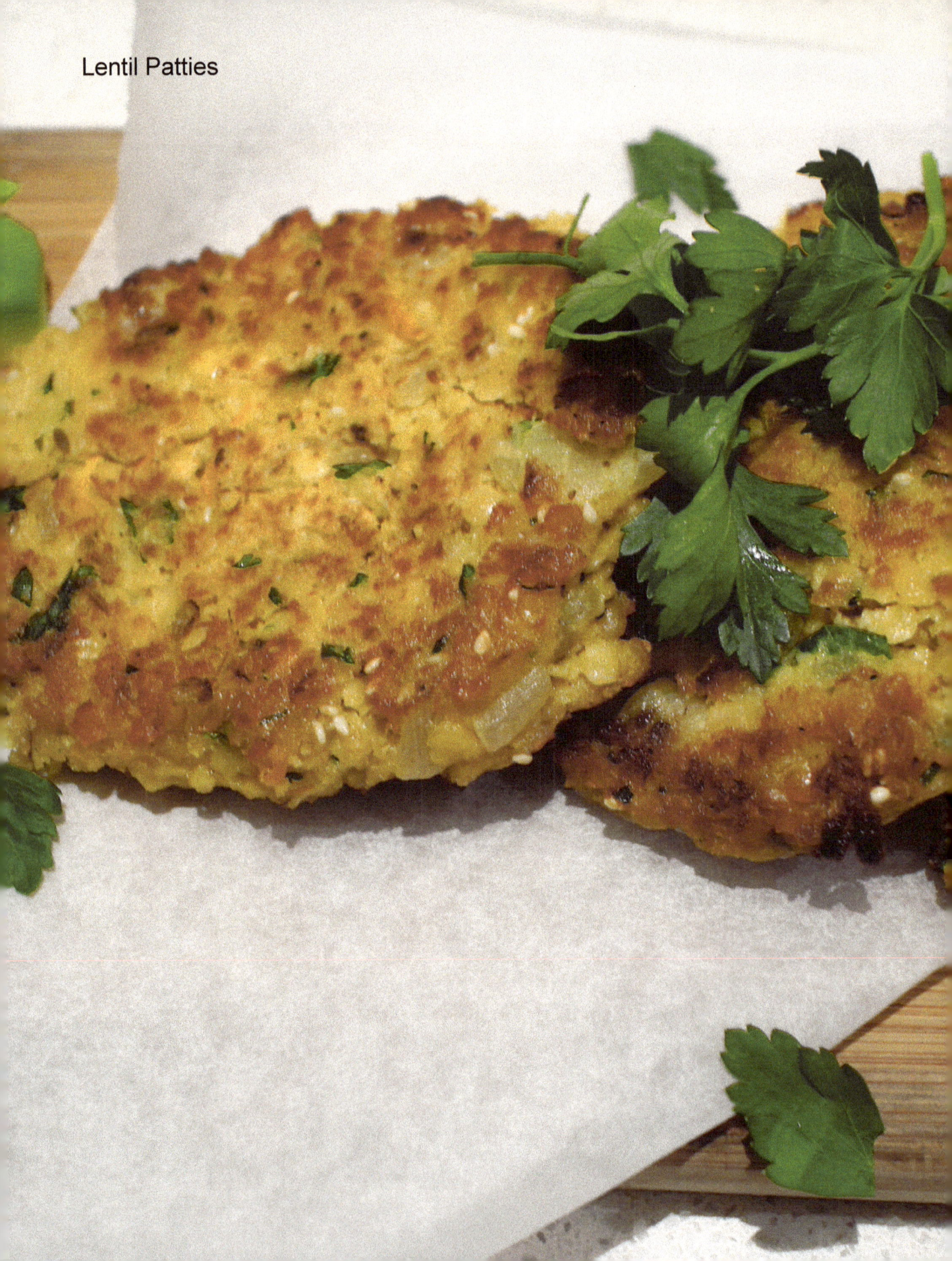

Lentil Patties

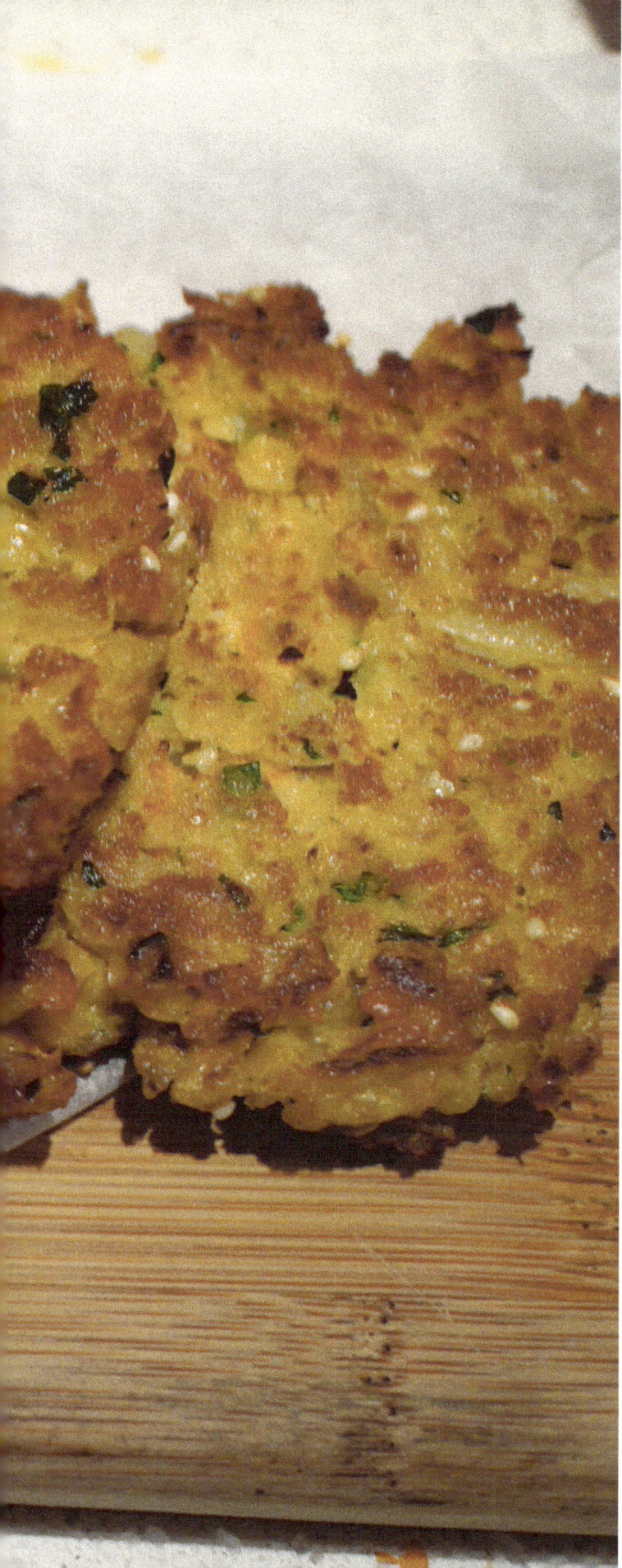

MAIN ENTRÉES

Heart-Healthy Bean Chili
Hummus and Veggie Wrap
Black Bean Burger
Tofu Thai Curry
Caribbean Curried Tofu
Baked Falafel
Tofu "Egg" Salad
Curried Bean Sandwich Spread
Coconut Chickpea Curry
Coconut Curry Eggplant
Seasoned Oven Fries
Roasted Vegetable Delight
Oats Walnut Balls
Chiles Rellenos
Dr. Cooper's Rosemary-Lemon Tofu Kabobs
Cashew Brown Rice Loaf
Oat-Nut Burgers
Spicy Tofu Burgers
Eggplant Roll-Ups
Eggplant Zucchini Bake
Mashed Cauliflower and White Beans
5-Grain Brown Rice Pilaf
Seasoned Vegetable Rice
Wild Rice and Mushroom Pilaf
Indian Rice
Seasoned Black Bean Brown Rice
Chickpea Avocado Spread
Lentil Walnut "Meatballs"
Pasta Primavera
Pasta with Vegetables
Veggie Wrap with Guacamole
Chickpea Curry
Lentil Patties
Walnut Balls
Sun-Dried Tomato, Black Bean and Rice Salad
Chinese Stir-Fry Vegetables
Mock Tuna Salad
Black Bean, Corn and Quinoa Salad
Quinoa Salad
Baked Mac & Cheese
Spicy Mexican Beans
Jamaican Stewed Peas

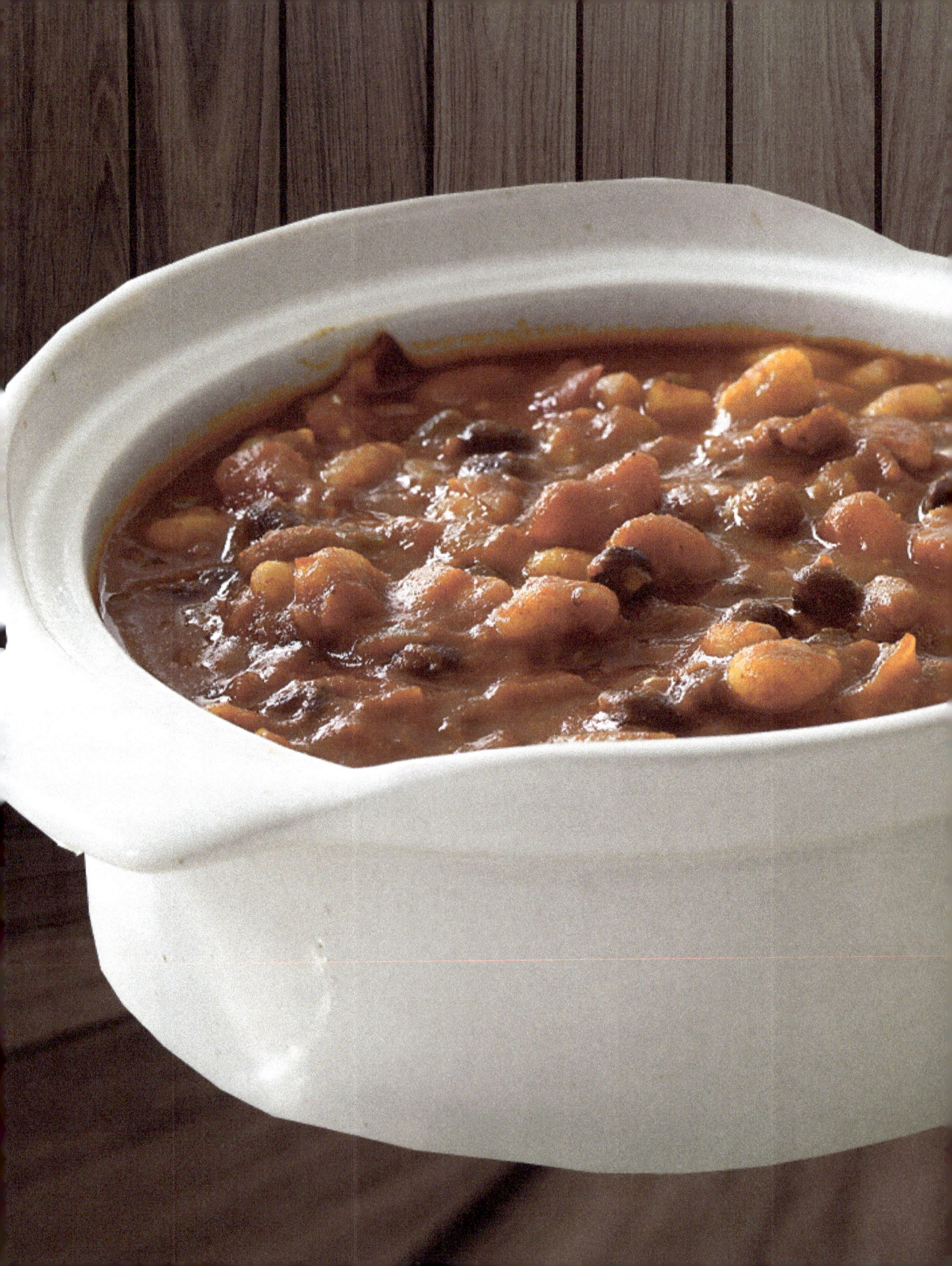

Heart-Healthy Bean Chili

1 tablespoon olive oil or vegetable oil
2 cups onions, diced
4 cloves garlic, mashed and then minced
1 cup carrot, chopped
2 cups vegetable broth
2 cups cooked kidney beans
2 cups cooked red beans
2 cups cooked black beans
1 cup frozen corn
3 cups cooked, chopped tomatoes
¾ cup of green bell pepper
1 tablespoon cumin powder
1 teaspoon dried oregano
3–4 bay leaves
1 teaspoon cayenne pepper
1 teaspoon sea salt, to taste

This dish is a great meat substitute. It is high in protein and fiber. It is ideal for those who are losing weight and will assist with keeping your blood sugar down if you are diabetic. Serve with fresh mixed vegetables or with baked sweet potato.

In a large, deep pot, add vegetable/olive oil and sauté onion, garlic, and onions for 3 to 5 minutes. Then add vegetable broth and the remaining ingredients and spices. Allow the mixture to cook for another 20 minutes.

Hummus and Veggie Wrap

- 2 (12-inch) whole-grain tortillas
- ½ cup hummus (refer to recipe on page 146)
- 1 cup spinach or kale
- 1 medium zucchini, cut in strips
- 1 large carrot, cut in strips
- ¼ cup black olives
- ½ cup tomato, sliced
- ½ cup avocado, sliced
- ½ cucumber, sliced

This dish is very quick and easy to prepare. There are different types of tortillas that you could use: sun-dried tomato, spinach, and whole wheat. You also have the option to add your favorite veggies.

Microwave the tortilla for a few seconds to make it pliable. Spread the hummus over the tortilla, and then layer on the assorted vegetables. Wrap the tortilla like a burrito and enjoy.

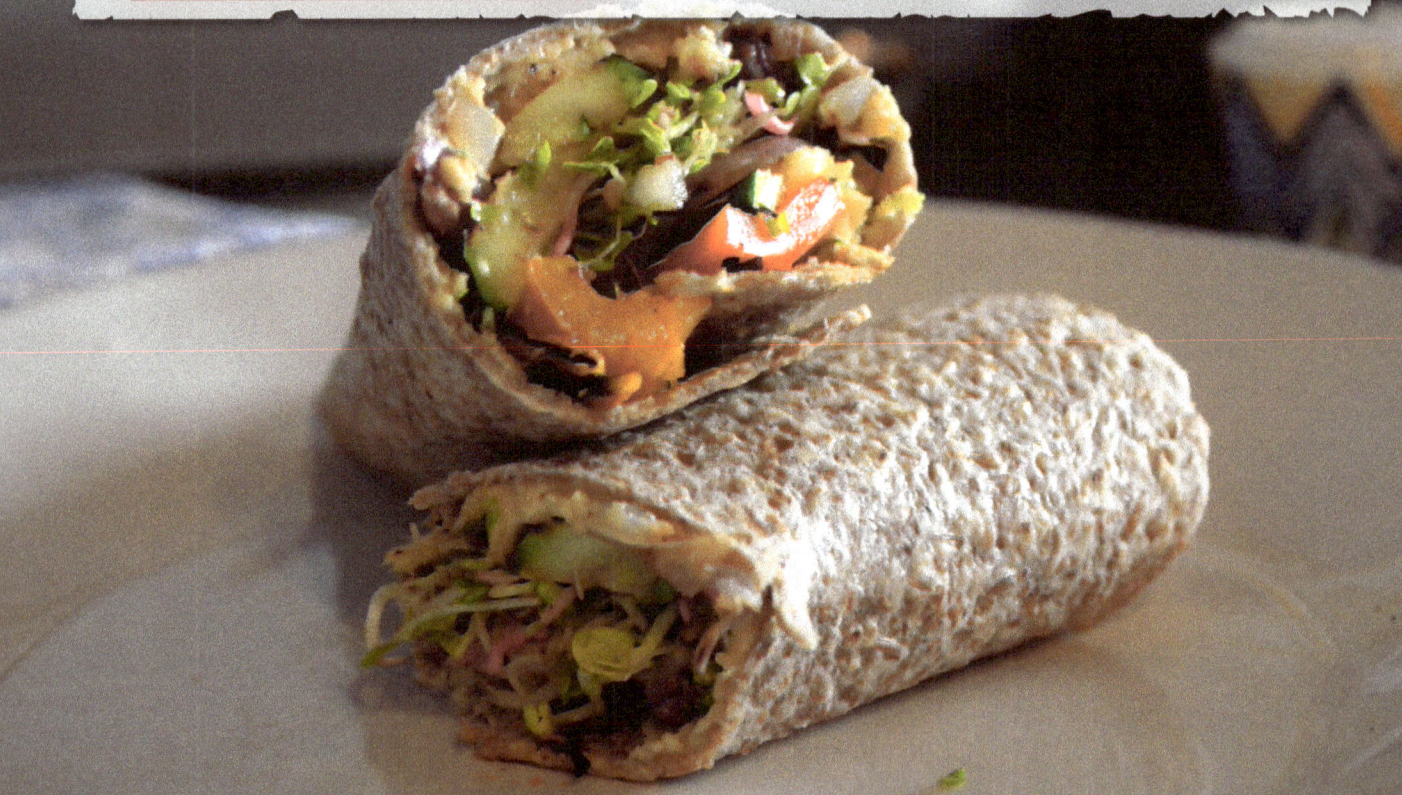

Black Bean Burger

1 (15-ounce) can black beans, drained
½ jalapeño, seeded and chopped
3 garlic cloves
½ medium onion, cut in wedges
⅔ cup rolled oats
½ cup frozen corn
1 tablespoon fresh cilantro, minced
2 teaspoon ground cumin
½ teaspoon curry powder
¼ teaspoon cayenne pepper
¼ cup bread crumbs
½ teaspoon salt or more to taste
Tomato
Mustard
Ketchup

This is a great burger to replace meat, which is high in saturated fat. If you want to keep your cholesterol down, then this is a great alternative for a healthy lunch meal.

In a medium-sized bowl, mash beans with fork and set aside. Place the onion, jalapeño, and garlic in a food processor and pulse 5 to 6 times. Add oats, corn, cilantro, cumin, curry powder, and cayenne. Season to taste with salt, and pulse about 10 to 12 times. Remove ingredients from food processor and add to bowl with mashed beans and stir well. Spray a small amount of oil into a skillet and heat to medium. Form the burger mixture into 4 equal patties. Cook the patties for 5 to 7 minutes on each side or until a golden crust develops and the patties are heated through. Remove the patties from the heat and place onto burger buns. Add sliced tomato, lettuce, mustard, and ketchup.

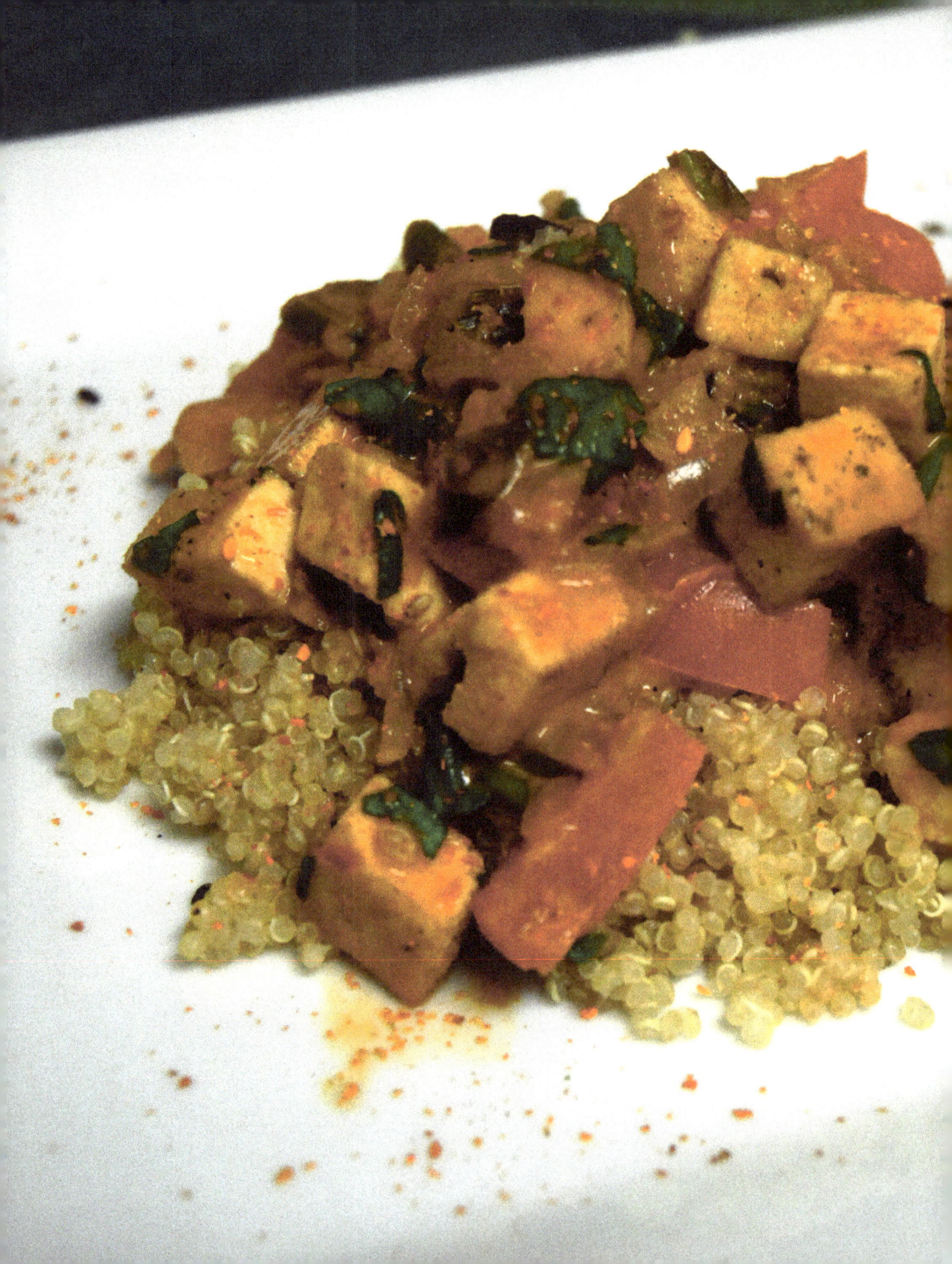

Tofu Thai Curry

1 (16-ounce) package of extra firm tofu, drained
1 tablespoon extra-virgin olive oil
1 medium onion, chopped
1 tablespoon garlic, mashed and minced
1 cup potato, cut in ½-inch cubes
½ cup carrot cut in ½-inch cubes
½ cup yellow or red bell pepper, julienned
½ cup fresh or frozen peas
1 teaspoon ground cumin
8 fresh basil leaves, chopped, or ½ teaspoon dry basil
1 tablespoon ginger, minced finely
1 teaspoon curry powder
1 teaspoon turmeric powder
1 (14-ounce) can coconut milk
1 ½ teaspoon salt or to taste

My patients at the wellness center love this dish. It is delicious and very easy to prepare and goes well with brown rice. Store leftover in the refrigerator. The dish is even more delicious 1 to 3 days after. Be careful not to overeat. This is a high-fat dish.

Preheat oven to 375 degrees Fahrenheit to begin baking the tofu. Spray a baking sheet with oil. Lay the tofu cubes out evenly and spray with oil. Then sprinkle with salt. Bake for about 20 minutes until golden brown. While the tofu is baking, prepare the curry. In a pot, sauté the onions, garlic, and other veggies over medium heat in olive oil until onions are transparent. Add ginger, curry powder, and turmeric. Then add coconut milk. Now incorporate tofu as well as all the other ingredients, cover, and allow to cook for 25 minutes or until veggies are cooked. Taste and add extra seasonings or salt. Enjoy!

Caribbean Curried Tofu

- 1 tablespoon vegetable oil
- 1 (12-ounce) package extra-firm tofu, drained and cubed
- 1 medium onion, chopped
- 4 cloves garlic, mashed and minced
- 2 teaspoons curry powder
- 1 teaspoon turmeric powder
- 1 tablespoon savory seasoning
- ½ cup carrots, sliced
- ½ cup potato, cubed
- 4 sprigs fresh thyme
- ¼ cup green onion, chopped
- 1 (14-ounce can) coconut milk
- 1 teaspoon Mrs. Dash
- ½ teaspoon salt or to taste

My daughter enjoys preparing this dish for large social or church events. Adding scotch bonnet pepper to this dish will give it the authentic Jamaican taste! Goes great with brown rice, roti, naan, or fresh mixed vegetables.

Heat oil in large skillet or wok over medium-to-high heat. Add tofu and braze until golden brown on all sides, stirring intermittently for about 10 to 15 minutes. Remove and set aside. Reduce heat to low-medium. Then add garlic and onion and sauté for 2 minutes. Then incorporate coconut milk, turmeric, curry, and the other ingredients. Return tofu to the skillet or wok. Allow it to cook for 15 to 20 minutes or until the carrots are tender. Taste and add extra spice if needed.

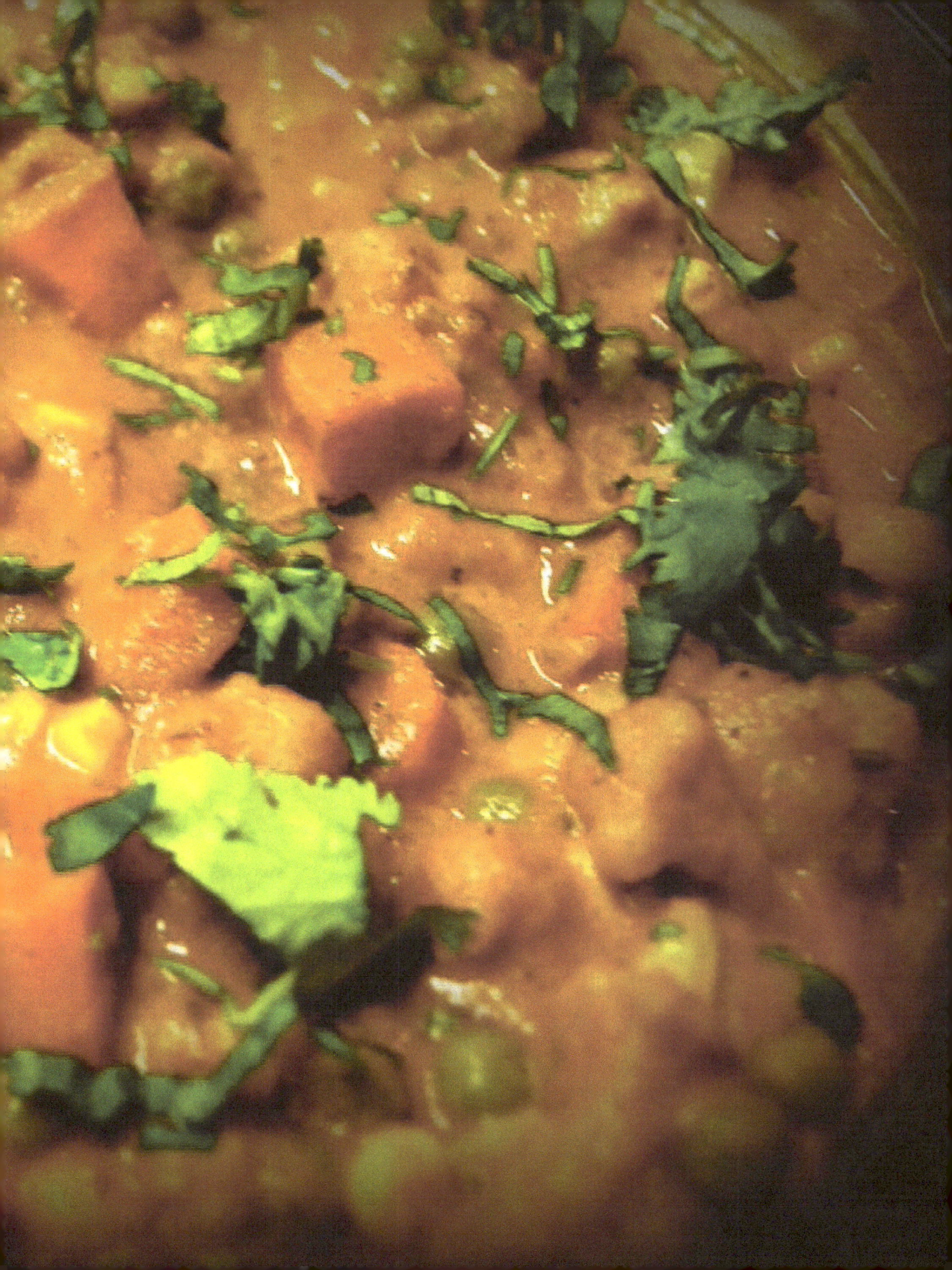

Baked Falafel

1 ½ (15-ounce) can garbanzo beans (chickpeas), drained, and ¼ cup liquid reserved
¼ cup fresh lemon juice
1 small onion, finely chopped
2 cloves garlic
¼ cup fresh cilantro
½ teaspoon dried basil
½ teaspoon dried oregano
1 teaspoon cumin
¼ teaspoon cayenne
½ teaspoon paprika
1 teaspoon salt
1 ½ cups whole wheat bread crumbs

Falafel is a well-known vegetarian dish that is served in a pita bread pocket with hummus and fresh vegetables. Feel free to add your special spices and herbs.

Preheat the oven to 350 degrees Fahrenheit. In a food processor, add the garbanzo beans, fresh lemon juice, onion, and garlic, and puree until smooth. Put the bean mixture in a large bowl and add all the other dry seasoning (oregano, basil, cumin, cayenne, paprika, and salt). Then, stir in the bread crumbs to hold the mixture together. Add more bread crumbs if the mixture is not holding together. Roll into 1-inch balls, and place them on a cooking sheet. Lightly spray the falafel with oil and bake in the oven for 10 to 15 minutes per side or until falafel are lightly browned. Test for doneness by pressing the outside with your finger. The falafel should come out moist inside and give to the pressure of your finger.

Tofu "Egg" Salad

- 1 pounds firm tofu, drained and crumbled
- ¼ cup Vegenaise
- 2 tablespoons prepared mustard
- ½ teaspoon ground turmeric
- 1 tablespoon soy sauce
- 1 teaspoon onion powder
- 1 teaspoon garlic powder
- 3 to 4 scallions, finely chopped
- ½ cup minced celery
- ½ cup green olives, chopped

This dish is very simple and easy to prepare. Feel free to add other vegetables and spices, such as bell pepper and shredded carrots. Serve as a spread on bread or stuff into pita bread.

Place the tofu in a bowl and mash with a potato masher. Add the Vegenaise (if desired), mustard, soy sauce, and turmeric. Mix well until the tofu takes on a bright-yellow color. Stir in the scallions, celery, and relish, if desired. Chill for an hour or more before serving.

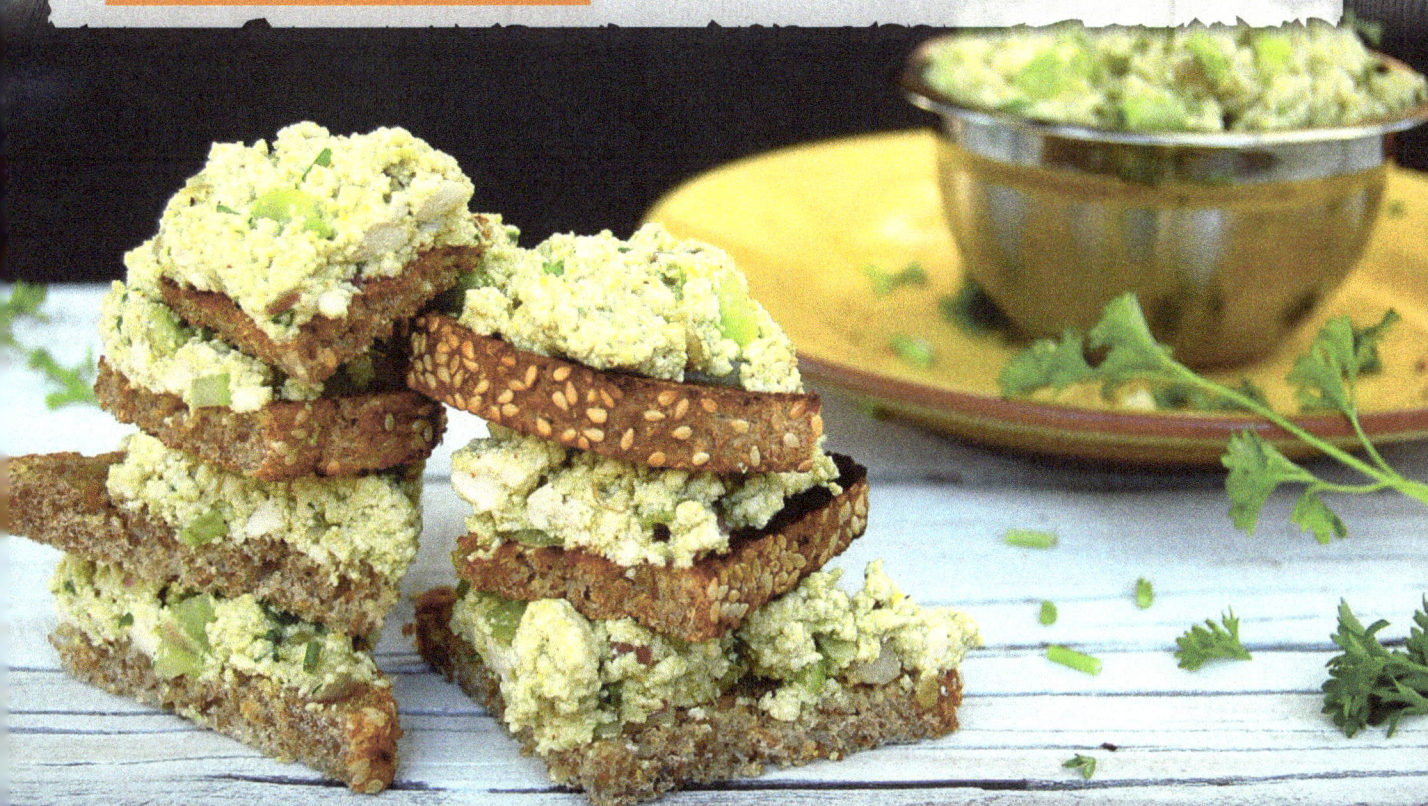

Curried Bean Sandwich Spread

- ¾ cup water
- 1 onion, finely chopped
- 1 green bell pepper diced
- ½ cup diced carrot
- 2 cloves garlic, mashed and then minced
- 1 teaspoon curry powder
- 1 teaspoon ground cumin
- ½ teaspoon thyme, dried
- 1 tablespoon savory seasoning (McKay chicken-style seasoning)
- 3 cups cooked white beans

This dish is very versatile. You can use it as a sandwich spread, stuffing for pita bread, or dip for your favorite veggies. Great dish for a social event.

Add water and vegetables to saucepan. Cook for 10 minutes. Then add all other ingredients, including curry power, turmeric, savory seasoning, and beans. Allow to cook for 12 to 15 minutes. Stir occasionally. Taste and add more seasoning as desired. Remove from the heat. Allow to cook. Then puree in a food processor. Enjoy!

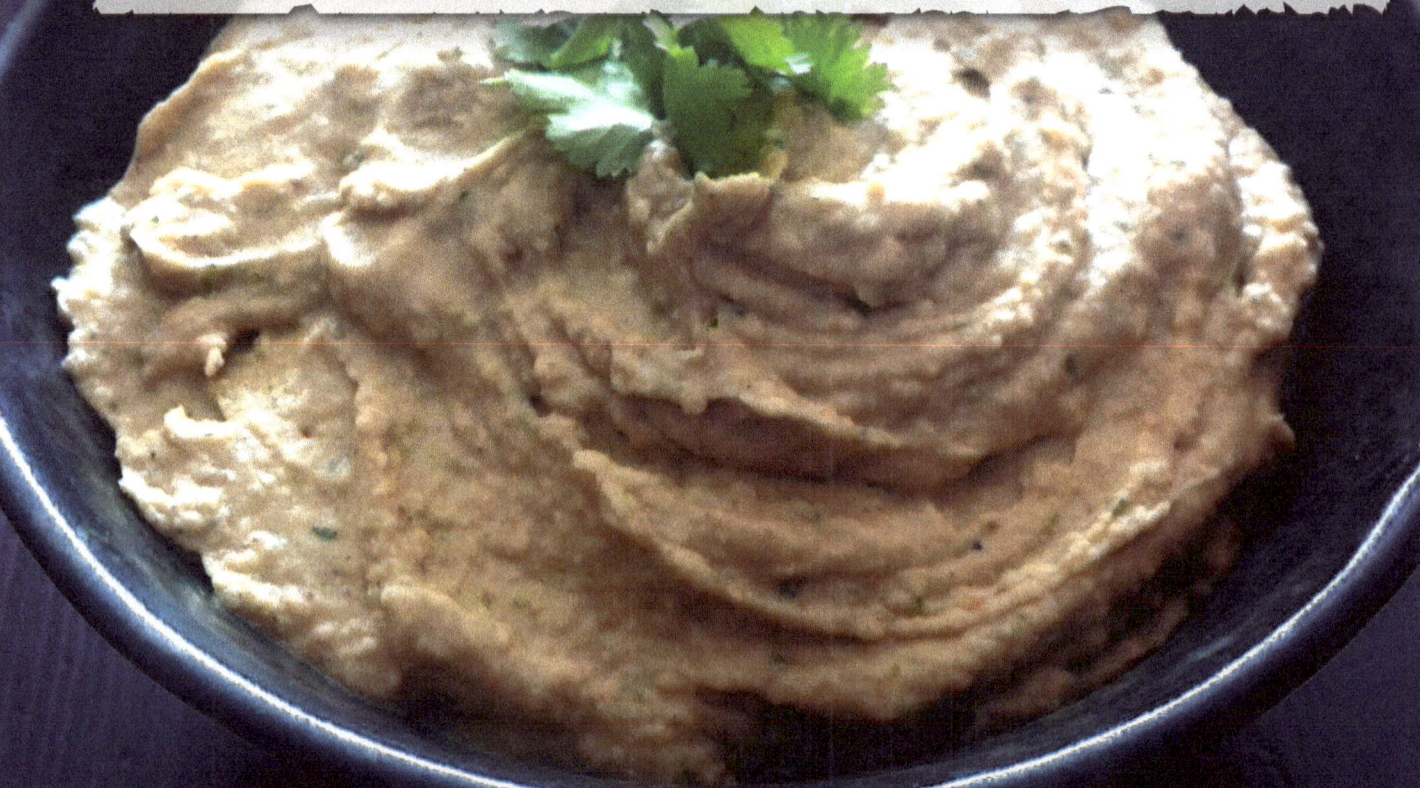

Coconut Chickpea Curry

1 cup coconut milk
2 teaspoons curry powder
2 teaspoons turmeric
½ cup chopped onions
2 cloves garlic, mashed and chopped
1 teaspoon thyme
1 teaspoon cumin
2 teaspoons savory seasoning salt
1 teaspoon sea salt (or to taste)
2 (15-ounce) cans chickpeas
1 small potato (cubed)
A dash of scotch bonnet or cayenne pepper (optional)

Chickpeas (garbanzo beans) are very high in fiber and a great protein source and can be used in many different menus. This dish can be enjoyed with baked sweet potato, brown (or wild) rice, mixed steamed vegetables. It can also be pureed and served as a sandwich spread or as a dip.

In a large, deep pot, first sauté a small amount of coconut milk, curry, and turmeric. Allow it to simmer for 2 to 3 minutes on low-to-medium heat. Then add onion and garlic, thyme, and other spices. Add potato and chickpeas. Add remaining portion of coconut milk and allow to simmer on low-to-medium heat for another 30 minutes or until potato is tender.

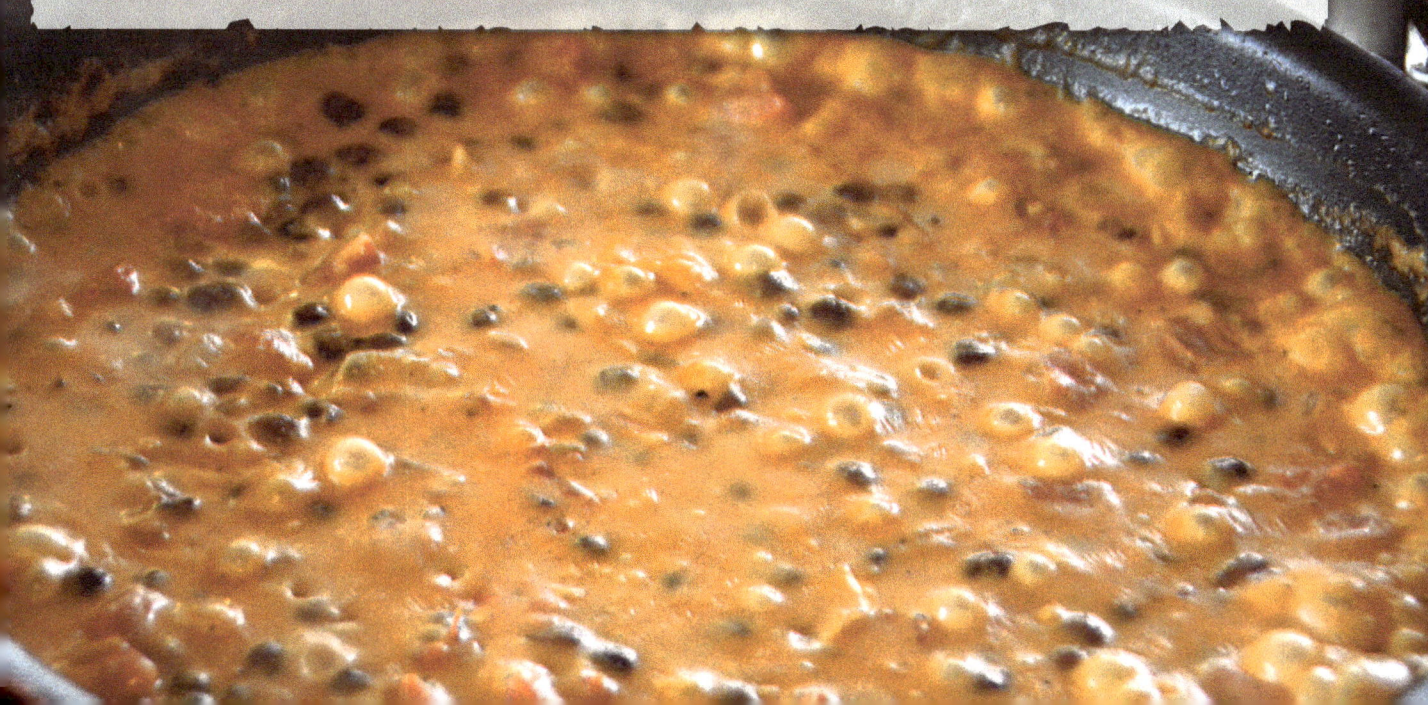

Coconut Curry Eggplant

- ½ cup coconut milk
- 2 teaspoons turmeric powder
- 2 teaspoons curry powder
- 1 medium onion, chopped
- 3 cloves of garlic, mashed and diced
- 1 medium green bell pepper, diced
- 2 large eggplant, cut in large cubes
- 1 teaspoon thyme
- 2 teaspoons savory seasoning salt
- 1 teaspoon salt, to taste

This is a great dish, simple and easy to prepare. It goes well with steamed, mixed veggies. It can also be pureed and served with whole wheat pasta.

Sauté curry powder and turmeric in coconut milk on low heat for 1 to 2 minutes. Then add onion, garlic, and bell pepper and simmer for another 2 minutes. Then add eggplant and the remaining ingredients. Allow to cook on low-to-medium heat for 30 minutes or until cooked. May be served with cooked brown rice or blend and use as a sauce over cooked pasta.

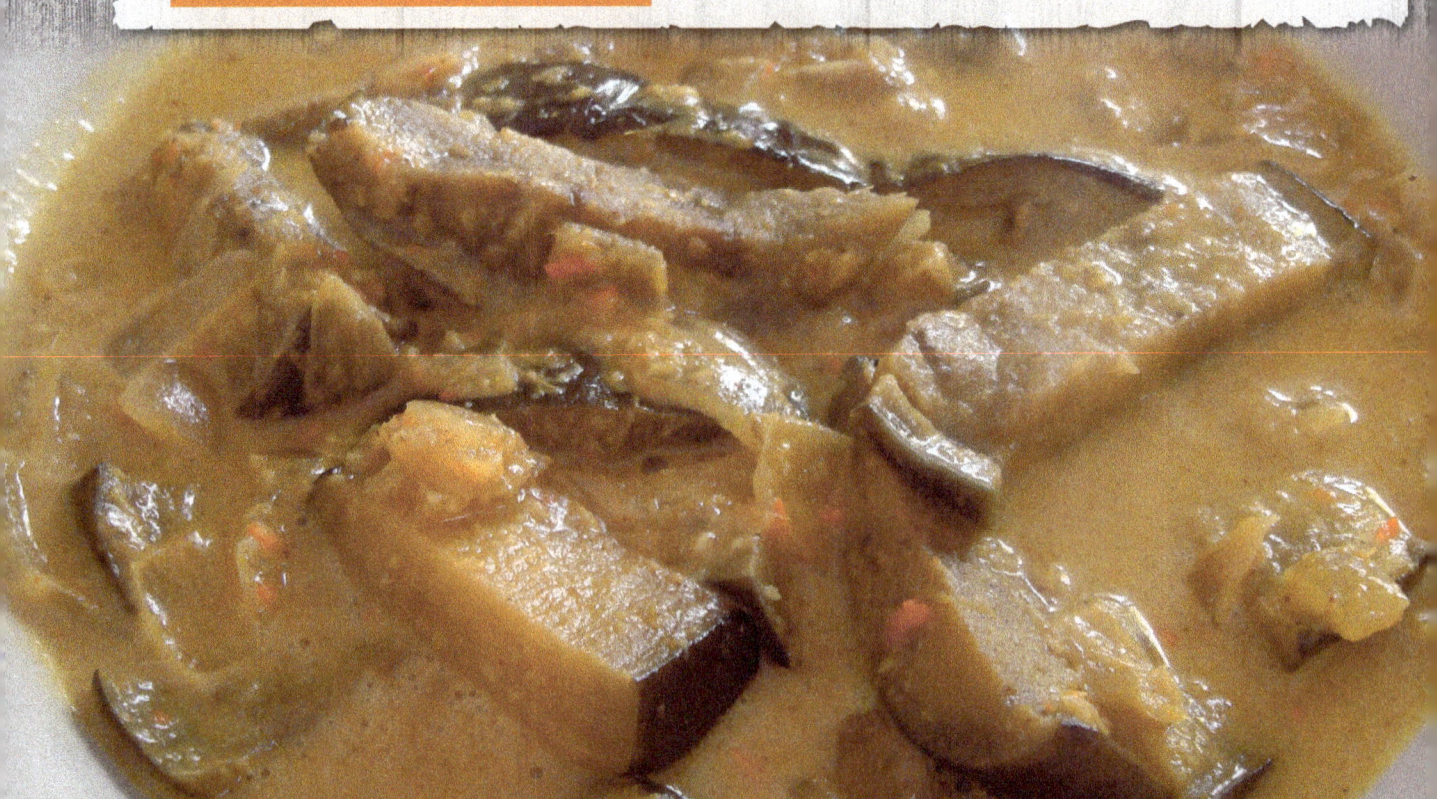

Seasoned Oven Fries

- 4 large potatoes
- 1 teaspoon Mrs. Dash
- 1 tablespoon McKay's seasoning
- 2 tablespoons soy sauce

Healthy replacement for French fries—tasty and delicious without the oil!

Thinly slice the potatoes lengthwise. Place the potatoes in a flat baking dish. Mix all the other ingredients together then pour over the potatoes and marinate for 1 hour, turning occasionally to make sure that all are coated. Preheat oven to 450 degrees Fahrenheit. Place the potatoes on a nonstick baking sheet. Bake for 45 minutes or until lightly browned, basting occasionally with dressing.

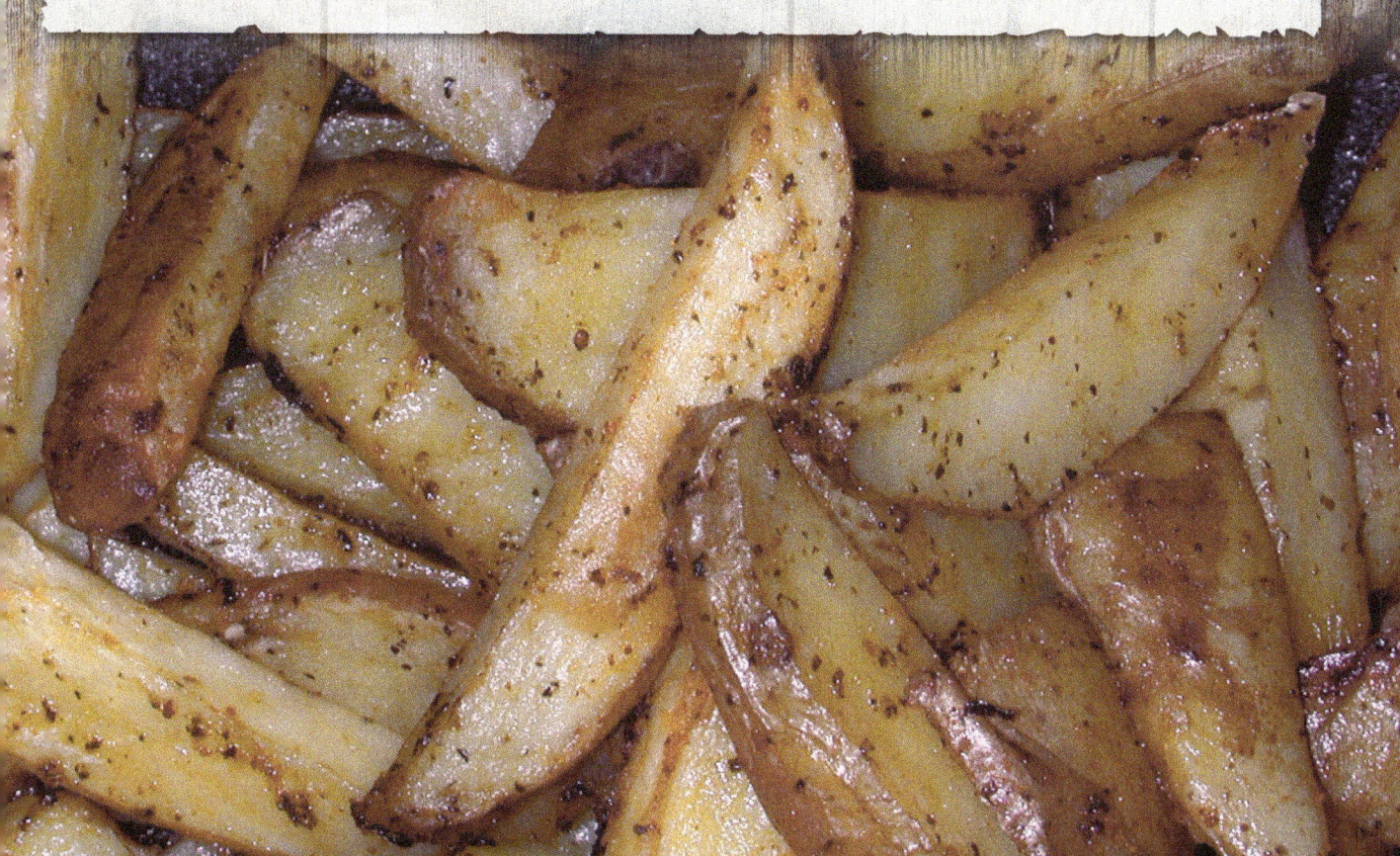

Roasted Vegetable Delight

- 1 zucchini, green
- 1 zucchini, yellow
- 3 cups broccoli
- 3 cups cauliflower
- 1 cup carrot
- 1 cup red pepper
- ½ cup diced onion
- 8 ounces of firm tofu
- 2 tablespoons Bragg's Amino Acids or soy sauce
- 1 package Lipton onion soup mix

This quick and easy recipe can be enjoyed at any meal. Leftovers are even more delicious.

All vegetables and tofu should be cut into small bite-sized pieces. Mix together all the ingredients in a large baking dish, cover, and bake at 400 degrees Fahrenheit for 10 minutes. Open and mix ingredients together. Then bake for another 10 to 15 minutes.

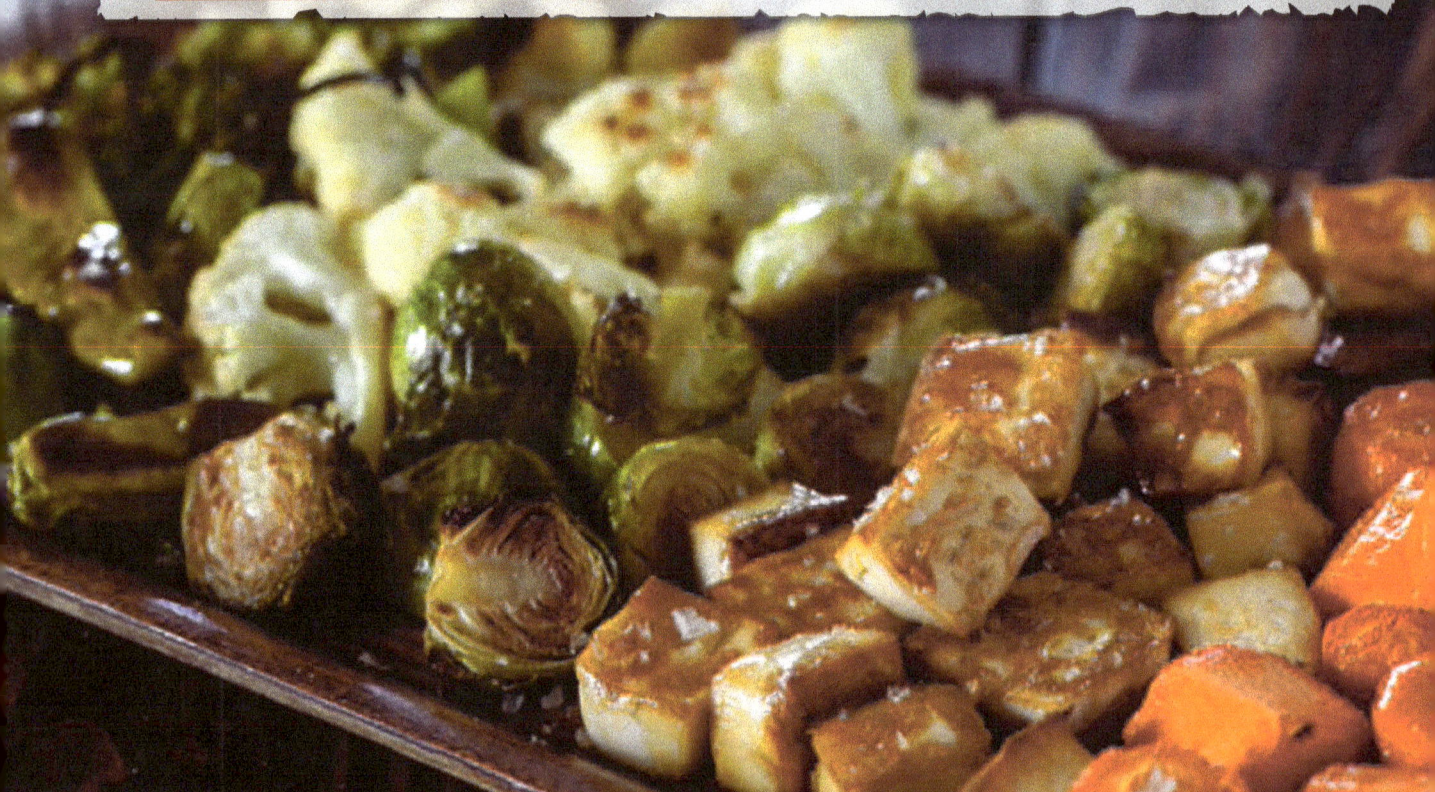

Oats Walnut Balls

- 4 cups water
- 1 cup chopped walnuts
- 1 cup chopped sunflower seeds
- ½ cup Bragg's Amino Acids or soy sauce
- 2 tablespoons olive oil (optional)
- ¼ cup nutritional yeast flakes
- 1 teaspoon garlic powder
- 2 teaspoons onion powder
- 2 cloves garlic, mashed & diced
- 1 medium onion, chopped
- 1 tablespoon dried basil
- 1 teaspoon thyme
- 1 teaspoon ground coriander
- 1 teaspoon sage
- 4 cups rolled oats

These no-meat meatballs are packed with fiber and protein while low in fat. You can add your special gravy, but it also goes well with marinara sauce.

Pour water in pot. Add all ingredients except rolled oats. Bring to a boil and then stir in rolled oats and cover. Remove from heat, cover, and set aside. When mixture is cooled, form 3-inch patties 1 ½ inch thick (form into balls). Place on oiled baking sheet and bake on each side for 15 minutes at 350 to 400 degrees Fahrenheit. Enjoy with your own sauce. Can be served with spaghetti.

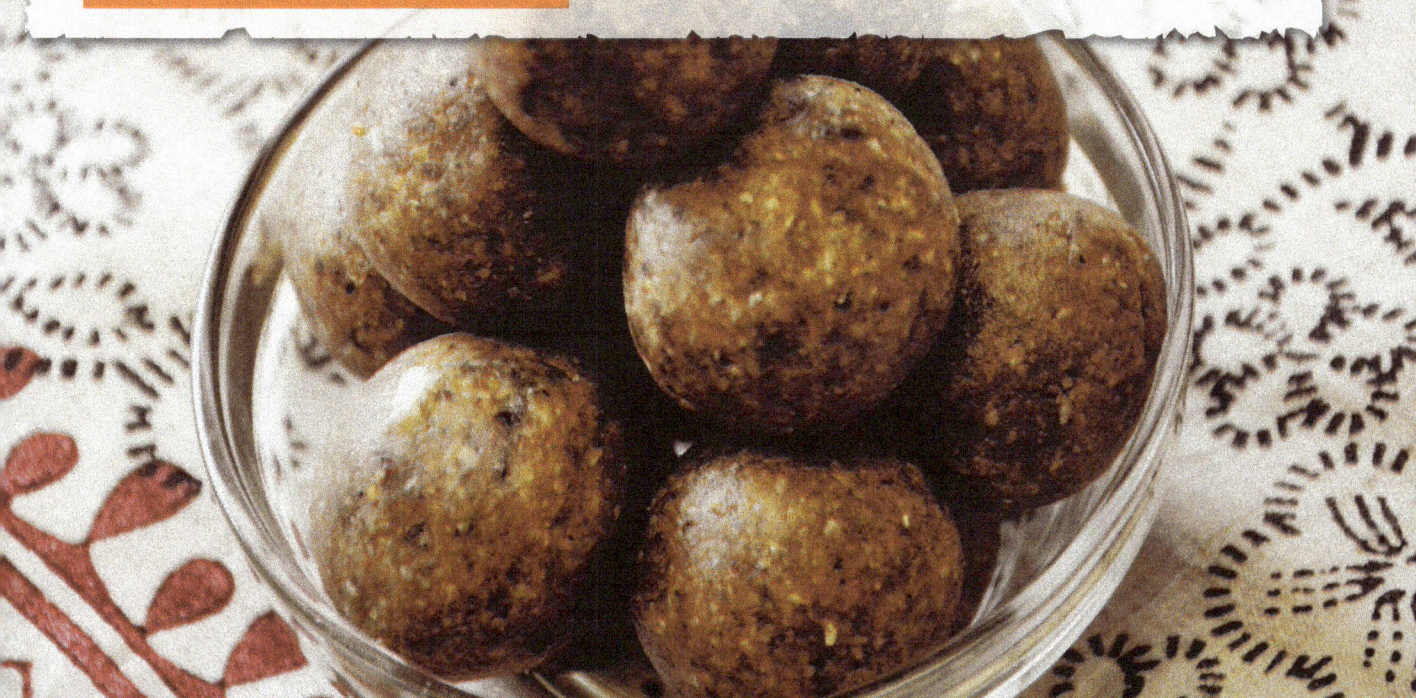

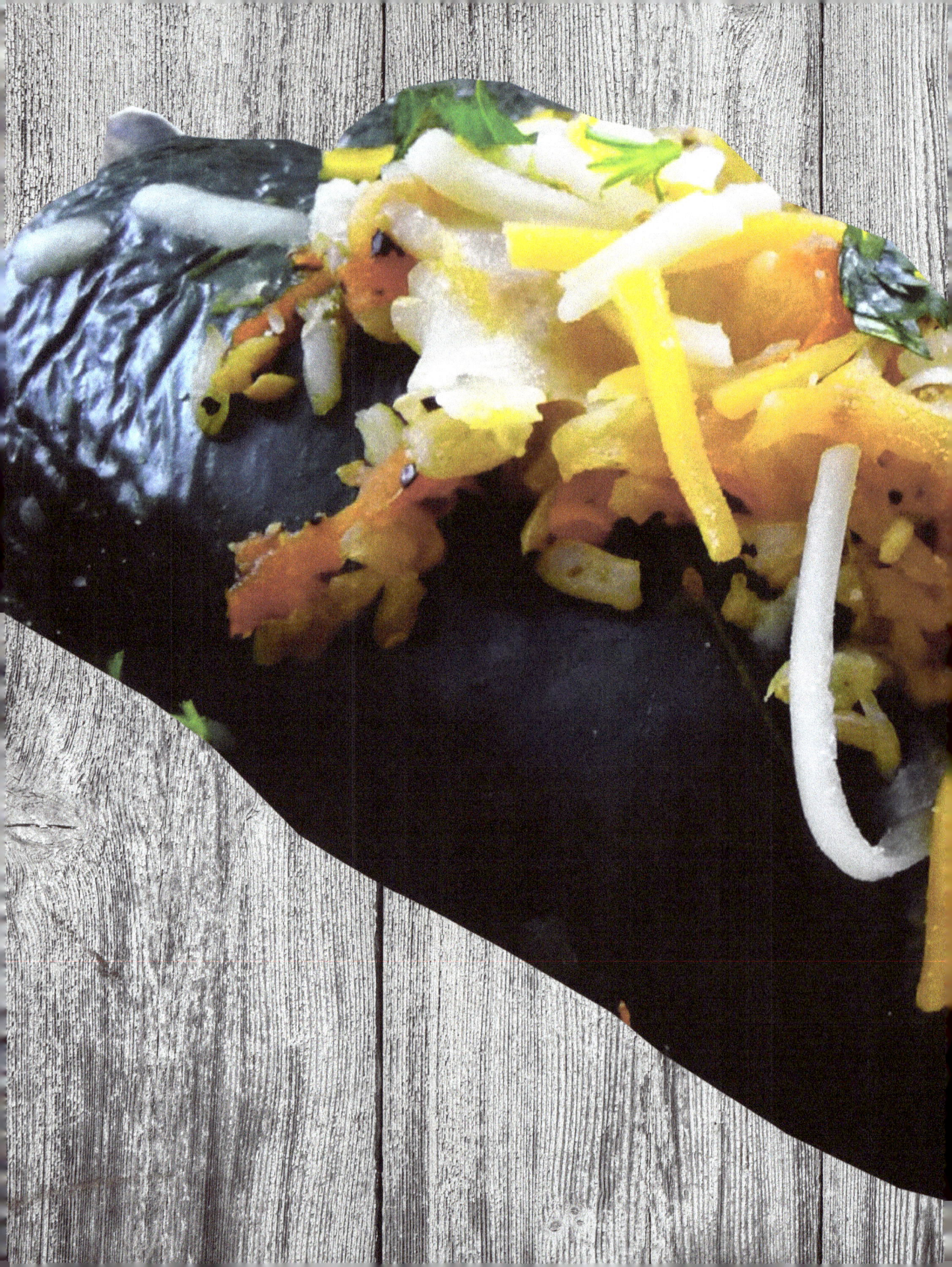

Chiles Rellenos

Olive-oil spray
1 large onion, finely chopped
3 cloves garlic, mashed and then minced
1 large green bell pepper, finely chopped
1 cup water
3 cups potatoes (cubed)
6 cups mixed vegetables (frozen corn, peas, and carrots)
2 small zucchini, finely chopped
1 (8-ounce) can tomato sauce
2 tablespoons chicken-style seasoning
2 teaspoons dried Mexican oregano
2 teaspoons ground cumin
10 small roasted poblano chilies, peeled, deveined
2 cups of soy veggie crumbles
4 sprigs fresh thyme
Cashew cheese sauce or shredded vegan cheese

This Mexican dish is delicious. The filling can be made with your favorite vegetables and spices.

Heat oven to 350 degrees Fahrenheit, then bake poblano peppers for 5-7 minutes, place in cold water, then peel and deveined and set aside. Spray oil in large skillet and heat on medium-to-high heat. Add onions, garlic, and bell pepper, potatoes, stirring frequently, and allow to cook for 7 to 9 minutes. Add other vegetables and a small amount of water. Then allow the mixture to cook for another 10 minutes. Add tomato sauce, seasoning, and vegetarian crumbles, cover, and allow to cook for 5 to 7 minutes. Taste and add more spices if needed. Spoon mixture into poblano chilies/peppers; place in shallow baking dish. Bake for 10-15 minutes. Top with cheese sauce.

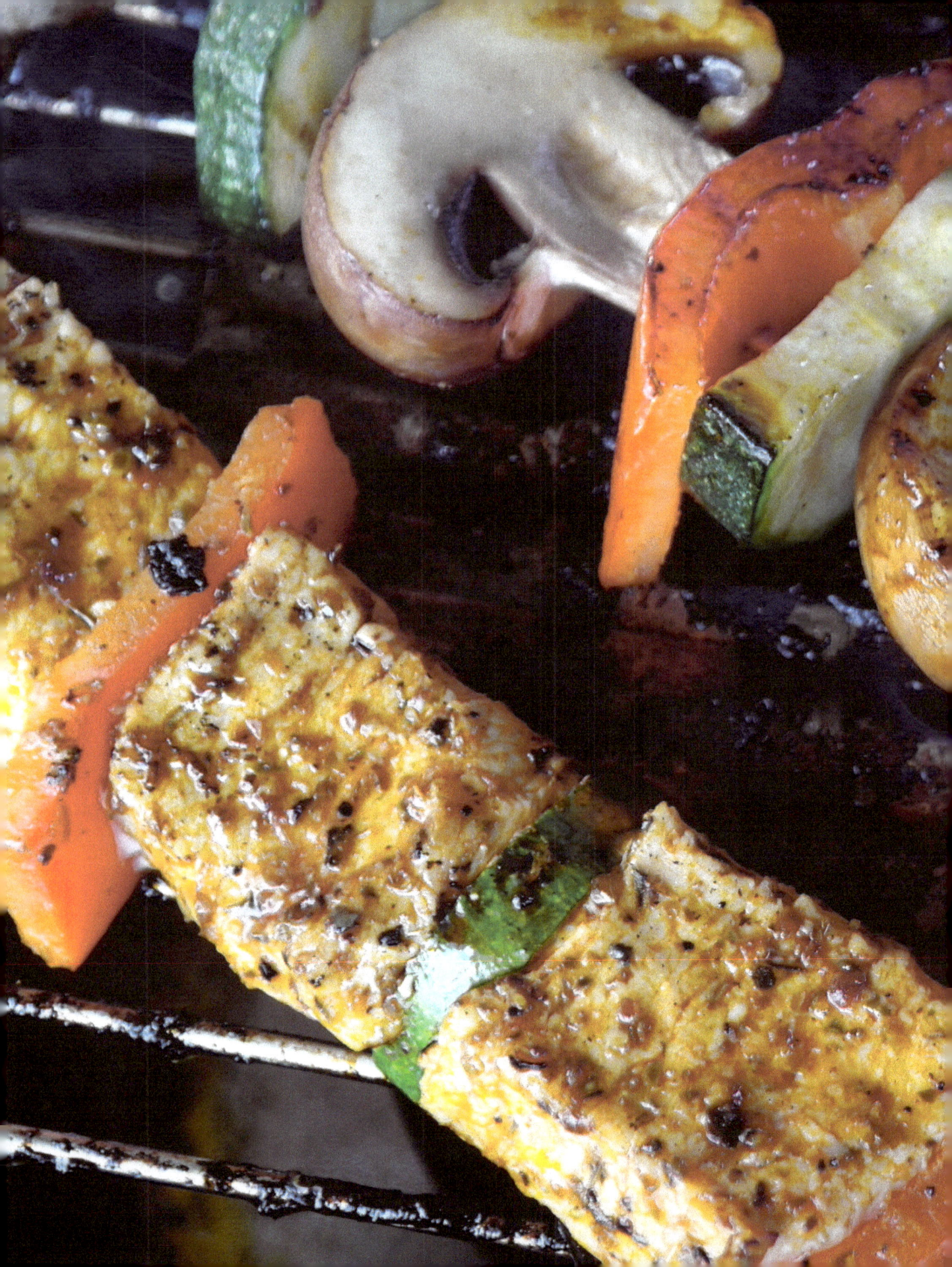

Dr. Cooper's Rosemary-Lemon Tofu Kabobs

4 small red potatoes, quartered
1 pack tofu cut in squares
2 teaspoons chicken-style seasoning
1 yellow onion
½ teaspoon dried rosemary
Dash of paprika
1 red bell pepper
2 tablespoons lemon juice
1 tablespoon olive oil
1 teaspoon grated lemon peel
½ clove garlic, minced
½ teaspoon salt

These are absolutely delicious, without the danger of saturated fat from beef or chicken. A great dish for parties or any social events.

Preheat broiler. Steam potatoes for 6 minutes or until crisp to tender. Rinse under cold water. Dry with paper towels. Sprinkle tofu evenly with chicken-style seasoning. Thread potatoes into 4 (10-inch) metal skewers, alternating with tofu and onion. Spray lightly with nonstick cooking spray. Sprinkle with rosemary and paprika. Place kabobs on baking sheet; broil 4 minutes. Turn over, and broil 4 more or until tofu is brown. Meanwhile, combine remaining ingredients in a small bowl. Spoon lemon mixture evenly over kabobs.

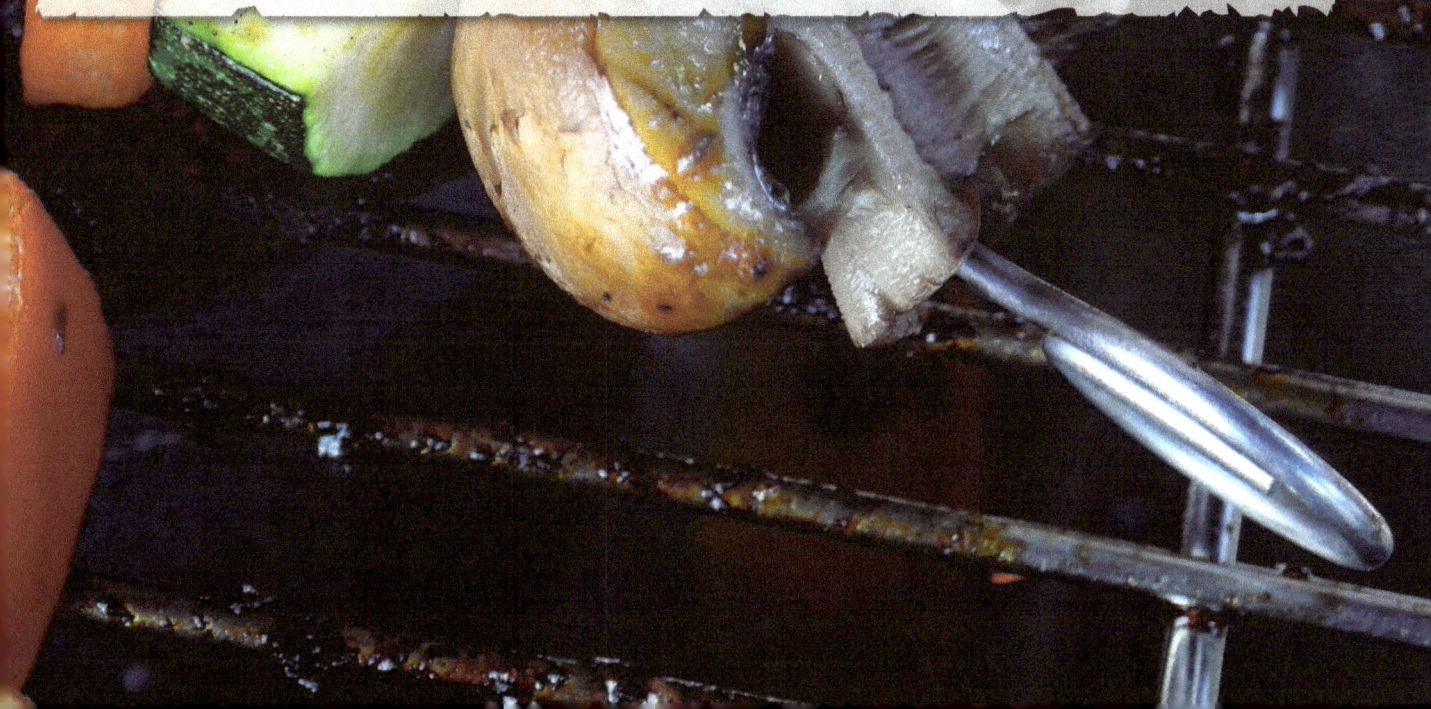

Cashew Brown Rice Loaf

2 cup cashews, raw
2 cups steamed brown rice
2 cups rich nut or soy milk
2 large onions, chopped
1 cup celery, finely chopped
¾ cup whole wheat bread crumbs
2 tablespoon Bragg's Amino Acids or soy
2 tablespoons thyme
2 teaspoons sage
2 tablespoons parsley, dried
1 teaspoon celery seed
1 teaspoon salt or to taste
1 teaspoon garlic powder
2 tablespoon nutritional yeast
2 tablespoons browning
2 tablespoons olive oil

This is quick and easy to prepare. Serve with cashew or mushroom gravy on a bed of green vegetable salad.

Place nuts and liquid ingredients in food processor or blender and chop. Add all other ingredients and continue to process. Spoon into baking loaf dish, cover with foil and bake for at least for 1 hour at 350 degrees Fahrenheit.

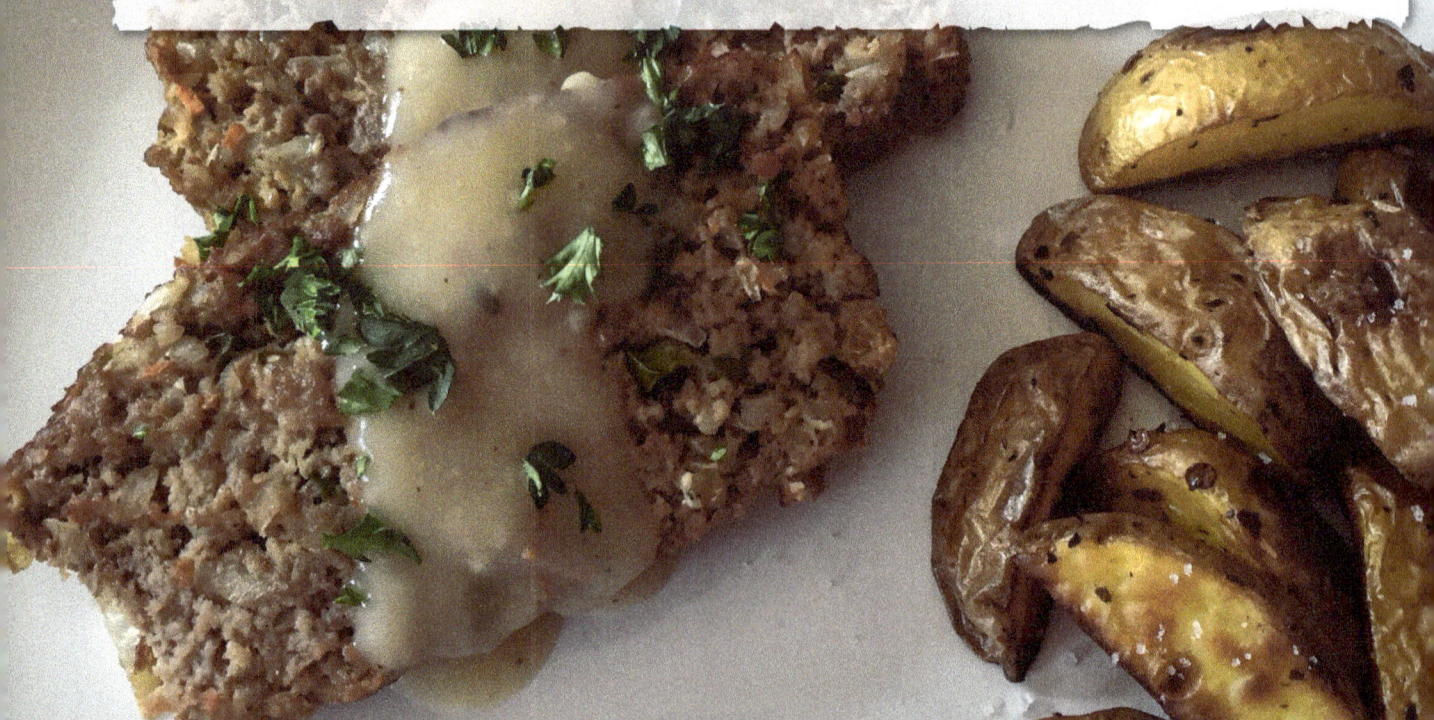

Oat-Nut Burgers

2 cups rolled oats
½ teaspoon onion powder
1 cup finely chopped walnuts
½ teaspoon coriander
½ teaspoon sage
1 tablespoon soy sauce
½ teaspoon garlic powder
½ teaspoon dried sage
1 small onion, finely chopped
2 cups hot water
1 tablespoon nutritional yeast

This burger patty is filled with fiber and good fat. Serve with tomato and lettuce on whole wheat bun or bread.

Place all of the ingredients in hot water, cover, and let rest for 20 minutes. Form into six or eight patties. Cook on a nonstick griddle over medium heat until browned on each side, 20 to 30 minutes.

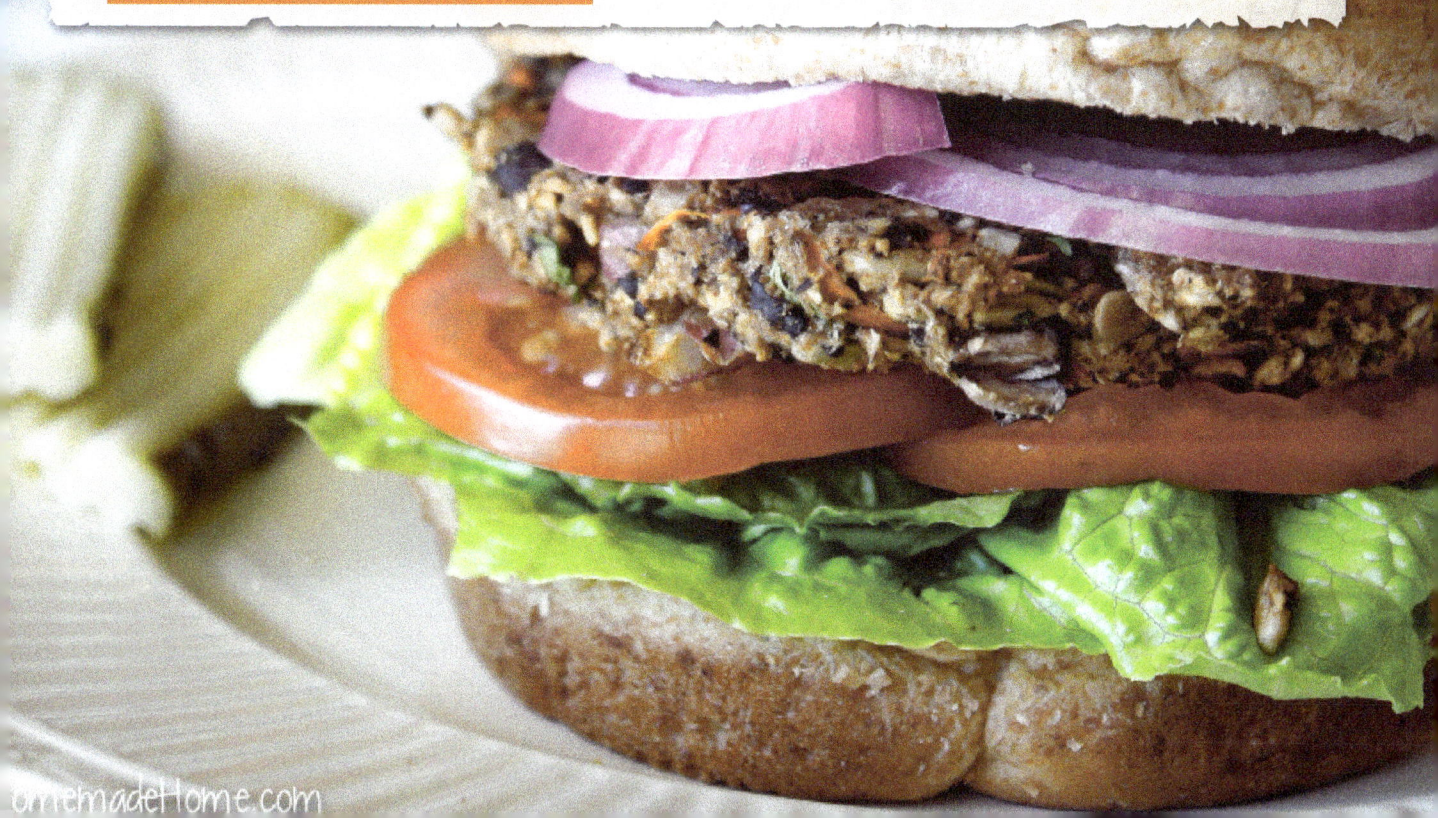

Spicy Tofu Burger

1 pound firm tofu, drained
2 cups rolled oats
2 tablespoons soy sauce
1 tablespoon cumin
1 tablespoon chili powder
½ teaspoon Mrs. Dash or Italian herbs
1 teaspoon garlic powder
1 teaspoon onion powder
1 teaspoon grated fresh ginger
1 small onion, finely chopped
2 tablespoons fresh thyme, finely chopped or minced

These burgers are tasty, high in protein, and low in calories, so enjoy!

Preheat the oven to 350 degrees Fahrenheit. Place the tofu in a large bowl and mash with a potato masher. Add the remaining ingredients and stir until well combined. Moisten your hands. Shape into eight patties and place on a nonstick baking sheet. Bake for 20 minutes on the first side; turn over and bake an additional 10 minutes. May also cook on stovetop using a slightly oiled nonstick skillet. Cook for 15 minutes on each side. Store the leftovers in the freezer and warm in microwave when needed.

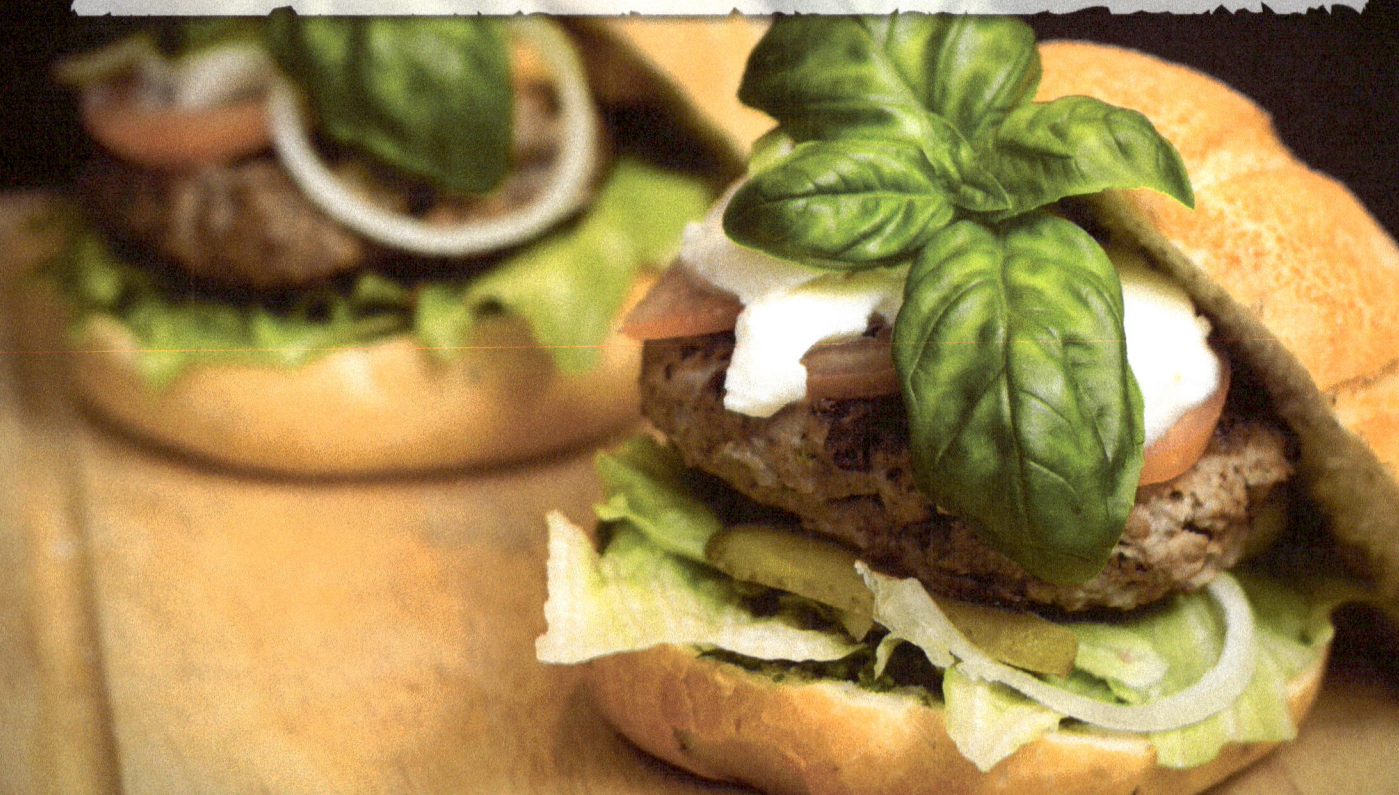

5-Grain Brown Rice Pilaf

1 medium onion, chopped
3 cloves garlic, mashed and diced
4 ½ cups vegetable broth or water, warmed
1 ½ cups long-grain brown rice
½ cup lentils
½ cup quinoa
¼ cup bulbar wheat
¼ cup couscous
1 tablespoon McKay's chicken-style seasoning
Salt, to taste

This is a complete dish, filled with complex carbohydrates, protein, and fiber.

Sauté in rice cooker or saucepan, half a cup of vegetable broth, onion, and garlic for 2 to 3 minutes. Stir in slowly the rice and grains for 2 minutes. Then add water or vegetable broth, salt, and McKay's seasoning and bring to a boil. Reduce heat, cover, and allow to simmer for 45 to 55 minutes. Remove from heat and allow to stand for another 10 minutes. This mixture could also be poured into a casserole dish, covered, and baked at 350 degrees Fahrenheit for 50 to 60 minutes.

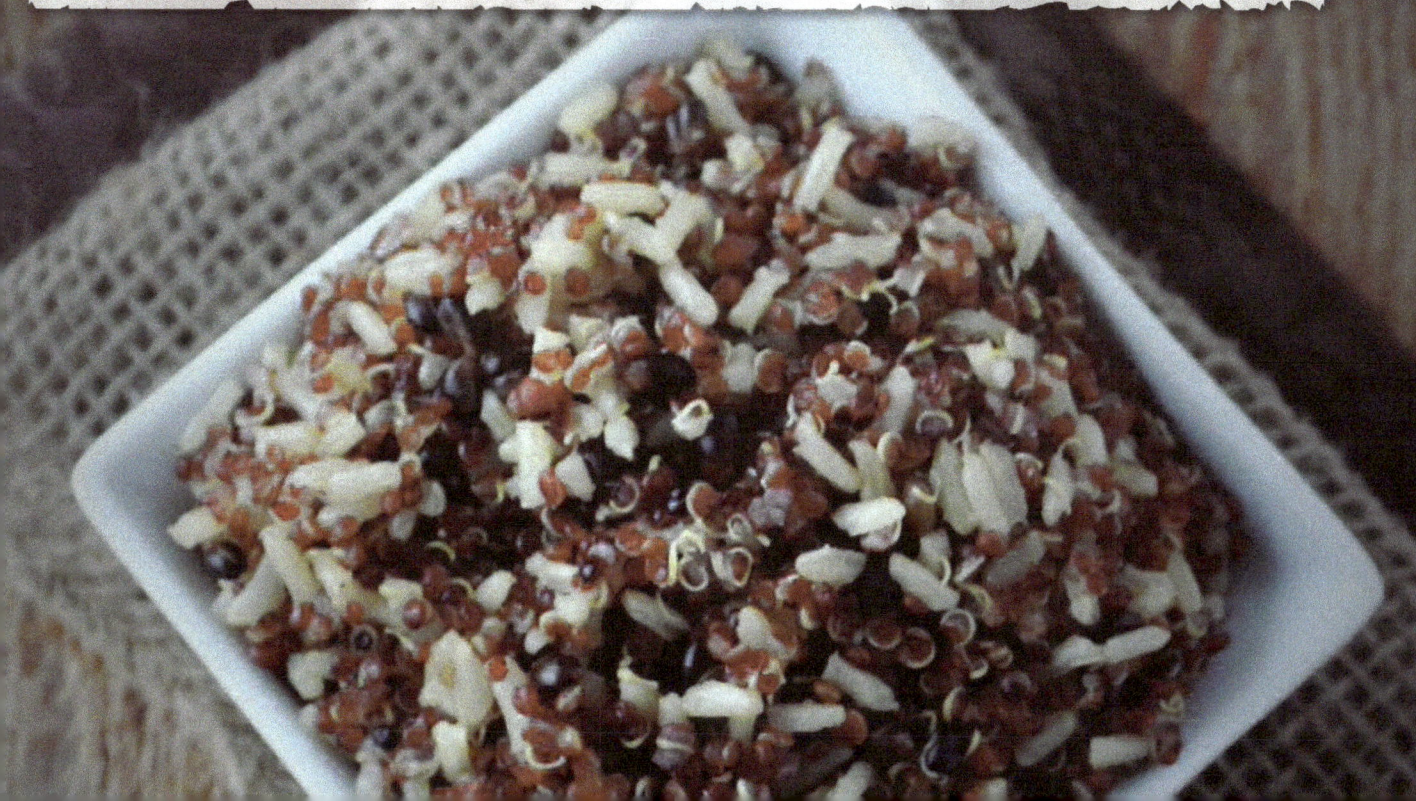

Eggplant Zucchini Bake

- 2 tablespoons olive oil
- 4 large zucchini (1-inch cubes)
- 2 medium eggplants (1-inch cubes)
- 2 cups cherry tomato (cut in halves)
- 1 small onion, chopped
- 1 tablespoon garlic powder
- ¼ cup basil, fresh
- ¼ cup parsley
- Salt to taste

Delicious and packed with vitamins and fiber, this is dish is great for everyone but is especially ideal for diabetic or those who are trying to lose weight.

Place oil in casserole dish and add zucchini, eggplant, and cherry tomatoes. Add other ingredients. Salt to taste and mix. Bake for 30 minutes, uncovered. Then cover with foil and bake for another 15 minutes.

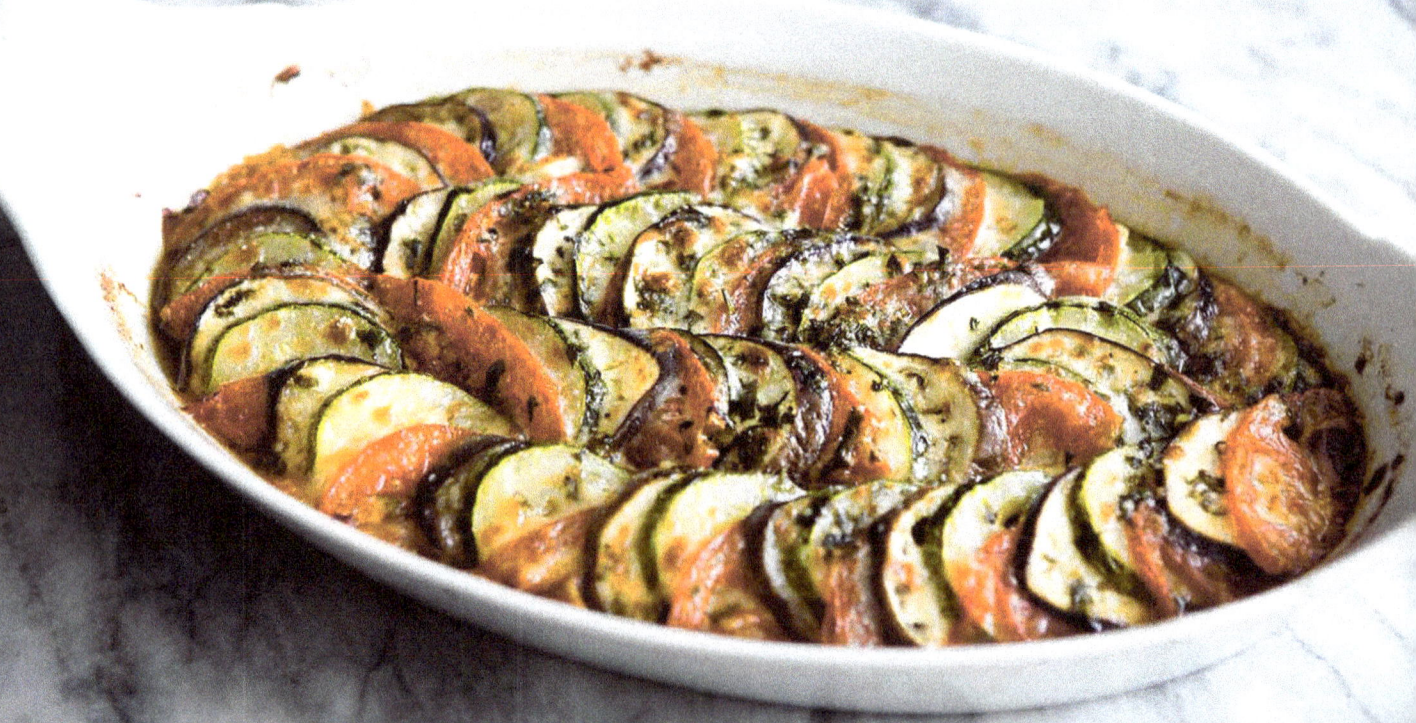

Mashed Cauliflower and White Beans

- 8 cups cauliflower florets, fresh or frozen
- 1 (15-ounce) can white or Lima beans
- ⅔ cup of cashew, raw (optional)
- 2 teaspoons onion powder
- 2 teaspoons garlic powder

This is a great dish for diabetics. It has complex carbohydrates, fiber, protein, and good fat.

In a medium-sized pot, cook cauliflower for about 6 minutes. Pat dry with paper towel. Do not allow the cauliflower to become cold. Warm the beans on medium heat. Then place in food processor with the cashews. Process for a few minutes, then add cauliflower and continue to process until smooth.

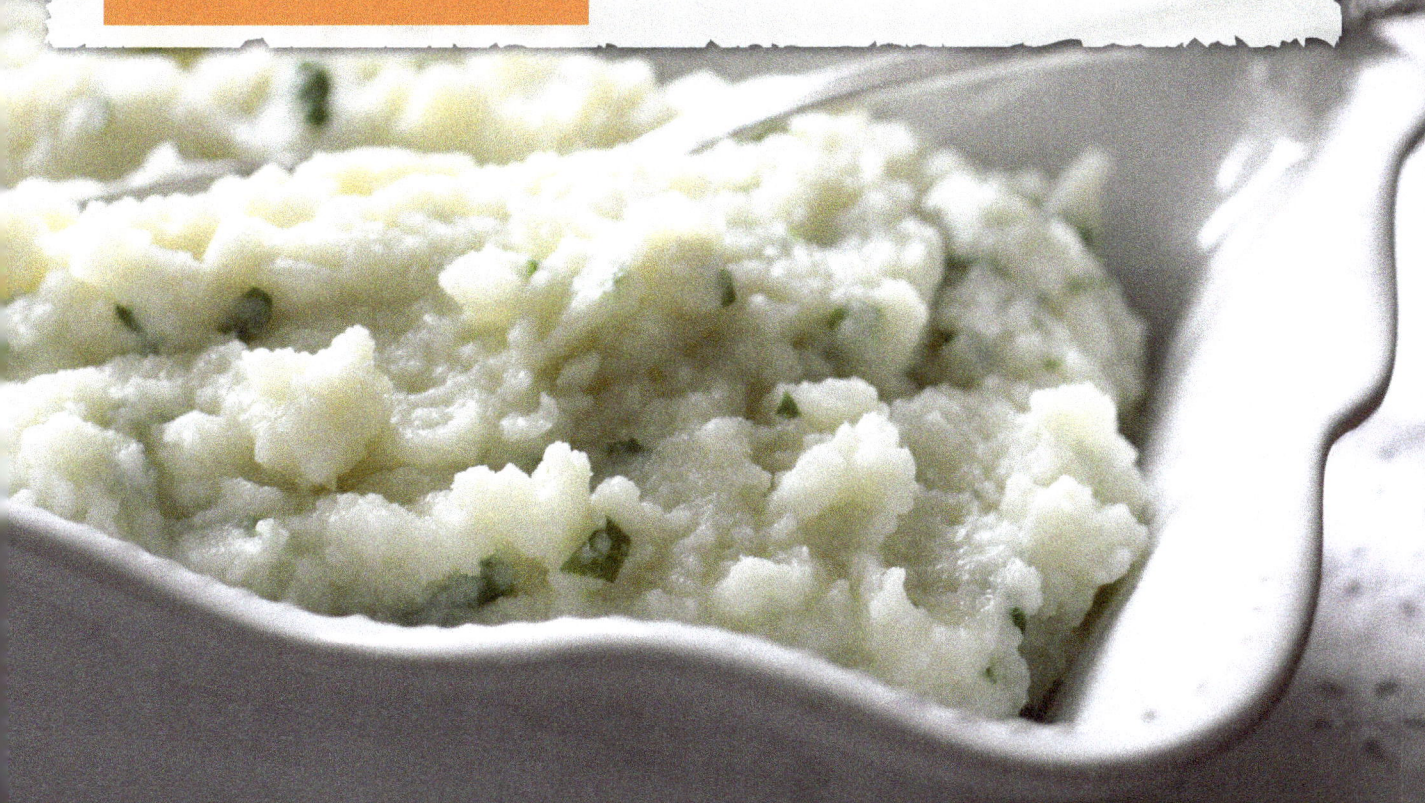

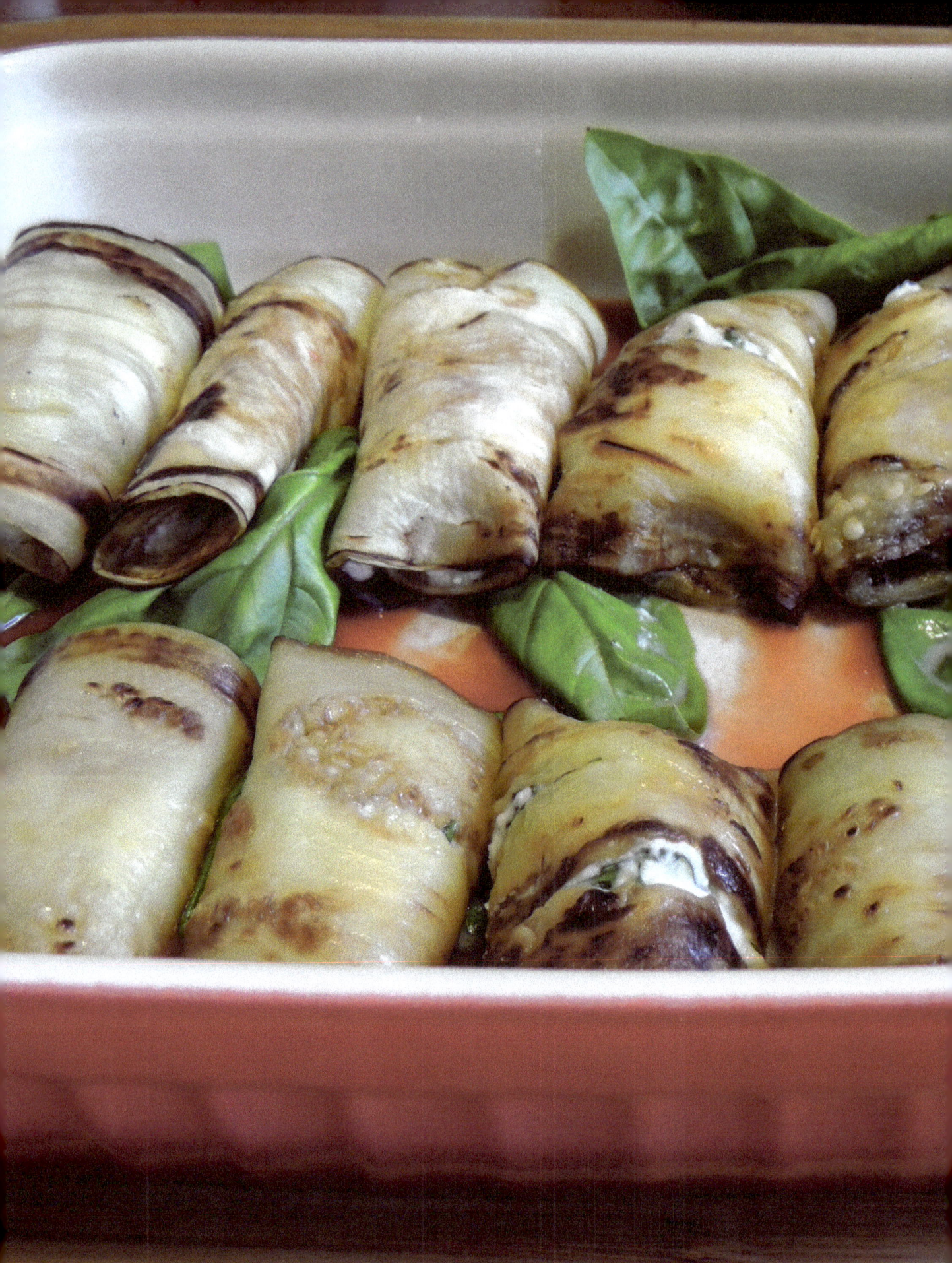

Eggplant Roll-Ups

- 2 large eggplants
- 1 ½ teaspoon salt
- 16-ounce package of firm tofu
- 32-ounce spaghetti sauce
- 1 tablespoon garlic powder
- 1 tablespoon onion powder
- 1 tablespoon rosemary
- 2 tablespoons Bragg's Amino Acids or soy sauce

A dish you can enjoy without the guilt of too many carbohydrates or too much fat. This dish is great for diabetics or for anyone who wants to lose weight.

Cut off both ends of the eggplants and then longitudinally slice, ¼ of an inch thick. Place slices on oiled baking sheet and then sprinkle salt to taste. Allow to bake for about 15 minutes on each side. In a large mixing bowl, place tofu, mashed or scrambled with a fork. Add powdered spices and rosemary and then mix well. Add Bragg's Amino Acids or soy sauce and mix (taste and add salt if needed). Place a full tablespoon of tofu on one end of each side of eggplant and roll. Add a thin layer of spaghetti at the bottom of the baking dish, and cover with spaghetti sauce. Cover with foil and bake for 45 minutes.

Seasoned Vegetable Rice

4 cups brown basmati rice, cooked
1 teaspoon extra-virgin olive oil
1 clove garlic, minced
1 small onion, chopped
2 to 3 teaspoons McKay's chicken-style seasoning
2 cups broccoli, finely chopped
2 cups carrots, shredded
¼ cup vegetable broth
Salt, to taste

This colorful dish goes well with beans or no-meat meatballs.

Cook the basmati rice according to the package directions. In a pot, over medium heat, sauté for 2 to 3 minutes garlic and onions in oil. Add vegetables and McKay's seasoning, then simmer for about 5 to 7 minutes. Additional vegetable broth may be added if needed. Add the cooked basmati rice and simmer for 7 to 10 minutes. Taste the mixture and add salt to taste. Serve with any protein dish of your choice.

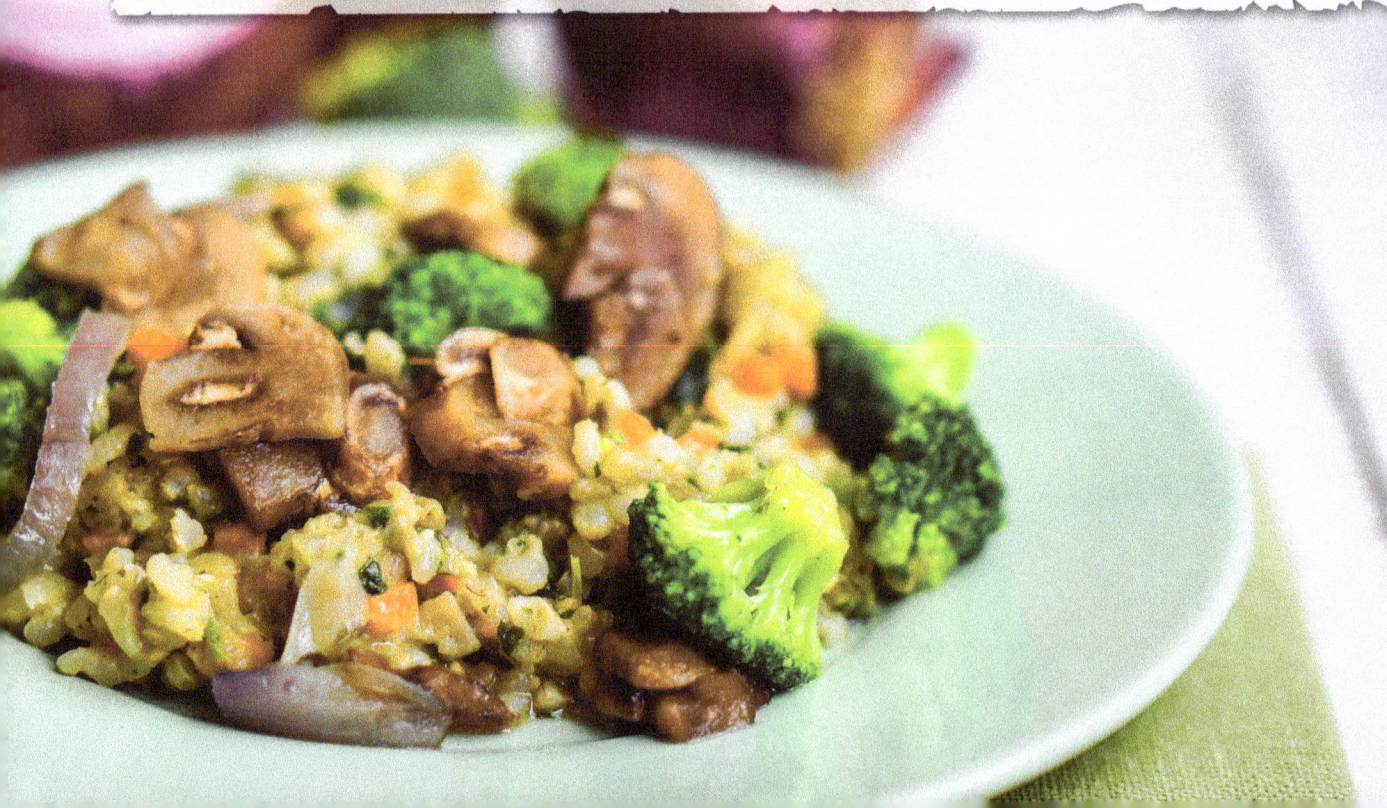

Wild Rice and Mushroom Pilaf

½ cup green onions, finely chopped

½ cup celery, chopped

3 cups sliced mushrooms

1 cup wild rice

1 ½ teaspoons McKay's chicken-style seasoning

3 cups pure water or broth

1 cup sliced almonds, lightly toasted

Wild rice has a low glycemic index; therefore, this dish will not significantly raise the blood sugar.

In a medium-sized covered pan, sauté the onions and celery in a little olive oil until tender. Stir in mushrooms, wild rice, almonds, and seasoning; sauté for 2 to 3 minutes. Carefully add the water or broth, and bring to a boil. Reduce heat, cover, and simmer for about 50 minutes until rice is tender and liquid is absorbed. Leave covered for 10 minutes. Fluff with a fork before serving and garnish with more almonds, if desired.

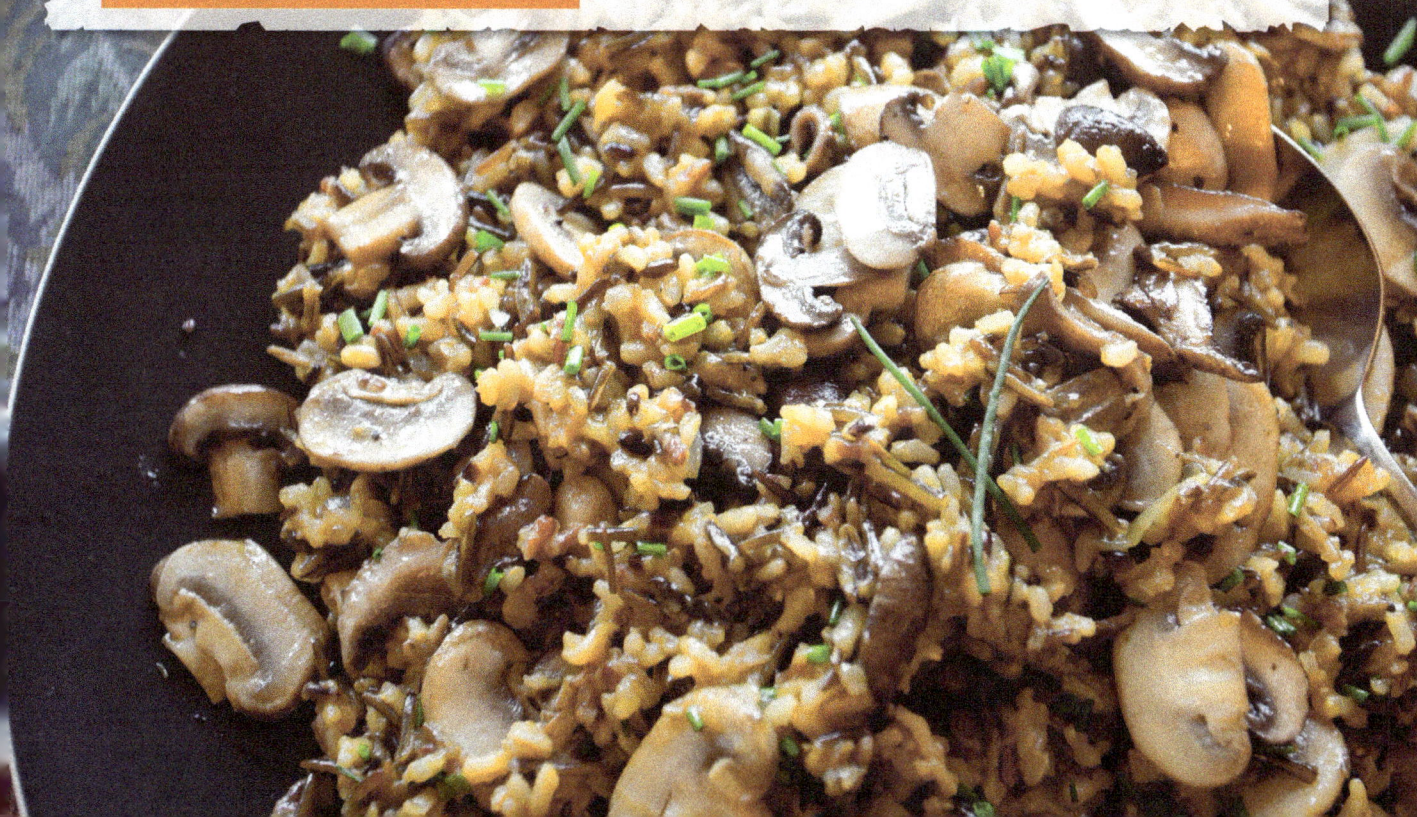

Indian Rice

1 medium onion, chopped
2 cloves garlic, mashed and diced
½ cup carrot, chopped
¼ cup slivered almonds
2 ½ cups boiling water
1 cup long-grain brown rice
½ cup frozen green beans
½ cup frozen corn
1 teaspoon cumin
¼ tablespoon ginger powder
2 teaspoons turmeric
1 tablespoon McKay's chicken-style seasoning
Salt, to taste

Add fresh vegetables to this delicious rice dish and enjoy.

Preheat the oven to 350 degrees Fahrenheit. Sauté the onion, garlic, and carrot for about 5 minutes. Add the rice and other ingredients, stirring together gently. Add the boiling water and pour into a 1 ½-quart casserole dish. Bake, covered, for 50 to 55 minutes. Lightly toast the almonds in a dry, nonstick skillet, and then stir them in with rice mixture. Serve with a bean salad or chickpea curry.

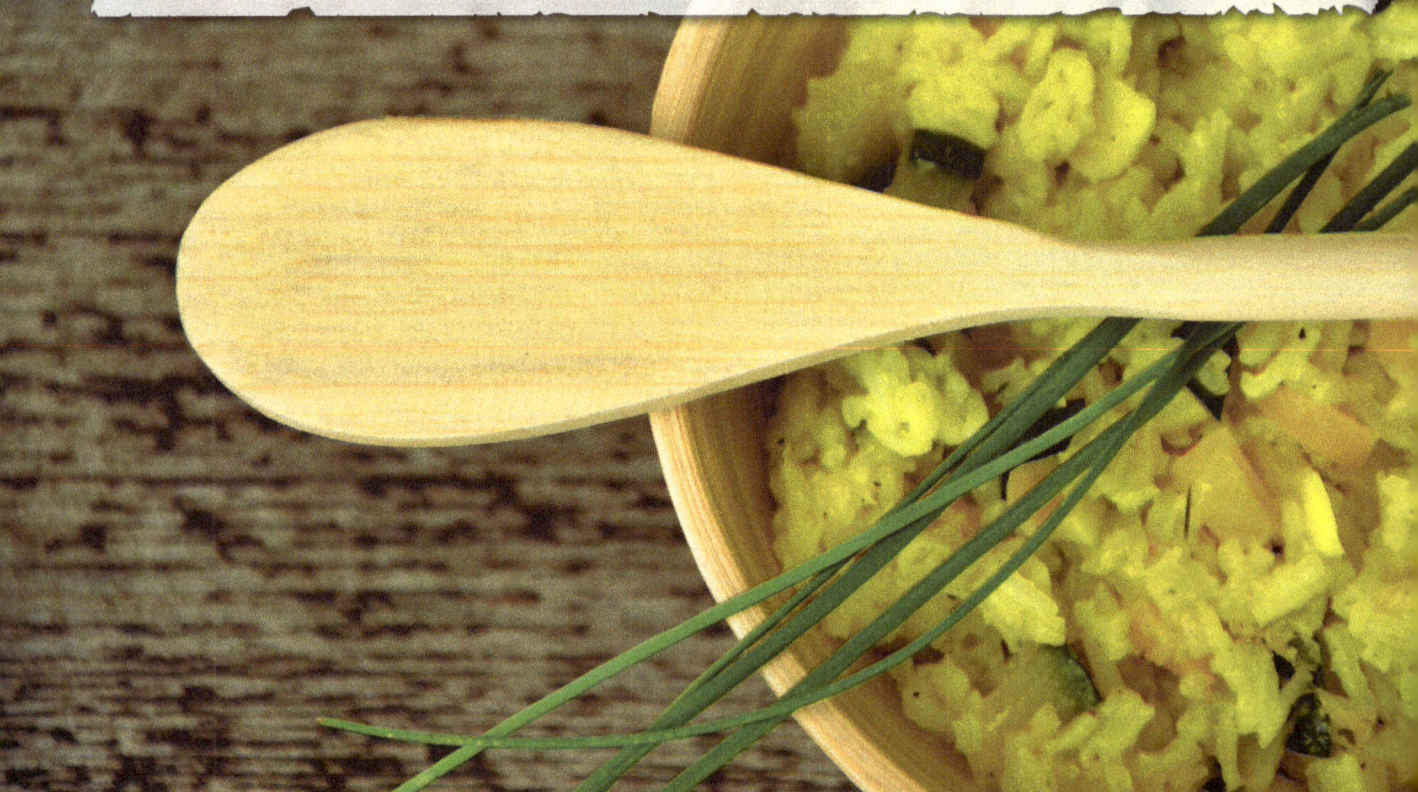

Seasoned Black Bean Brown Rice

1 medium onion, chopped
3 cloves garlic, mashed and diced
2 cups long-grain uncooked brown rice
1 (15-ounce) can black beans
4 cups water
2 teaspoons thyme
1 tablespoon McKay's chicken-style seasoning
1 tablespoon Mrs. Dash, salt-free seasoning

If you enjoy black beans, then this is a great dish for you.

Preheat oven to 350 degrees Fahrenheit. On low heat, sauté for 2 to 3 minutes the onion and garlic in a small amount of water. Add in the rice, black beans, and other ingredients. Continue to sauté for another 3 minutes. Now add the 4 cups of water. Pour mixture in a casserole dish, cover, and place in preheated oven at 350 degrees Fahrenheit for 60 minutes. Use as a main dish or serve with a fresh vegetable salad.

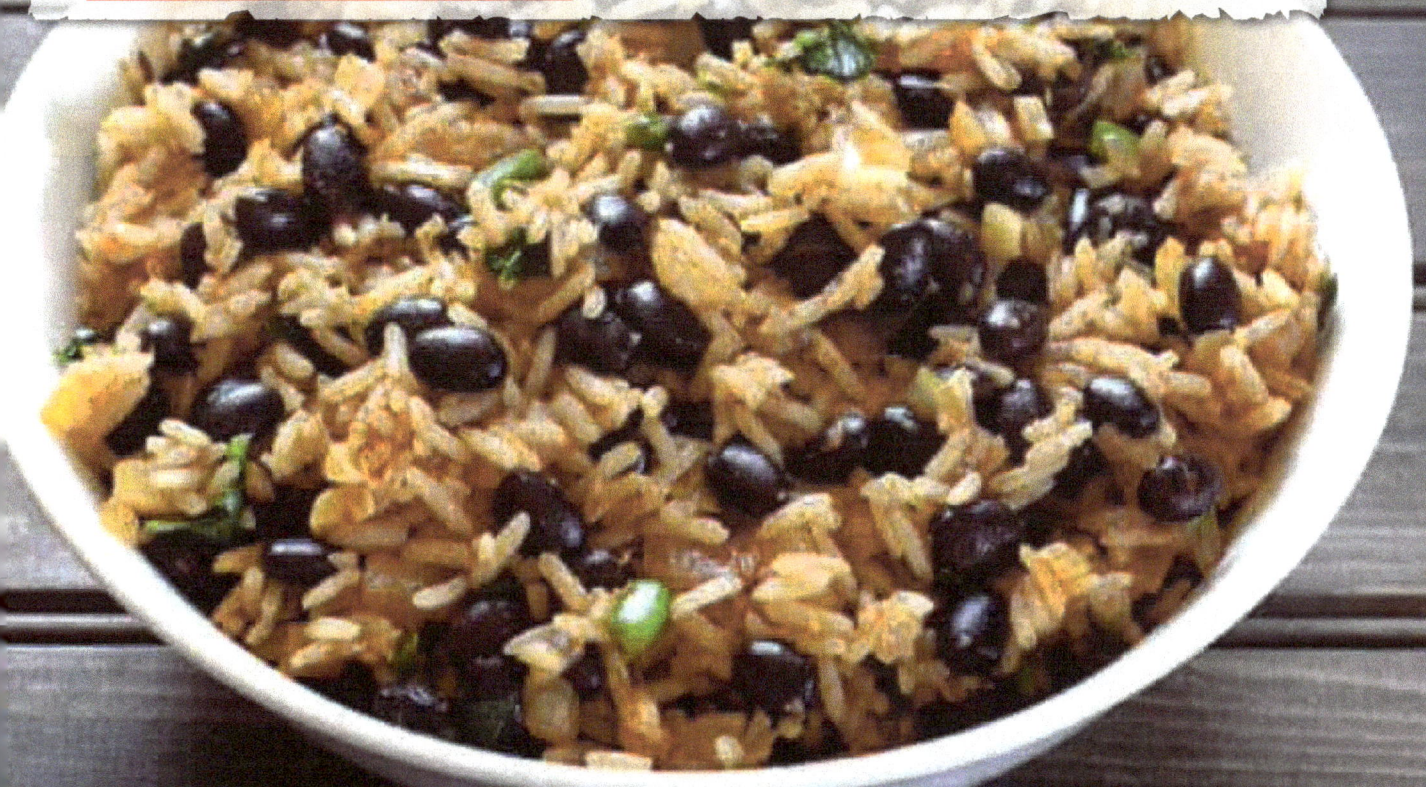

Chickpea Avocado Spread

- 1 medium avocado
- 15 ounce chickpeas
- 1 tablespoon lemon juice
- ½ sweet onion
- Salt to taste

This spread make a wholesome and delicious sandwich. Just add tomato, spinach leaves, and alfalfa sprouts.

Remove peel and seed from avocado. Drain and rinse chickpeas. Add all the ingredients to the food processor and process until smooth. Can be used as sandwich spread or dip.

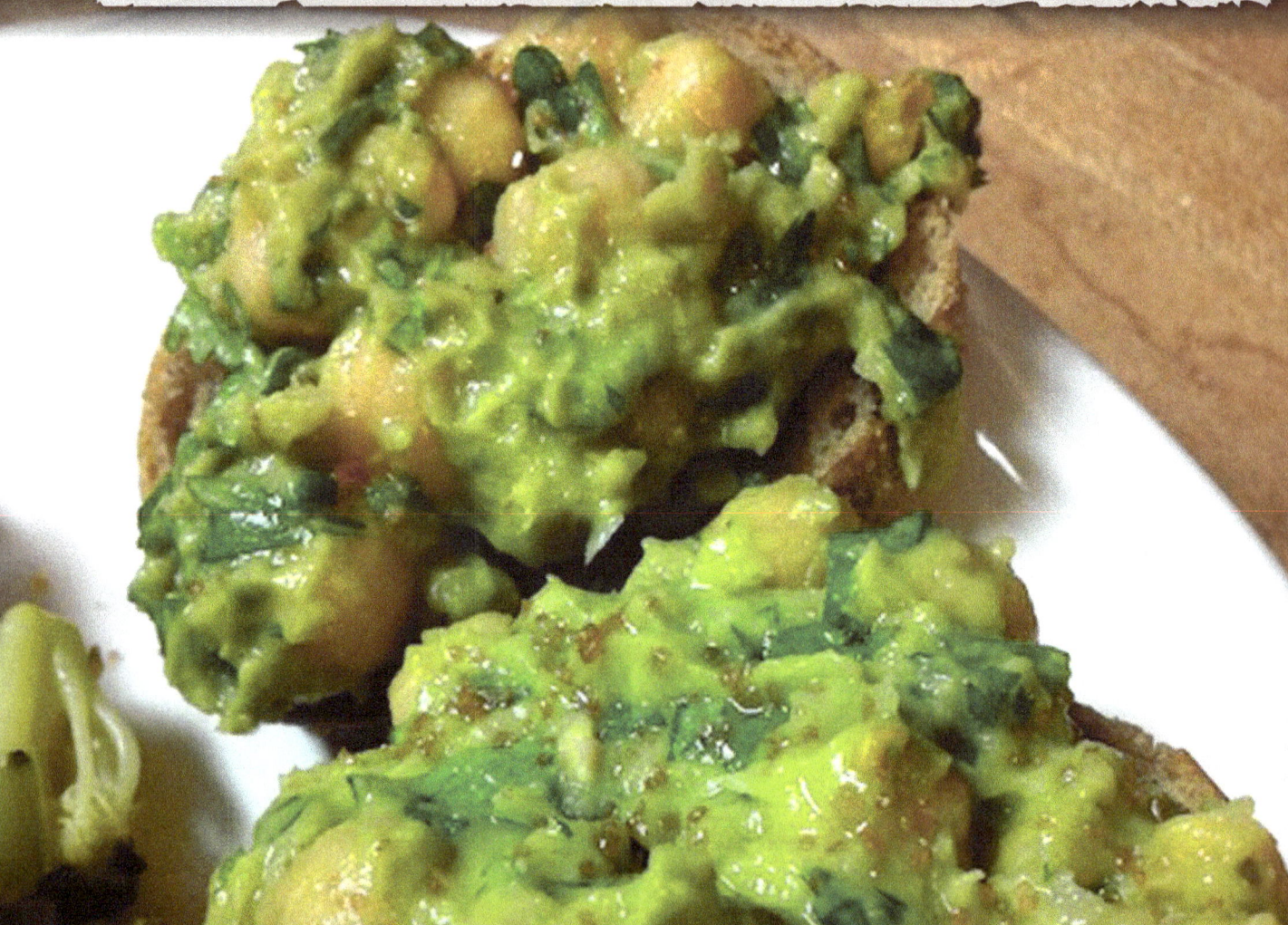

Lentil Walnut "Meatballs"

1 cup soaked lentils (cover in water and soak overnight)
¼ cup of walnuts, chopped
½ cup onion, chopped
1 teaspoon thyme
1 teaspoon cumin
2 tablespoons tahini
1 teaspoon garlic powder
½ cup oat flour
1 teaspoon sage
1 teaspoon salt
1 teaspoon fresh basil, finely chopped

These look and taste better than meat. Cook in tomato sauce and serve over whole wheat spaghetti. (Refer to Tomato Sauce recipe on page 140.)

Pour off the water and then blend lentil to a paste. Place lentils in a bowl. Add all the other ingredients and mix together. Form small balls and then place them on a baking tray. Preheat oven to 200 degrees Fahrenheit, and bake for approximately 20 to 25 minutes.

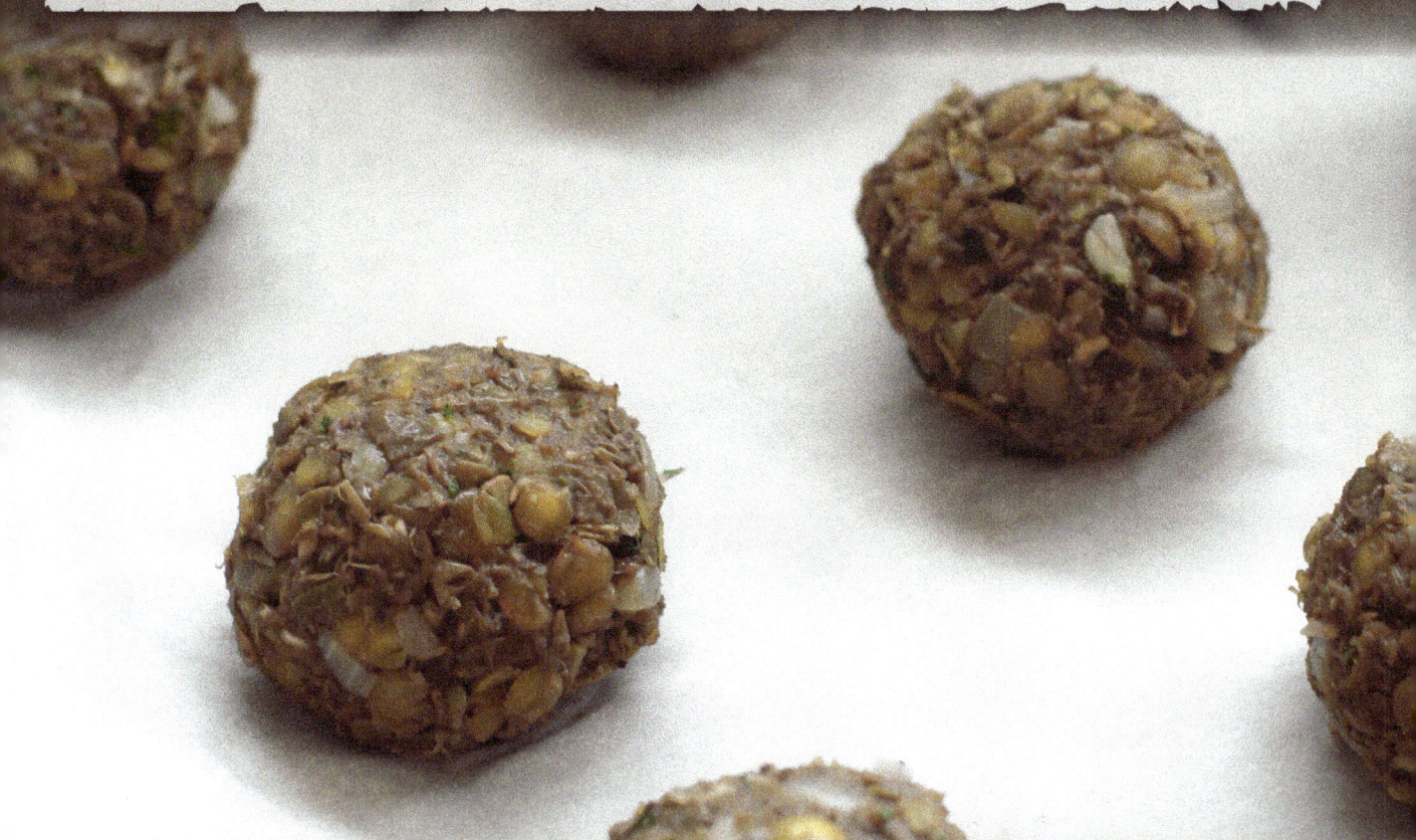

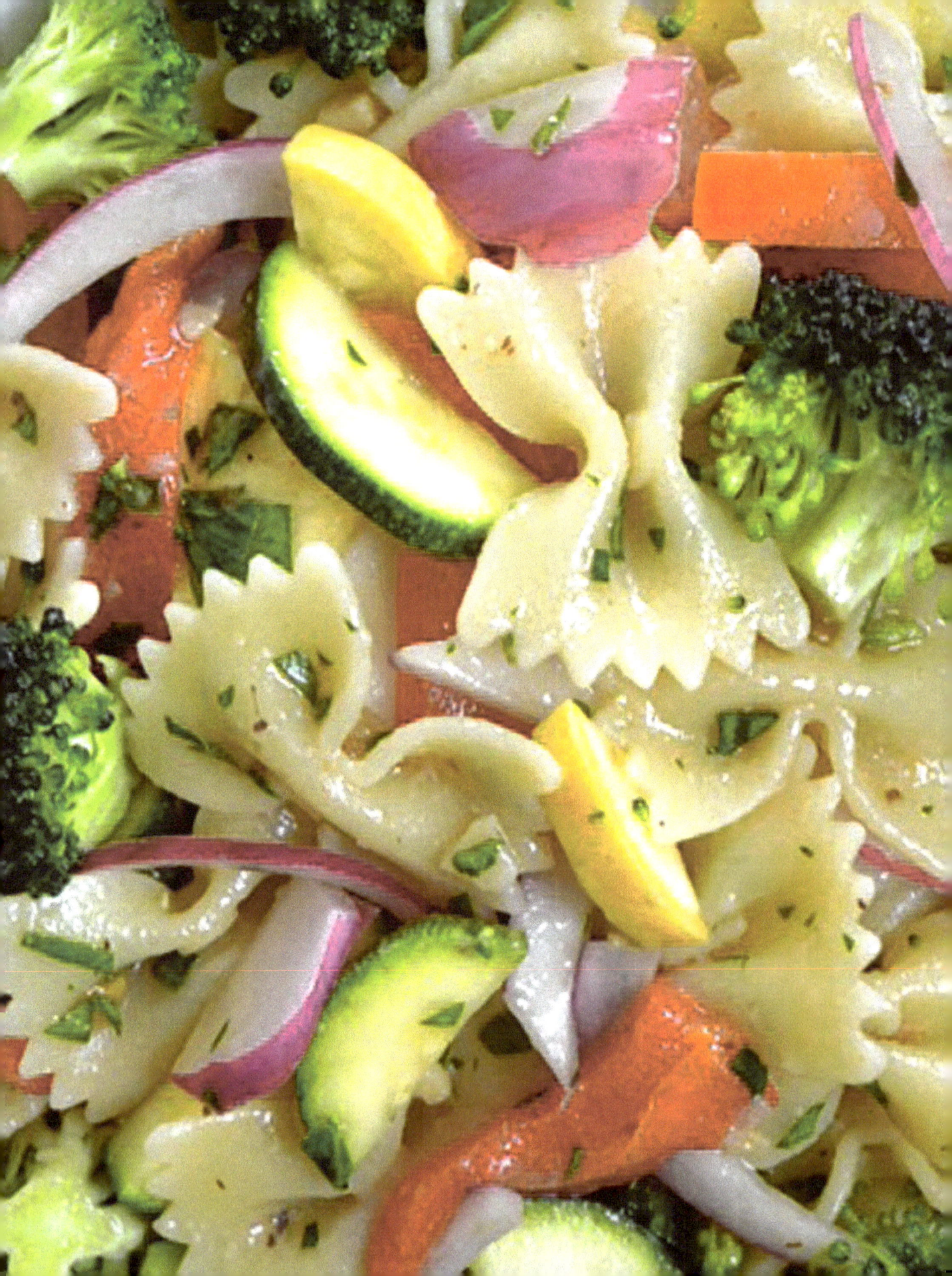

Pasta Primavera

1 tablespoon olive oil
½ cup onion, thinly sliced
2 cloves garlic, mashed and then minced
½ cup red or yellow bell pepper, sliced
½ cup carrot, julienned
2 cups cauliflower florets
1 bunch broccoli florets
1 medium zucchini, sliced
1 teaspoon salt or to taste
1 cup tomatoes, diced
1 box (16 ounces) pasta, cooked, using instructions on package
1 recipe Alfredo sauce
¼ cup nondairy parmesan cheese or nutritional yeast flakes (optional)

Another great source of vitamins and phytochemicals. This dish will empower you as you seek to keep diseases in retreat! Be careful not to overcook your veggies. Too much heat will destroy some of the nutrients in these foods.

In a large saucepan, heat oil over medium heat. Add onion, garlic, carrot, and bell pepper. Cook until softened (about 4 minutes). Add cauliflower, broccoli, zucchini, and salt. Stir occasionally. Cook until vegetables are ready (about 5 minutes).

Prepare pasta using instructions from the package. Add pasta and sauce to the vegetables. Gently mix together and cook until heated through. Top with tomatoes and nondairy parmesan cheese.

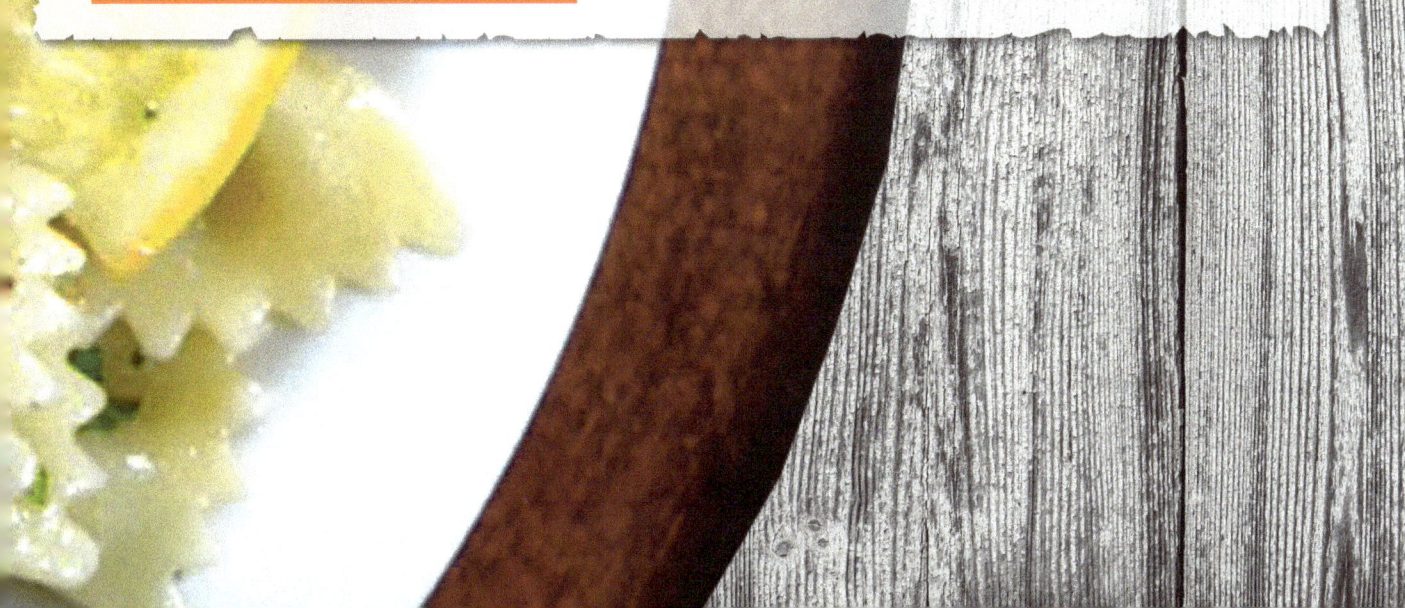

Pasta with Vegetables

2 tablespoons olive oil
½ cup red onion, diced
2 cloves garlic, mashed and minced
4 stalks celery, diced
1 cup carrot, julienned
1 pound fresh asparagus or green beans, cut in 1-inch pieces
1 medium zucchini, thinly sliced
1 cup leafy greens
3 tablespoons Bragg's Amino Acids or soy sauce
2 cups vegetable broth
½ tablespoon cornstarch
1 package (14 ounces) whole-grain angel hair pasta, cooked using directions on package
2 cups tomatoes, chopped
6 to 8 leaves fresh basil or 1 teaspoon dried basil
½ teaspoon dried oregano

Be creative and use the vegetables that you enjoy. Using vegetables of many colors will give different vitamins, minerals, and phytonutrients, which are all essential for disease prevention or reversal.

Heat oil in wok over medium heat. Add onion, garlic, celery, and carrots. Cook until softened, stirring occasionally, about 7 to 8 minutes. Add asparagus, zucchini, and salt. Cook until vegetables are just softened, about 4 minutes. Whisk cornstarch and broth together in a small bowl. Add broth and remaining ingredients to wok. Bring to a boil over high heat and cook until thickened.

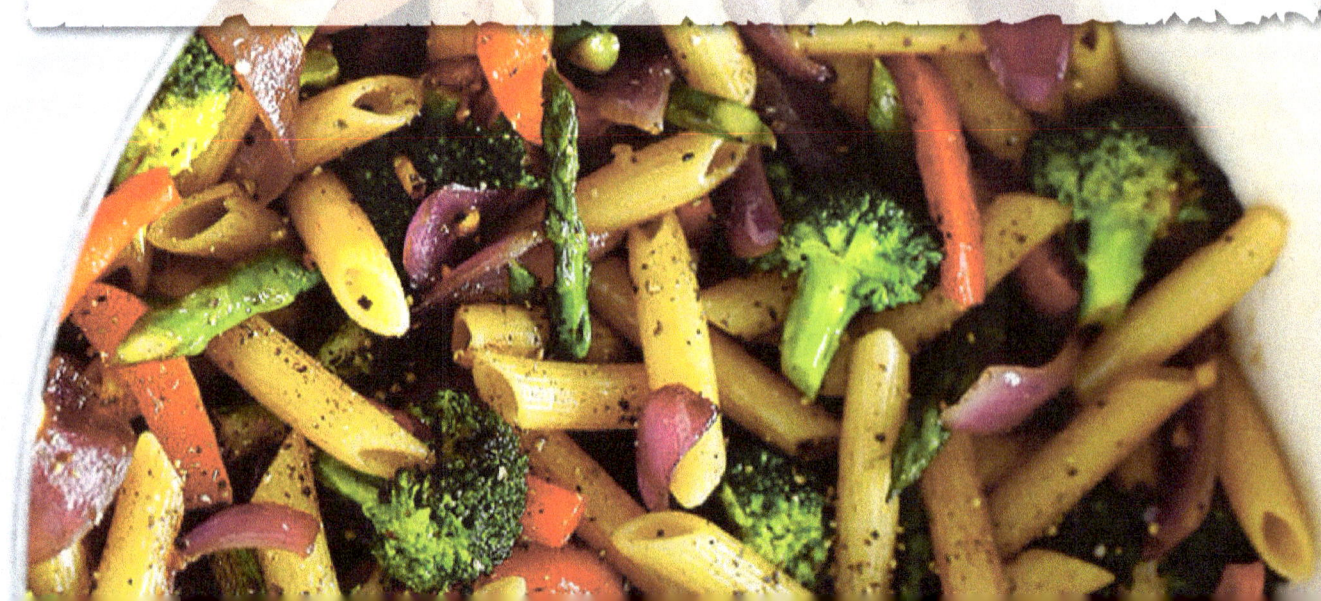

Veggie Wrap with Guacamole

- Finely grate any vegetables
- Carrots
- Cabbage
- Butternut squash
- Slice any of the following
- Sweet peppers
- Onions
- Mushrooms
- Sprouts of your choice
- Nuts of your choice
- One batch of tahini sauce
- One batch of guacamole

Here is another meal in which you want to use your creativity. Choose veggies that you enjoy. Prepare veggies ahead, and then the rest is easy. This is a complete meal with vegetables, protein, carbohydrates, and good fat.

Bake wrap for 15 seconds in a very hot pan (without oil) to prevent from breaking when rolling. Spread guacamole in a rectangle in the middle of the tortilla. Put your choice of vegetable on the guacamole, and fold like an envelope, leaving the top side open. Put some tahini sauce on, close your envelope, and enjoy.

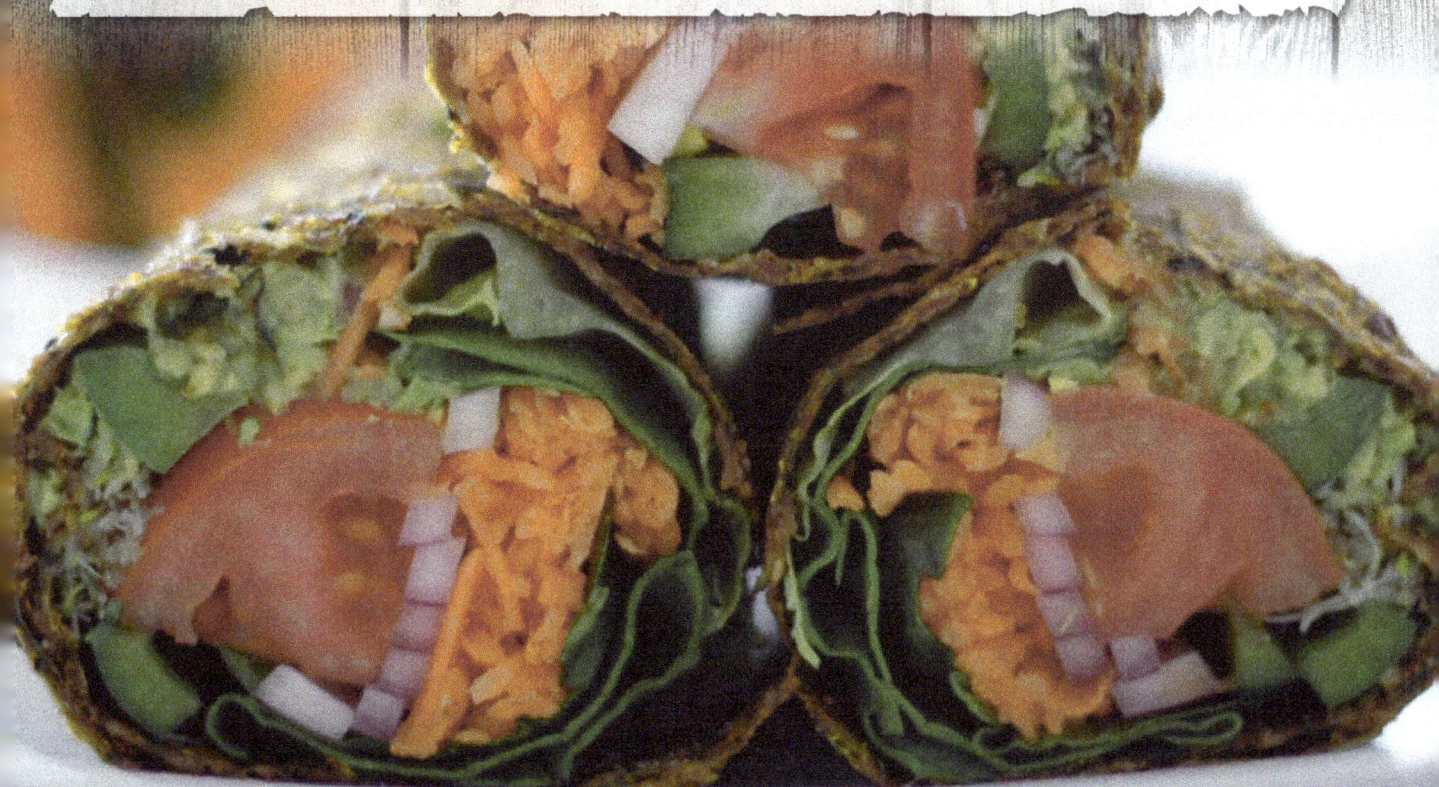

Chickpea Curry

2 tablespoons olive oil
1 onion, chopped
2 cloves garlic, mashed then minced
2 teaspoons fresh ginger root, finely chopped
2 teaspoons cumin
1 teaspoon ground coriander
1 teaspoon sage
Sea salt to taste
1 teaspoon cayenne pepper
1 tablespoon ground turmeric
2 (15-ounce) cans chickpeas
½ cup water

This is another recipe the patients at Cooper Wellness Center of McAllen enjoy. It goes well with steamed brown rice. It is somewhat spicy, so feel free to decrease the amount of ginger or cayenne pepper that the recipe calls for.

Heat oil in a large saucepan over medium heat. Add onion and spices. Sauté until tender. Then add beans and water. Cook for 20 minutes.

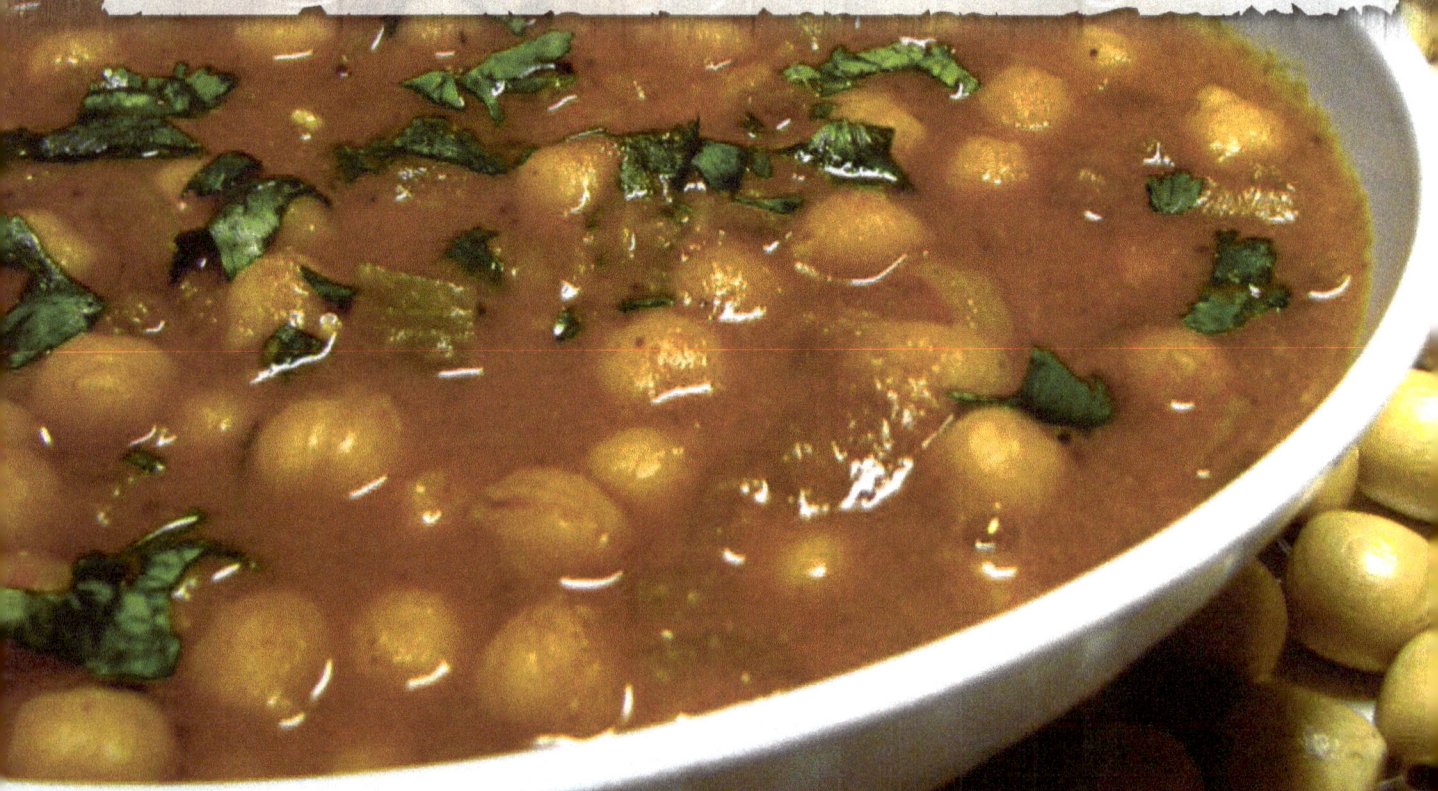

Lentil Patties

- 2 cups cooked red lentils, drained
- ½ cup onions, finely chopped
- 1 teaspoon dried thyme
- 1 cup finely ground chia seeds
- ¼ cup brown rice flour or oatmeal flour
- 2 teaspoons sea salt
- 1 teaspoon garlic powder
- 1 teaspoon onion powder
- 1 ¼ teaspoon sage
- 1 cup grated carrots
- 1 cup pecans
- 175 grams tiny mushrooms, drained and chopped
- 1 cup water or milk
- 1 cup celery, finely chopped

These are absolutely delicious. You will not miss the meat. Serve on a bun or with gravy over rice or baked potato or with mixed vegetables.

Line your baking pan with parchment paper or spray your pan with oil. Mix all the ingredients together and make patties. Put patties on the baking pan. Bake at 350 degrees Fahrenheit for 30 minutes. Turn them over after 20 minutes. Hint—use an ice cream scoop and make balls instead of patties and bake.

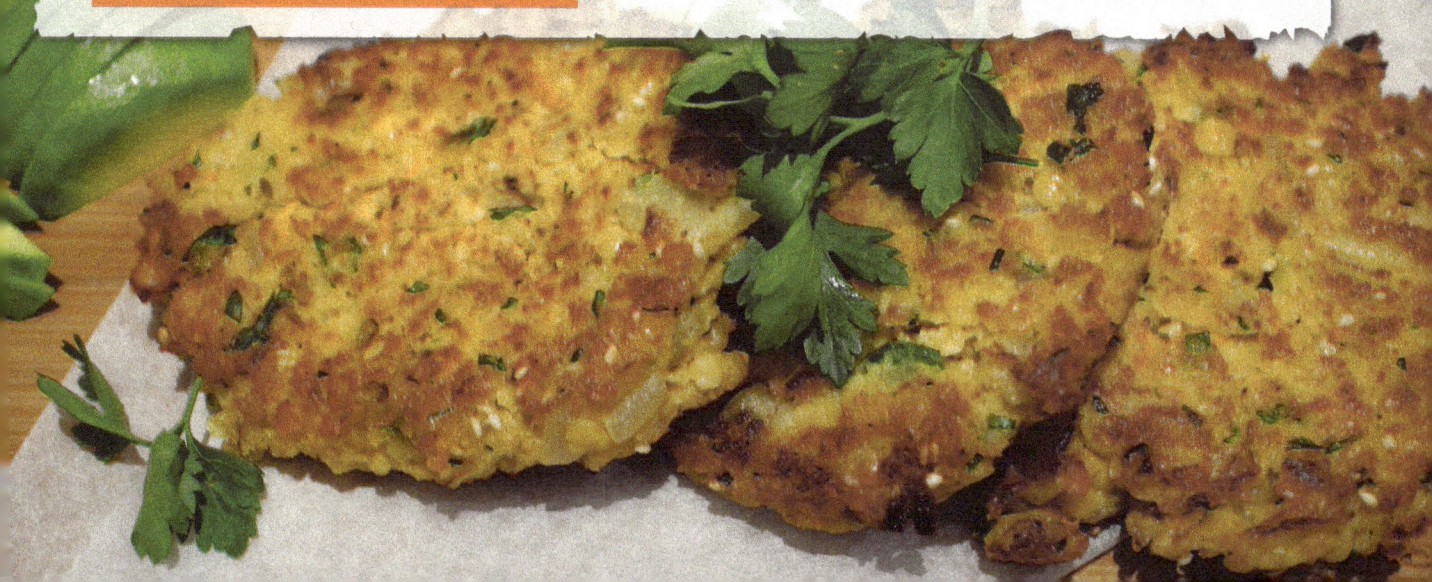

Walnet Balls

- 4 cups water
- 4 cups rolled oats
- 1 medium onion, finely chopped
- 4 garlic cloves
- ½ cup raw sunflower seeds
- ½ cup Bragg's Amino Acids
- ½ cup walnut, chopped
- ¼ cup olive oil
- 1 tablespoon molasses
- ½ cup nutritional yeast
- 1 tablespoon Italian seasoning
- 1 teaspoon ground coriander
- 1 teaspoon dried sage

These are very delicious and can be served with spaghetti with sauce.

This recipe makes 24 balls.

Boil 4 cups of water. Mix the hot water with all the other ingredients and let it sit in the bowl for 10 minutes. Shape into balls. Put in the baking dish and bake at 350 degrees Fahrenheit for 20 to 30 minutes. These walnut balls taste better the next day. Freeze well.

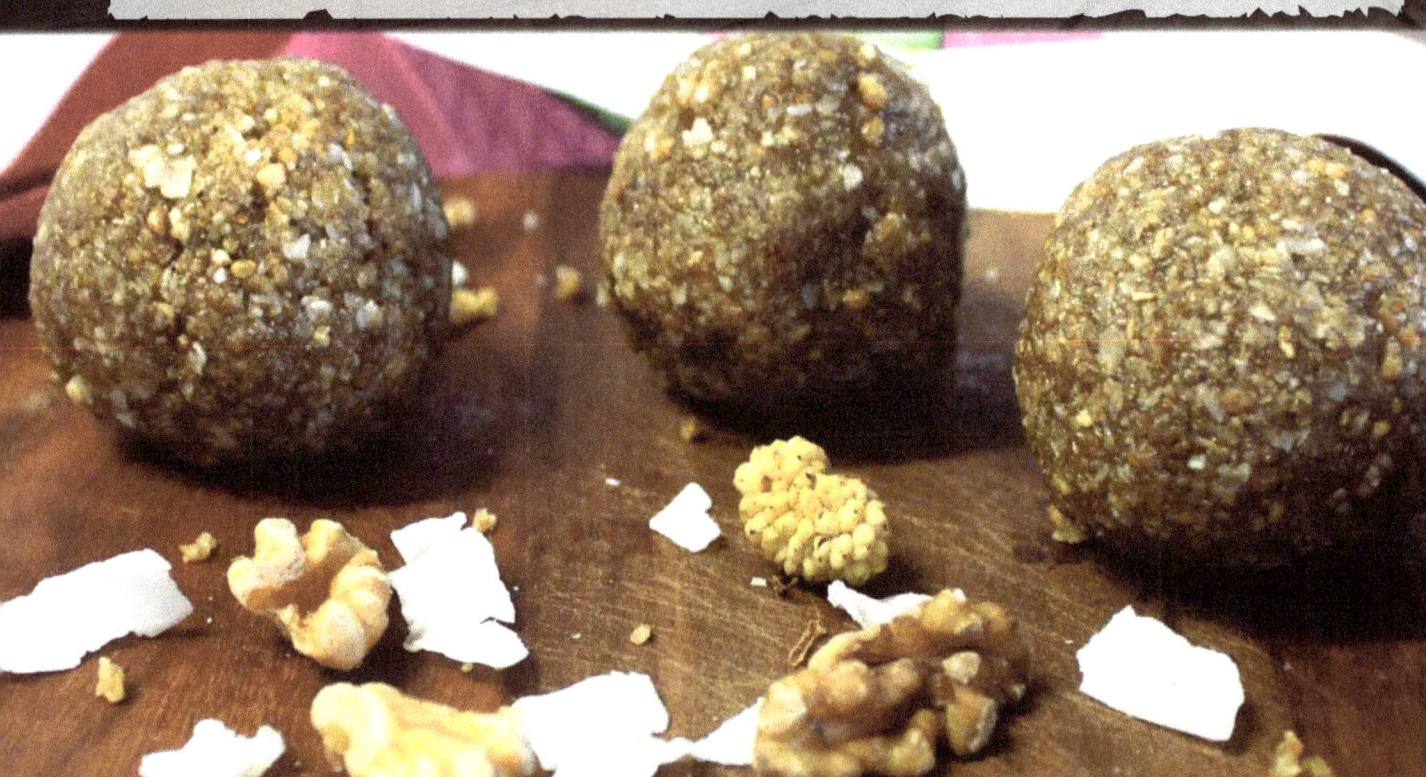

Sun-Dried Tomato, Black Bean and Rice Salad

- 2 ½ cups long-grained brown rice, cooked
- ½ cup marinated sun-dried tomatoes, coarsely chopped
- 1 ripe avocado, diced
- ½ cup black bean, cooked
- 1 stalk celery, finely chopped
- ¼ cup almond slivers
- 3 leaves fresh basil, julienned
- 1 tablespoon fresh lemon juice
- 1 tablespoon garlic powder
- 1 tablespoon diced red onion
- 1 teaspoon salt

This very delicious dish is packed with protein, fiber, complex carbohydrates, and good fat. Goes well with raw vegetables and may prevent diabetes, heart disease, and obesity.

In a large mixing bowl, combine all ingredients and mix well.

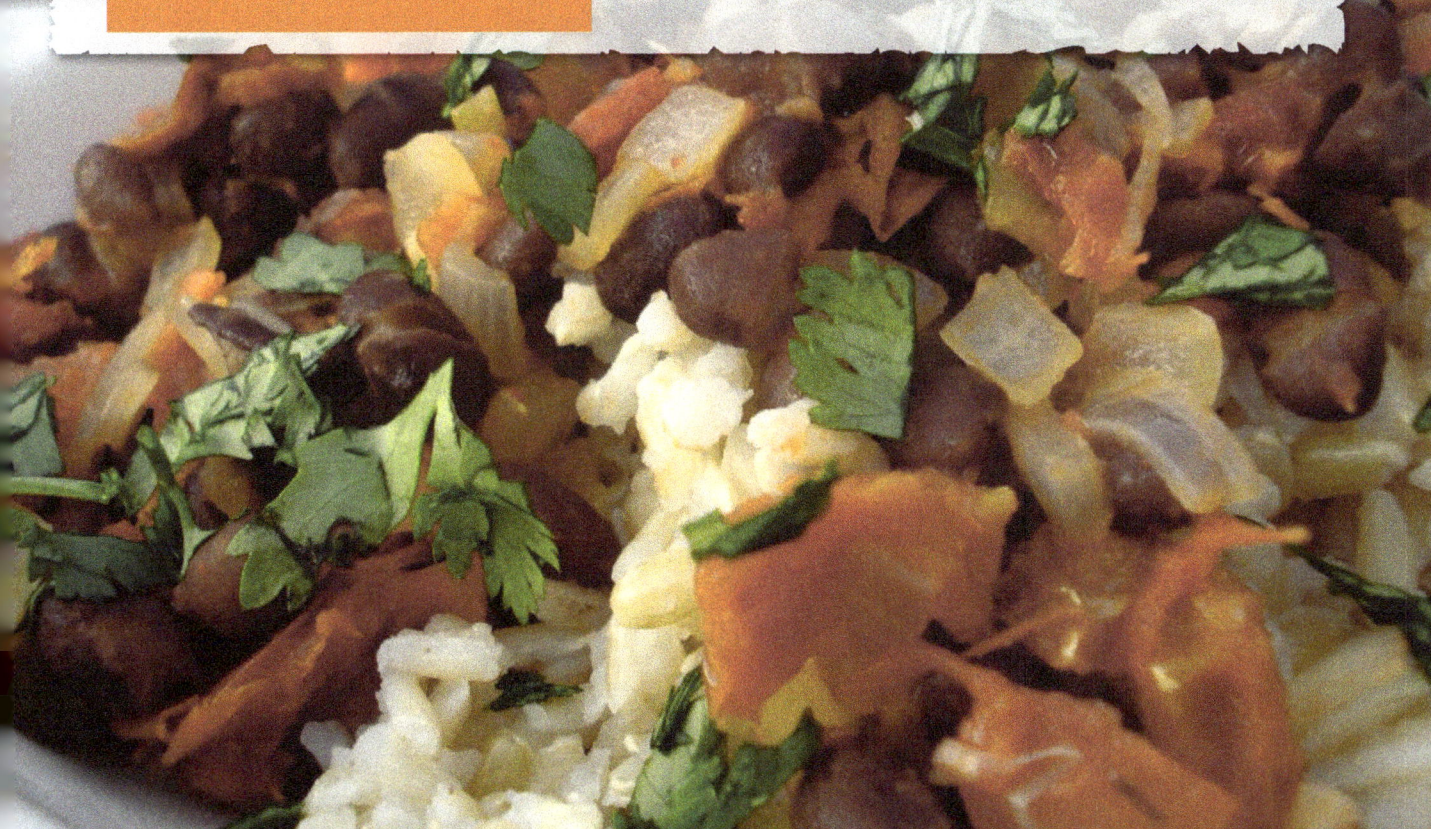

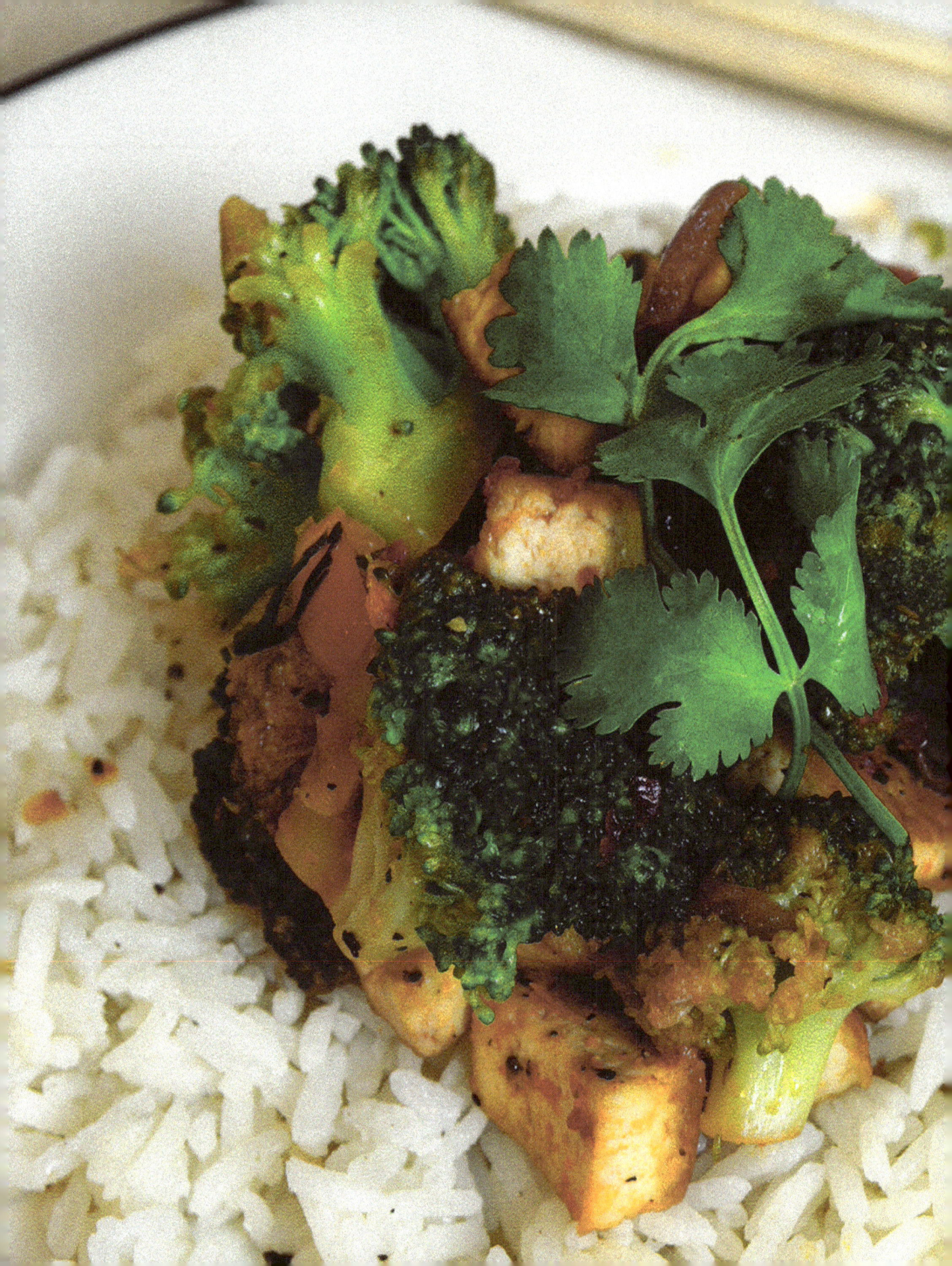

Chinese Stir-Fry Vegetables

Olive-oil spray
1 pound (16 ounces) tofu, firm, cut into bite-sized cubes
1 medium to large onion, sliced
⅔ cup carrots, julienned
1 cup cauliflower florets
¼ cup water
⅔ cup celery, cut in 3-inch pieces
1 cup broccoli florets
½ cup bean sprouts
⅔ snow pea pods
1 can water chestnuts
1 can baby corn cobs
⅔ cup bok choy, chopped
2 tablespoons chicken-like seasoning of your choice, to taste
2 tablespoons Bragg's Amino Acids or soy sauce

This dish is very colorful with many different vegetables. This indicates that you will receive various nutrients from this one dish. Serve with brown rice.

Spray small amount oil in wok or nonstick skillet and then place it on medium-to-high heat. When oil is hot, add tofu. Slightly braze tofu, allowing each piece to become slightly brown. Then remove and place aside. Now add onion to wok or skillet and sauté for 2 minutes. Then add vegetables. First, add the carrots and the cauliflower and allow to cook for 3 to 5 minutes. May need to add a small amount of water. Now add the other vegetables. Stir intermittently, allowing all the vegetables to be cooked evenly for 3 minutes. Add tofu, chicken-style seasoning, and Bragg's Amino Acids or soy sauce. Continue to stir and allow to cook for 2 minutes more. Take care not to overcook the vegetables.

Mock Tuna Salad

- 1 (15-ounce) can of chickpeas, drained
- ¼ cup reduced-fat Vegenaise
- ⅓ cup celery, finely chopped
- 2 tablespoon sweet onion, finely chopped
- ½ tablespoon nutritional yeast flakes
- 1 teaspoon low-sodium soy sauce

This is a great dish for a party or any social event. It is delicious and easy to prepare. It may be served on whole wheat bread with lettuce. Leftovers can be stored in the refrigerator for 3 to 4 days.

In a medium-sized bowl, mash the chickpeas with a fork and combine with the rest of the ingredients.

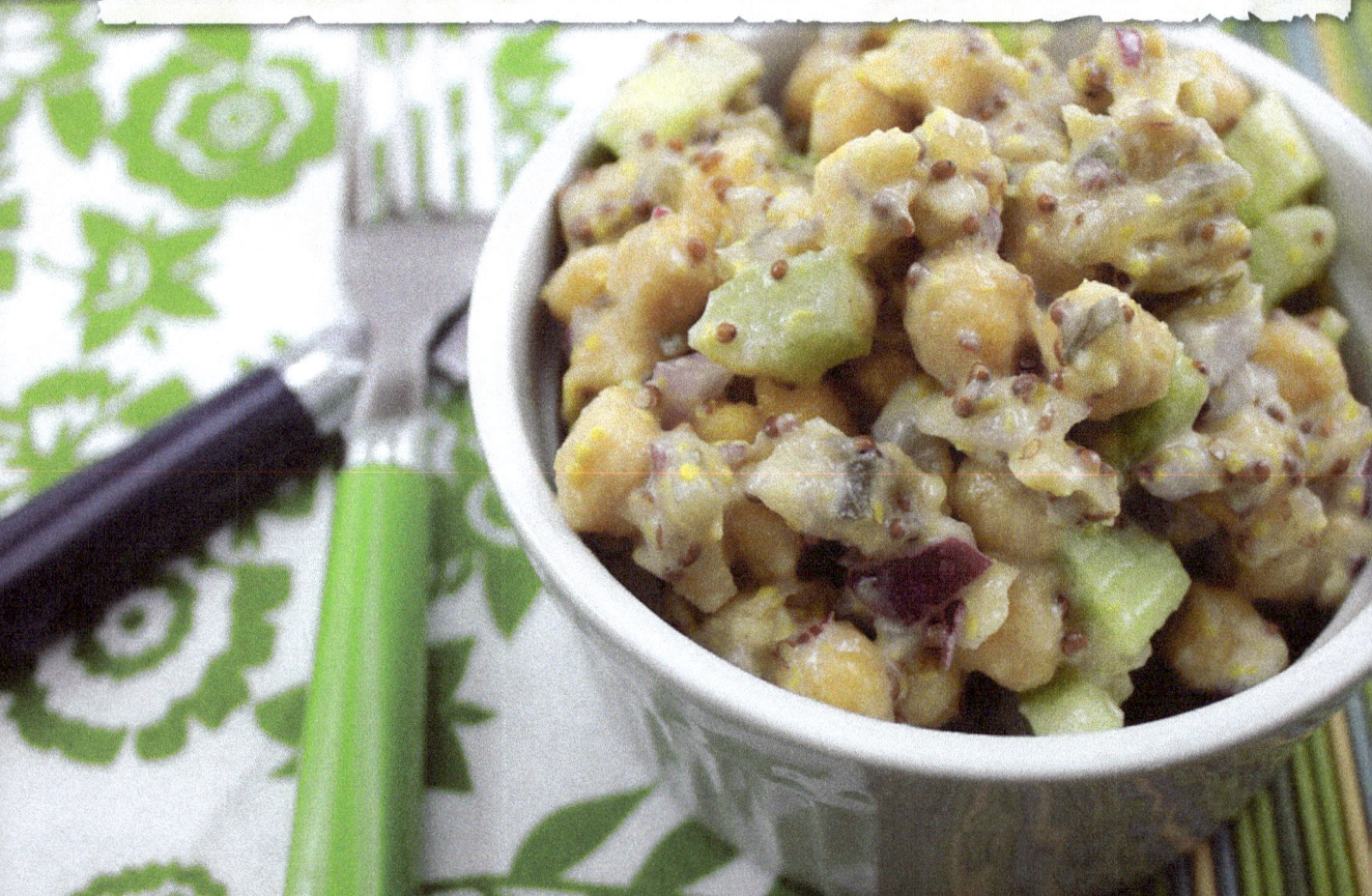

Black Bean, Corn and Quinoa Salad

- 1 tablespoon extra-virgin olive oil
- 1 onion, chopped
- 3 cloves garlic, minced
- ¼ cup quinoa, uncooked
- 1 ½ cups vegetable broth (low sodium)
- 1 tablespoon ground cumin
- ¼ tablespoon cayenne pepper
- Salt to taste
- 2 cups frozen corn kernels
- 2 (15-ounce) cans black beans, rinsed and drained
- ½ cup fresh cilantro, chopped
- 2 tablespoons lime or lemon juice
- 1 jalapeño, seeded and diced finely (optional)

Quinoa is a whole grain that has a high-protein and high-fiber content. It is great for those seeking to stay healthy.

Over the medium heat, heat oil in a saucepan and sauté the onion and garlic until they're soft and translucent. Add the quinoa to the pan and cover with vegetable broth. Season with cumin, cayenne pepper, and salt. Then bring the mixture to a boil. Cover, reduce the heat, and simmer for 20 minutes, stirring occasionally. Add the frozen corn to the pan and continue to simmer for 5 more minutes. Mix in the black beans, cilantro, lime juice, and optional jalapeño and cook until beans are heated through.

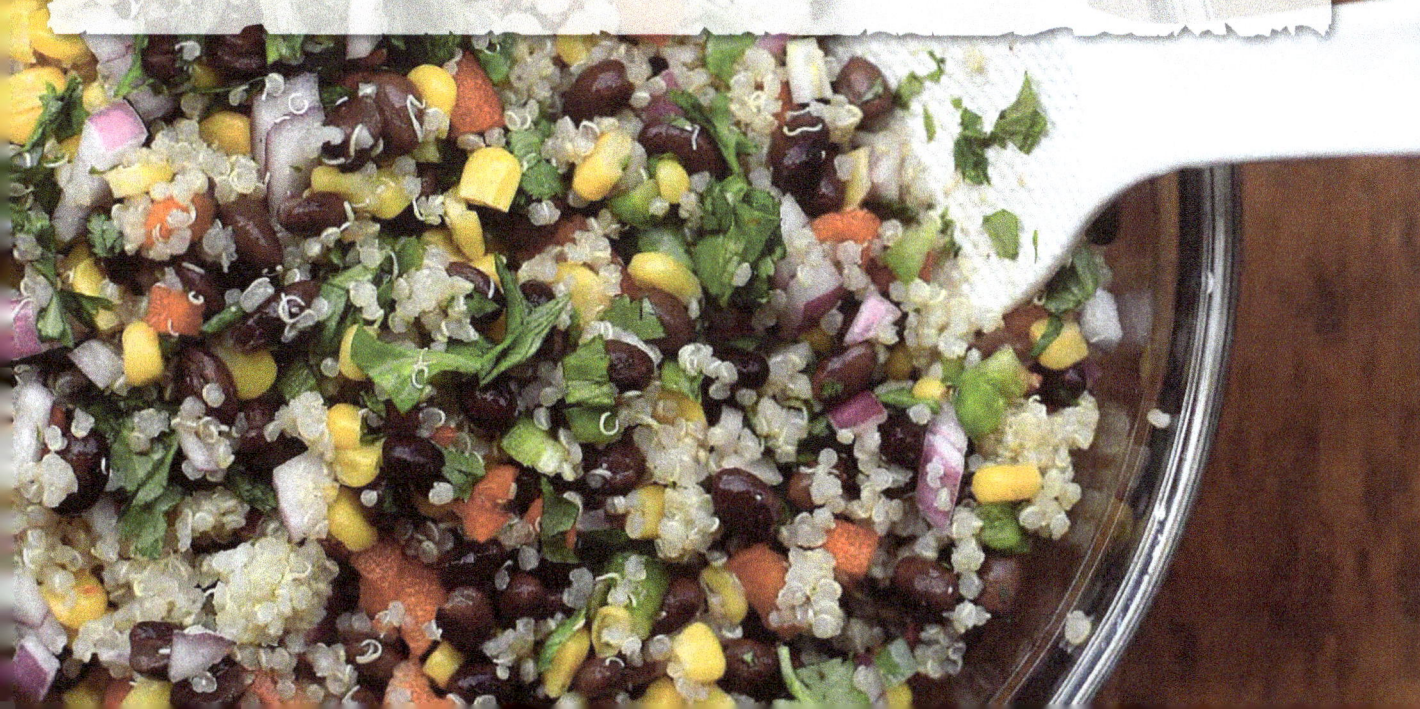

Quinoa Salad

- 2 cups quinoa
- 4 cups water
- 1 green bell pepper, chopped
- ¼ cup chopped red onion
- ½ cup seedless grapes in halves
- 1 cup cherry tomatoes in halves
- 1 medium cucumber (cubed)
- ¼ cup walnuts (optional)
- ¼ cup fresh mint (chopped)

This is a salad that everyone enjoys. It is packed with minerals, vitamins, healthy fat, and complex carbohydrates. All these nutrients will help to keep diseases in retreat.

Rinse the quinoa well before cooking. Place the quinoa and water in a saucepan. Bring to a boil, cover, and reduce the heat. Simmer for about 15 minutes or until the liquid is absorbed. Then allow quinoa to cool. Combine the chopped vegetables in a bowl, including the fresh chopped herb of your choice. Mix well. Add the cooked quinoa. Toss gently and add dressing of your choice. Toss again and add pepper to taste. Cover and chill for at least 2 hours before serving.

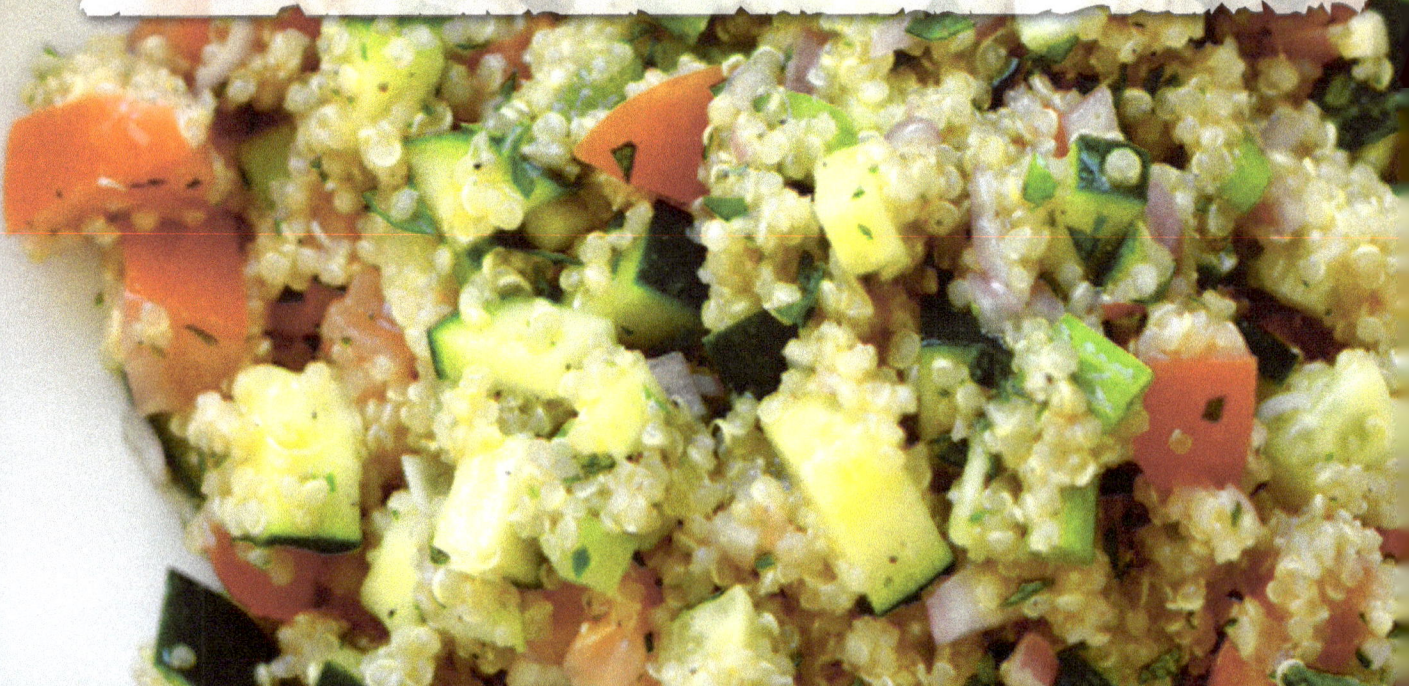

Baked Mac & Cheese

½ cup of raw cashew
1 pack firm tofu
¾ cup nutritional yeast flakes
3 cups of water
1 large red bell pepper
2 tablespoons Bragg's Amino Acids
1 teaspoon turmeric
2 tablespoons of lemon juice
3 tablespoons of olive oil
4 cloves garlic (mashed)
1 large onion (chopped)
1 tablespoon savory seasoning
1 ½ teaspoons sea salt
2 tablespoons cornstarch
6-7 cups of wholegrain macaroni (cooked)

Blend cashew nuts with water. Then add the remaining ingredients and blend until smooth. Place cooked macaroni in a casserole dish and liquid mixture and bake for 40-50 minutes.

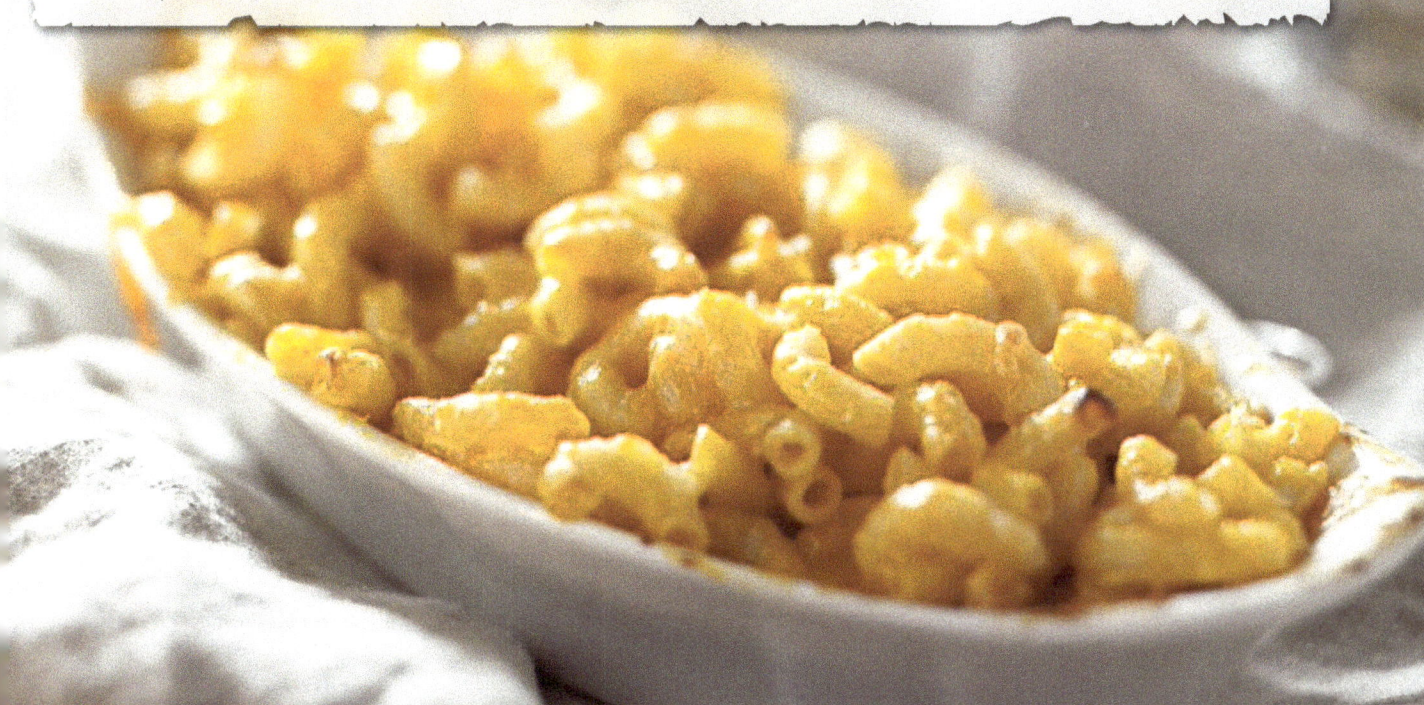

Spicy Mexican Beans

- 1 onion, finely chopped
- 2 cloves garlic
- 2 (15-ounce) cans pinto beans
- 1 teaspoon cumin
- 2 teaspoons chili powder
- 1 teaspoon cayenne powder
- 3 tablespoons water

May use as filling for tacos, burritos, or enchiladas or served as a side dish.

Place saucepan on medium heat. Sauté the onion and garlic in 2 tablespoons water for 3 minutes. Lower heat and then add the other ingredients and stir. Allow to cook for about 8 to 10 minutes. Remove from heat and allow to form a few minutes. Place beans in a food processor and pulse a few times until desired consistency is achieved.

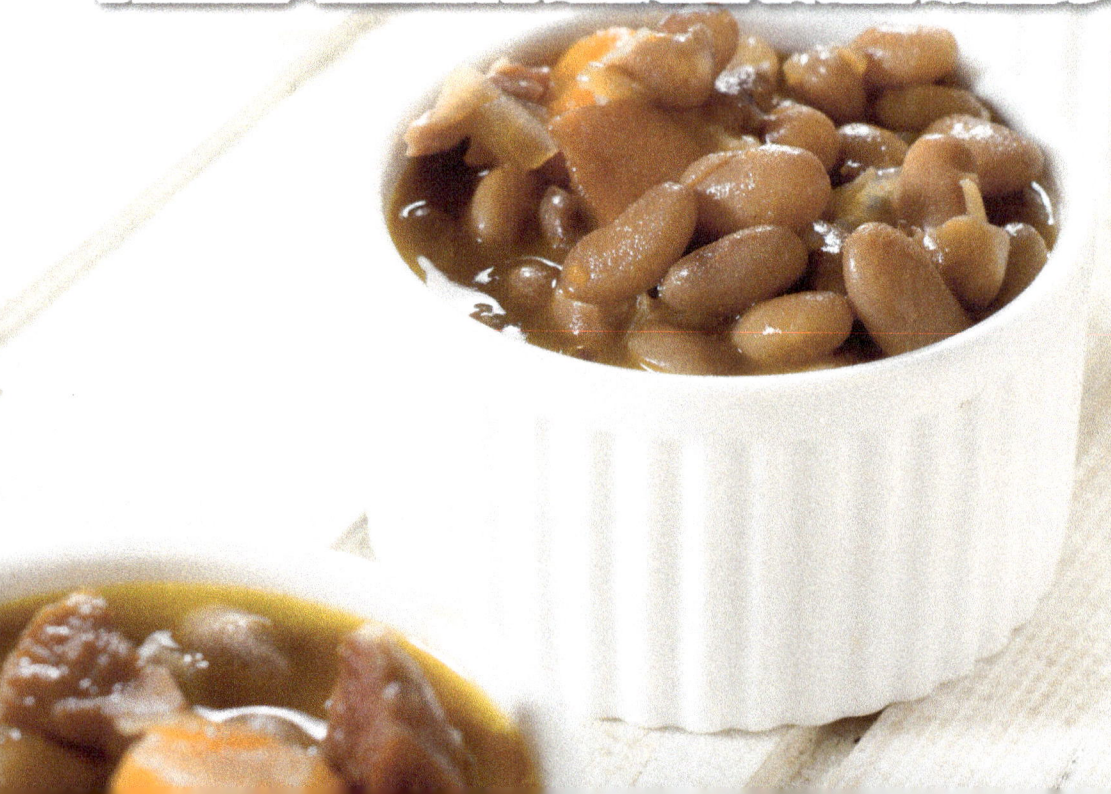

Jamaican Stewed Peas

- 2 cups dry red kidney beans
- 1 large onion, chopped
- 2 stalks scallion, mashed and chopped
- 4 cloves garlic
- 3 sprigs fresh thyme, chopped
- 2 teaspoons savory seasoning salt
- 1 (15-ounce) can coconut milk
- 2 tablespoons vegetable or olive oil

This dish is high in protein and fiber and goes well with rice, potatoes, or steamed mixed veggies. A great dish for diabetics, the high fiber content promotes blood sugar control.

Place beans in 8 cups water and soak overnight. Pour water off. Add 6 cups water and cook for about 2 hours until tender. Add all the other ingredients and allow to simmer on low-to-medium heat for 1 hour until cooked. Serve with seasoned brown rice and fresh vegetable salad.

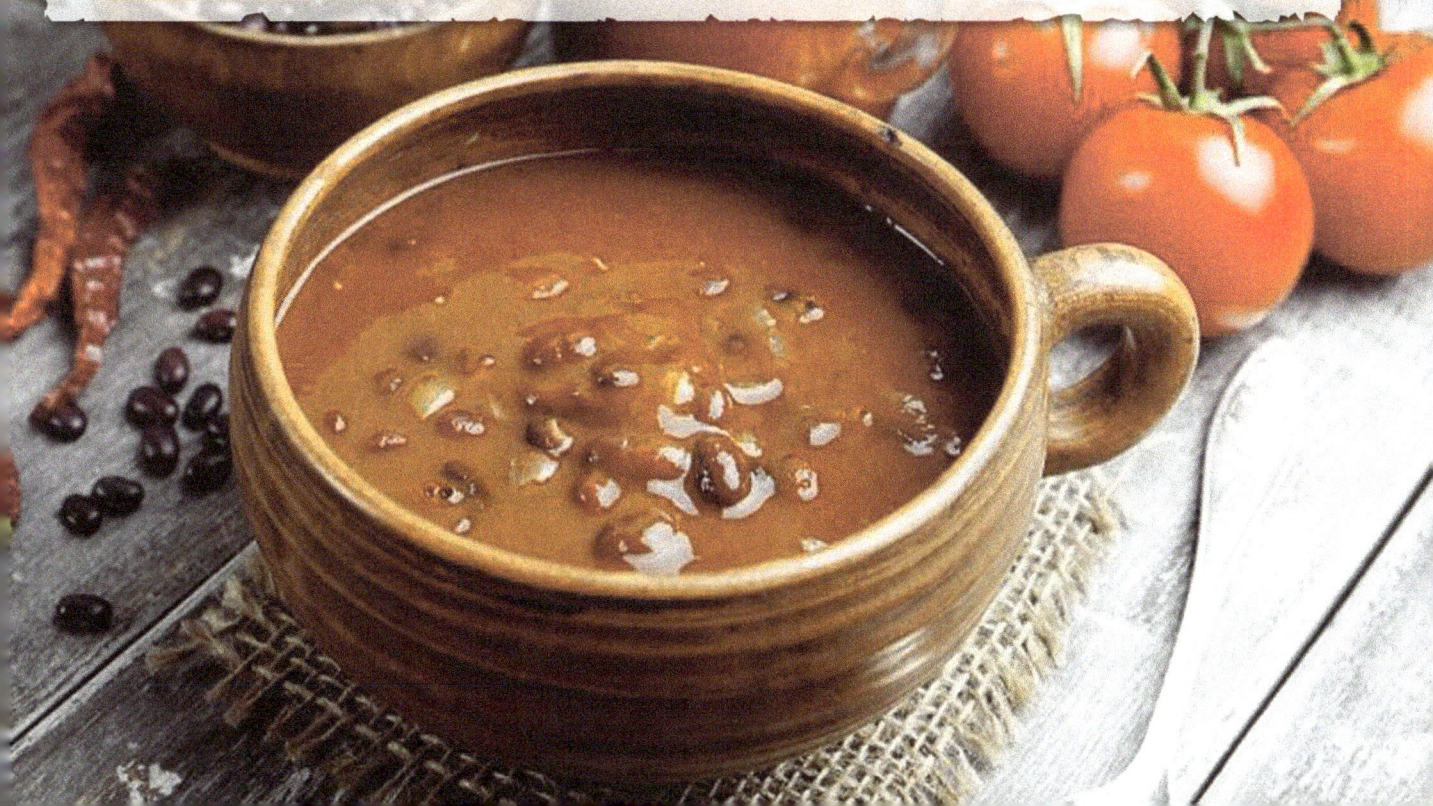

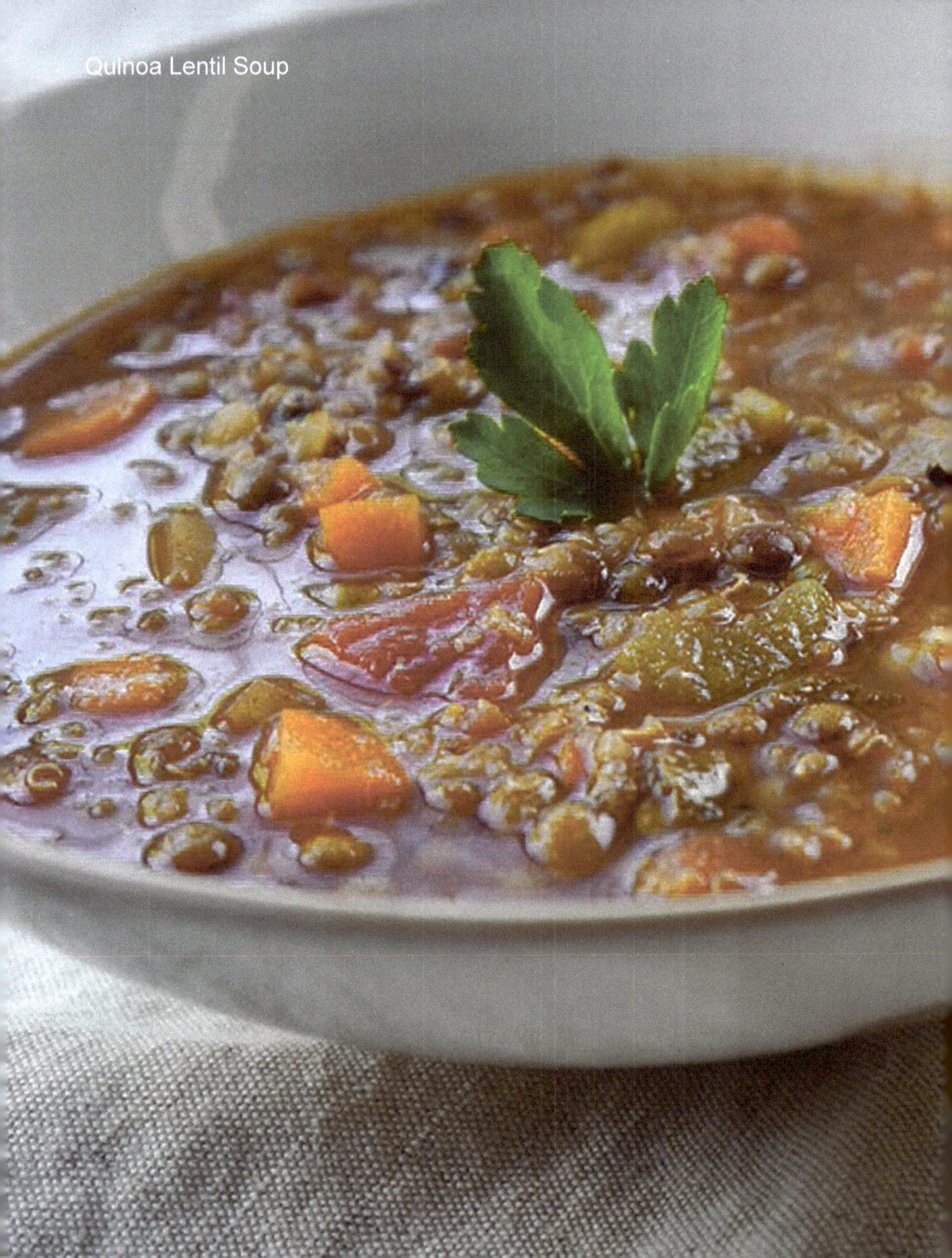
Quinoa Lentil Soup

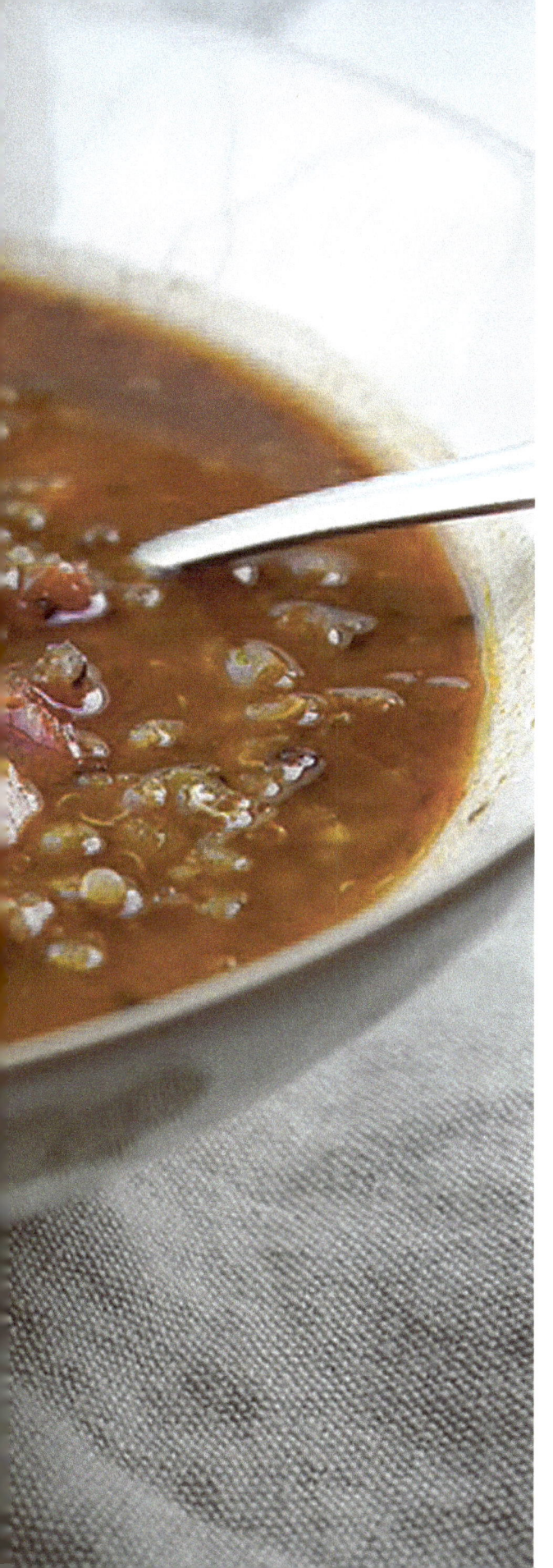

SOUPS

Corn and Potato Chowder

Quinoa Lentil Soup

Thai Coconut Curry Soup

Creamy Potato Broccoli Soup

Kale and White Bean Soup

Italian White Bean Soup

Zucchini and Cauliflower Soup

Split Pea Soup

Italian Minestrone Soup

Lentil Soup with Vegetables

Indian Lentil Soup

Jamaican Kidney Bean Soup

Spinach Kale Soup

Cream of Pumpkin Soup

Lentil Stew

Easy Green Pea Soup

Summer Soup

Cream of Broccoli Soup

Corn and Potato Chowder

3 cups water
3 cups potatoes
⅓ cups carrots, diced
1 cup green onion, chopped
1 ½ teaspoons sea salt
1 ½ teaspoons rosemary
1 teaspoon all-purpose or McKay's chicken-style seasoning
3 cups creamed or liquefied fresh corn
1 tablespoon nut butter, blended with corn
¾ cup green pepper, chopped

In a soup pot, bring all ingredients except corn to a boil. Reduce heat and simmer to almost tender. Add blended corn and nut butter. Simmer for 8 to 10 minutes more. Garnish with fresh minced parsley, chives, or dill weed. Serve with soup crackers or breadsticks.

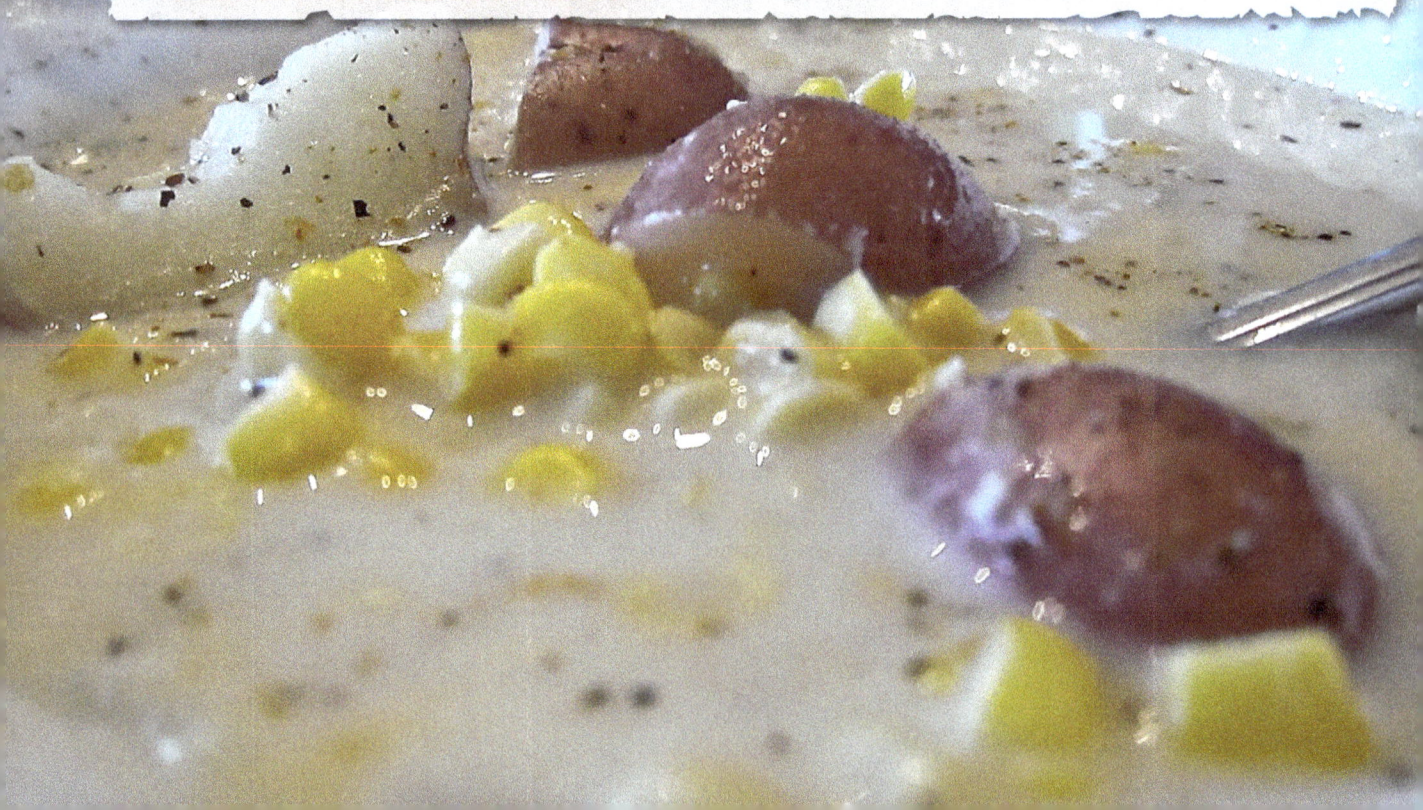

Quinoa Lentil Soup

2 cup quinoa
4 cups lentils, cooked
8-10 cups water
2 cups corn
3 cups cabbage, chopped in large pieces
2 cups carrots, thinly sliced
3 cloves garlic, mashed and then minced
2 cups onions, chopped
5 tablespoons chicken-like seasoning
1 teaspoon Mrs. Dash seasoning
4 sprigs thyme
1 cup celery, chopped

This recipe is simply delicious and healthy. It is packed with fiber, protein, vitamins, and minerals. Just an ideal dish for disease reversal!

Place all ingredients in a large pot and cook for about 30 minutes or until carrot is cooked. Serve hot.

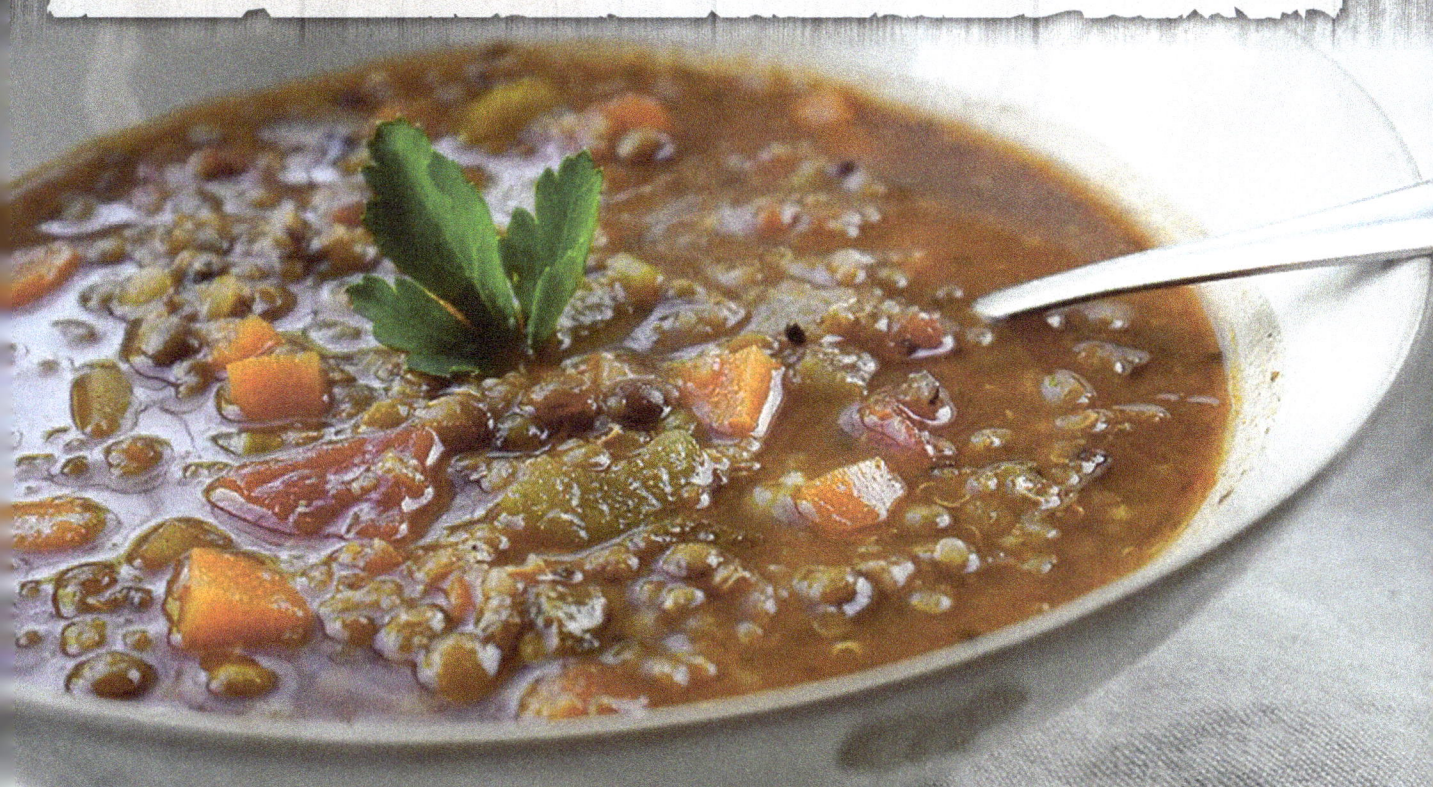

Thai Coconut Curry Soup

1 large onion, chopped
1 clove garlic, mashed and minced
1 red or orange bell pepper, chopped
¼ head cauliflower, chopped
2 red potatoes, diced
⅓ head cabbage, chopped
1 cup green beans, diced
1 cup carrot, cubed
2 cans coconut milk
4 cups water or vegetable broth
2 tablespoons curry powder
1 teaspoon turmeric
1 tablespoon olive oil
2 tablespoons McKay's chicken-style seasoning or other savory seasoning
½ teaspoon salt
1 tablespoon fresh grated ginger
½ teaspoon turmeric

Place oil in a large pot on medium heat, sauté onion and garlic for 2 minutes. Then add all vegetables. Now add the coconut milk and water or vegetable broth, and bring to a boil. Now incorporate the remaining ingredients, reduce heat, cover pot, and allow to cook until vegetables are tender. Taste and add salt, if desired. May garnish with chopped green onion.

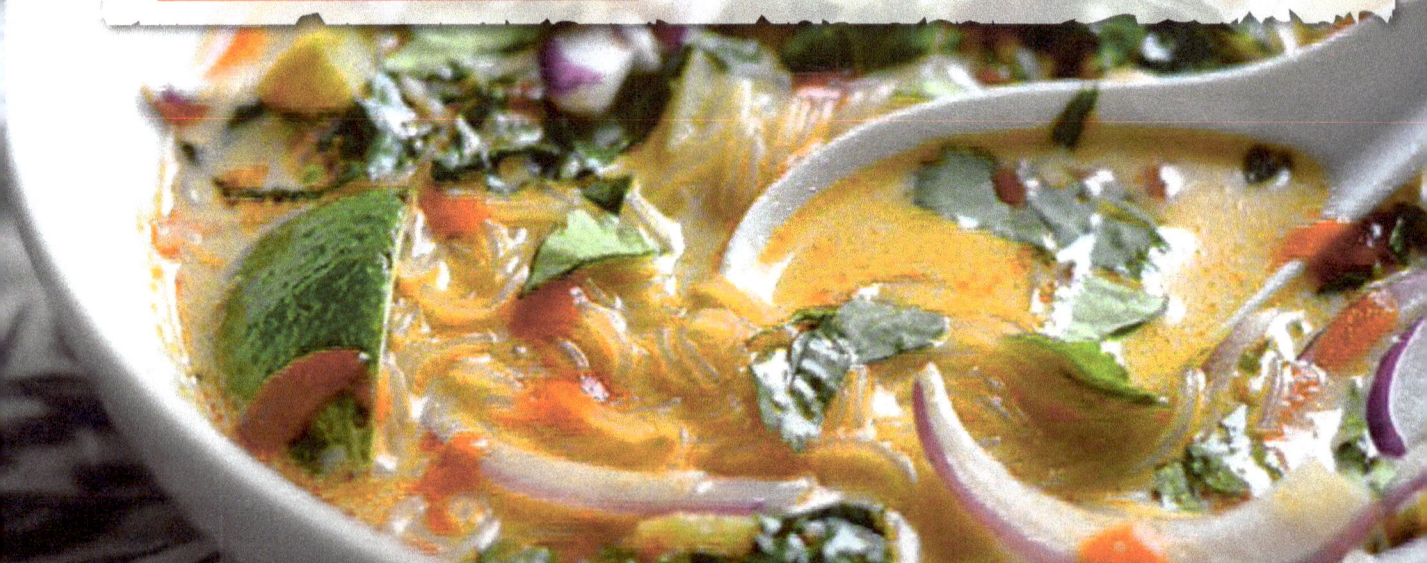

Creamy Potato Broccoli Soup

- 2 cups onion, chopped
- 7 cups of water
- 2 ½ pounds potatoes, peeled and diced
- 3 cups broccoli florets, cooked
- 1 cup raw cashews
- 2 tablespoons McKay's chicken-style seasonings
- 2 teaspoons garlic powder
- 1 teaspoon salt or to taste
- 1 tablespoon fresh thyme, chopped

In a large pot, sauté onion in small amount of water. Then add six cups of water, add potatoes, cover, and allow to cook on medium-to-high for 15 minutes. Remove outer skin from broccoli stems and add broccoli to soup. Blend cashew nuts in 1 cup of water until smooth. When potatoes are cooked, add cashew mixture to pot. Also, add all the spices and other ingredients. Stir occasionally and allow to cook for another 5 minutes. Remove ½ the soup (potatoes and broccoli) and blend. Then return this blended mixture to pot. Serve hot.

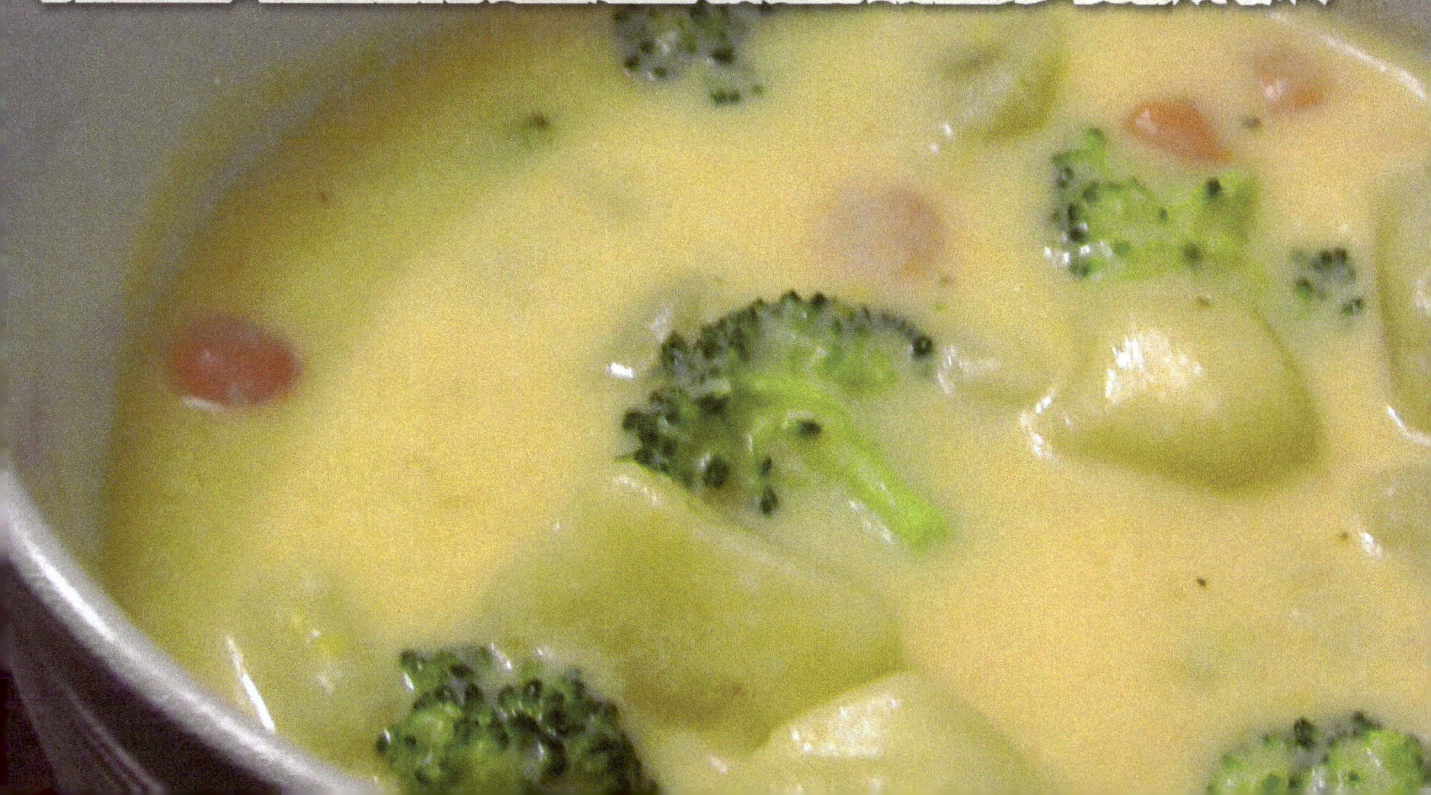

Kale and White Bean Soup

Olive oil spray
1 medium onion, diced
4 cloves garlic, minced
8-10 cups vegetable broth (low sodium)
4 cups kale, ribs removed, chopped
2 large carrots, sliced in ¼-inch coins
1 (15-ounce) can Italian-style diced tomatoes
1 teaspoon, fresh thyme, chopped
2 (15-ounce) cans white beans, drained and rinsed
1 teaspoon Italian seasoning
Salt, to taste

Soups are usually filling and supply only a few calories. This dish is packed with protein, fiber, vitamins, minerals, and antioxidants.

In a large pot, cook the onions with olive oil over medium heat for about 3 minutes. Add the garlic and cook for 2 minutes more. When the onion and garlic are translucent, add the vegetable broth, kale, tomatoes, carrots, Italian seasoning and thyme. Then cover. Cook until carrots and kale are tender, about 15 to 20 minutes. Add the white beans, salt to taste, and cook until beans are heated through. Serve hot.

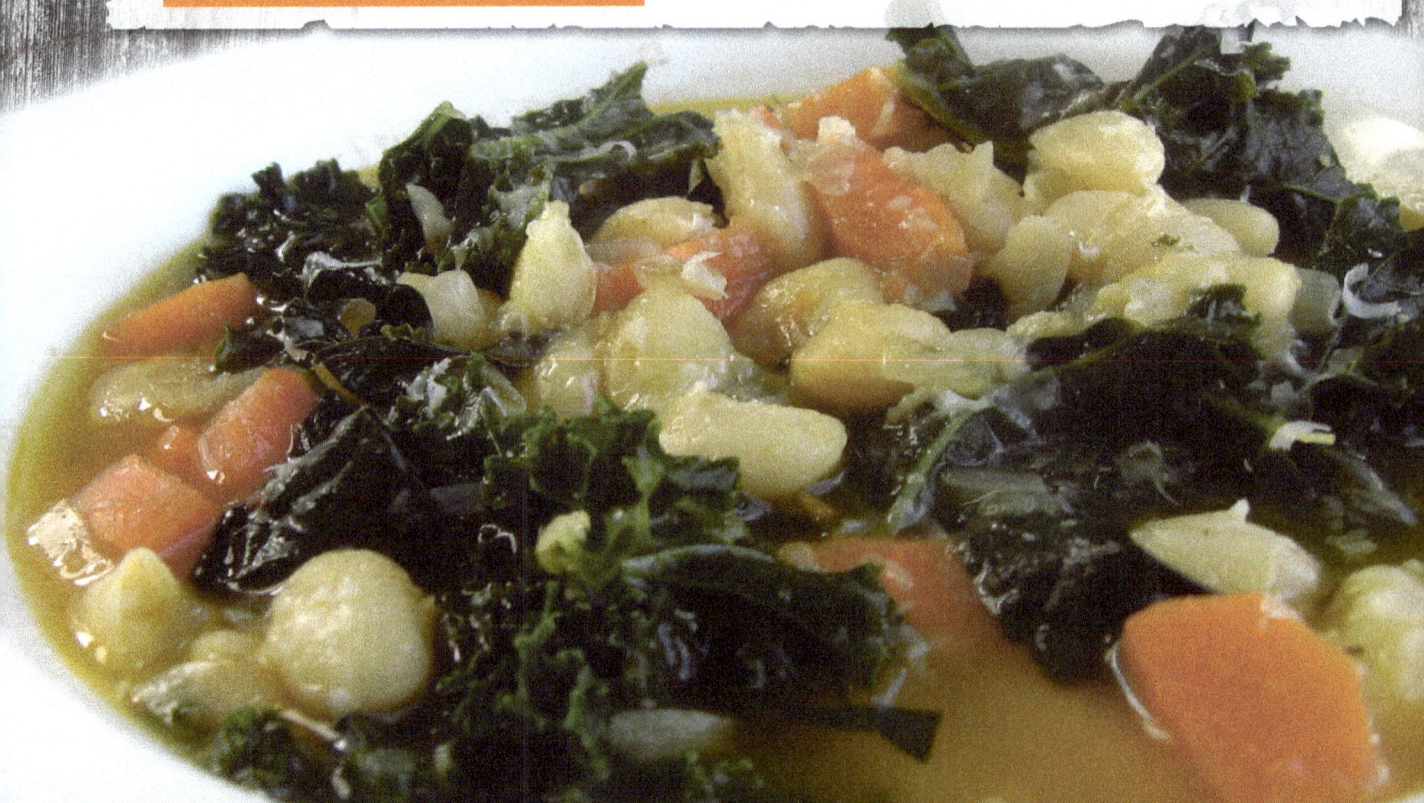

Italian White Bean Soup

1 teaspoon extra-virgin olive oil
2 cloves garlic, minced
4-6 cups water
1 (32-ounce) can great northern beans, liquid reserved
1 to 2 teaspoons McKay's chicken-style instant broth and seasoning
¾ cup of celery, chopped
¾ cup of carrots, chopped
1 teaspoon fresh thyme, chopped

This is another great recipe. Feel free to incorporate the vegetables and spices that you enjoy. Serve hot.

In a medium-sized pot, sauté the garlic in olive oil for 2 to 3 minutes. When the garlic is cooked, add the remaining ingredients and simmer for 10 minutes more.

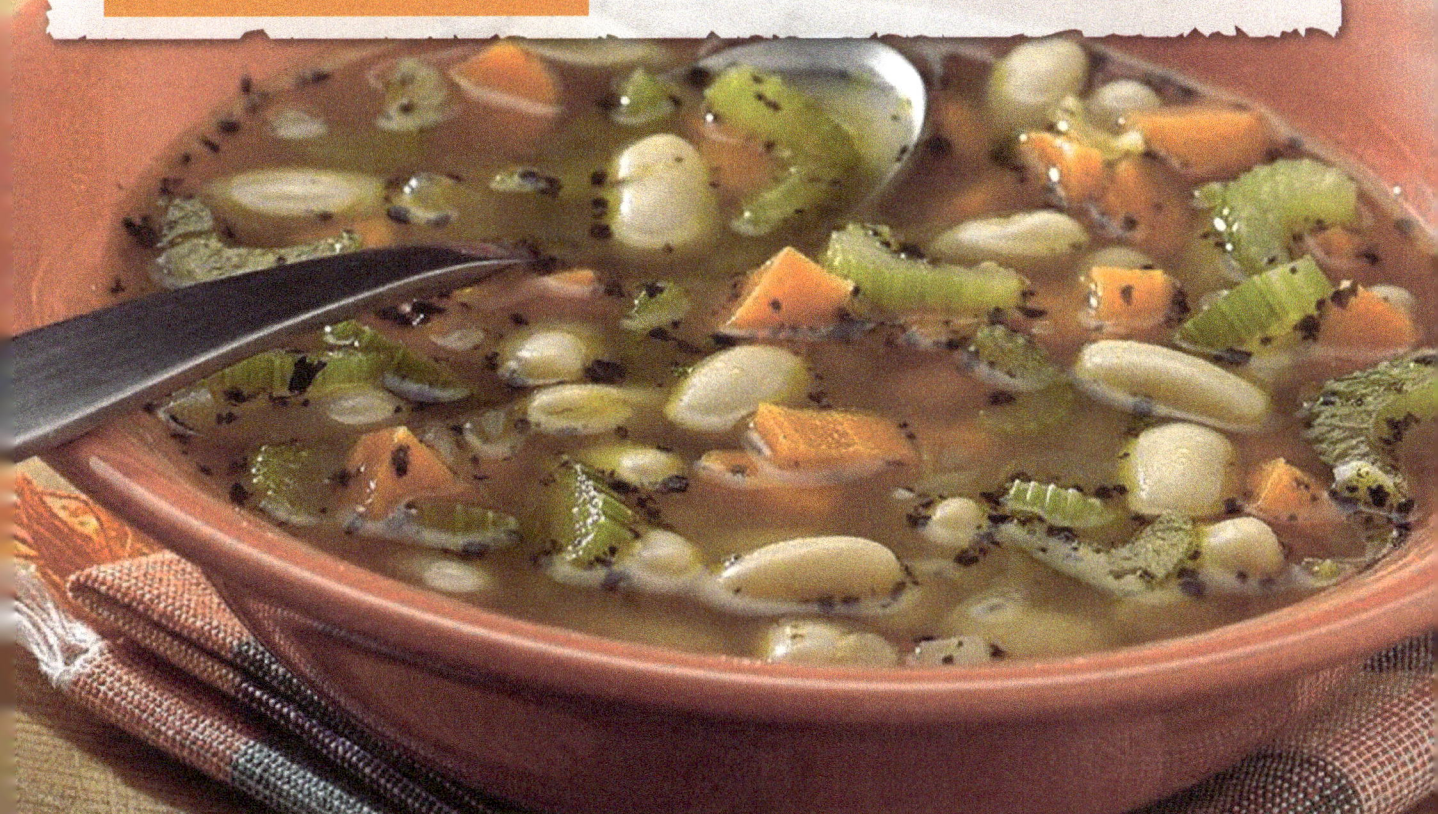

Zucchini and Cauliflower Soup

- 4 medium zucchini, chopped
- 5 cups water/vegetable broth
- 1 small onion, chopped
- 2 cloves garlic, mashed and minced
- 2 tablespoons savory seasoning
- ½ cup soy milk or ¼ cup soymilk powder
- 1 teaspoon fresh thyme, chopped
- 3 cups cauliflower florets, chopped

This is a great vegetable, and low in calories, so enjoy and keep the weight off. This dish is also great for those who want to keep their blood sugar down. These vegetables have very low glycemic index values.

Place the zucchini, cauliflower, water, onion, garlic, and thyme in a saucepan and cook over medium heat until the vegetables are tender, about 15 minutes. Add the remaining ingredients. Blend the soup in batches in a blender or food processor until smooth. Serve at once, or reheat just before serving.

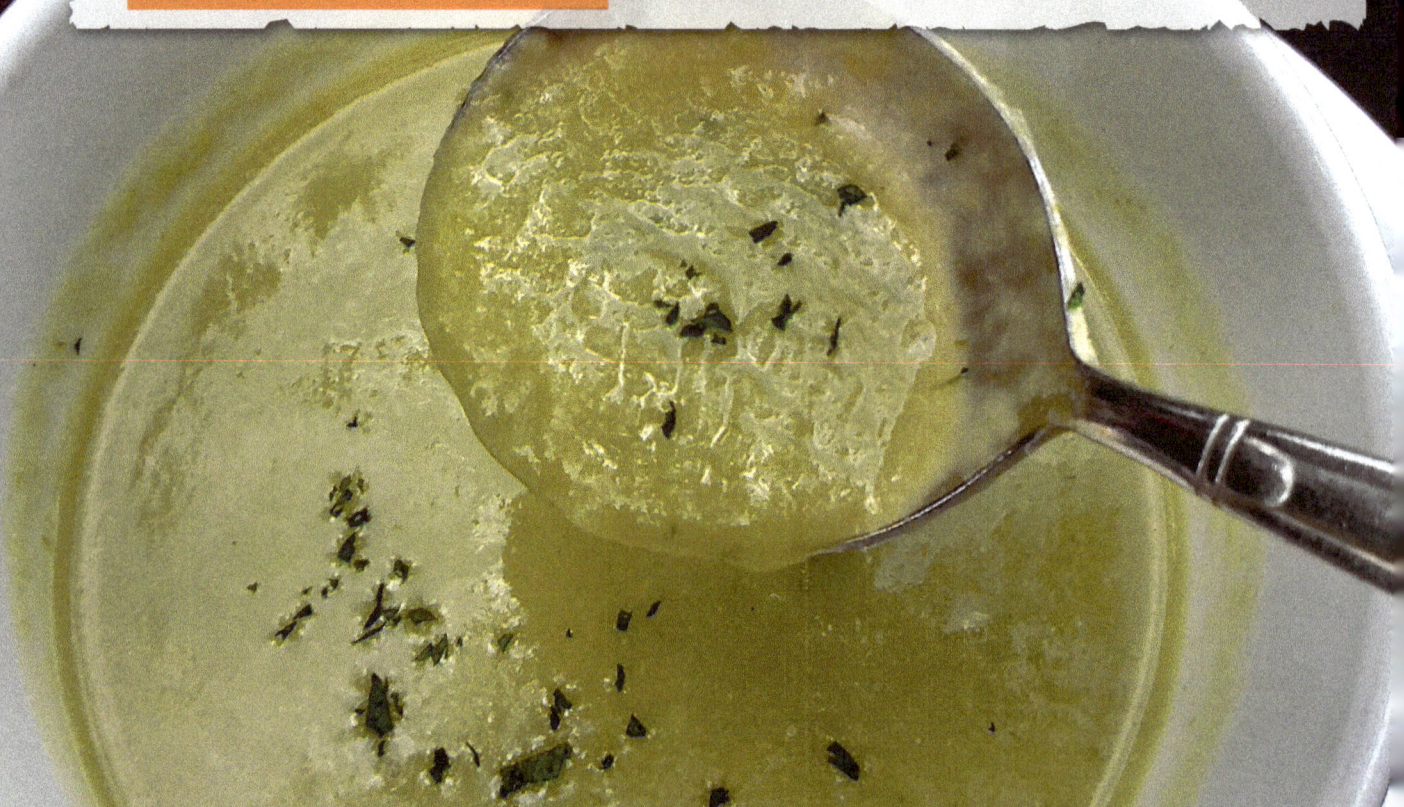

Split Pea Soup

2 cups split peas
4–5 cups water
2 tablespoons pearl barley
2 carrots, sliced or diced
2 celery stalks, diced
1 onion, chopped
½ teaspoon sea salt or to taste
2 cloves garlic, mashed then minced
3 sprigs fresh thyme
½ teaspoon Mrs. Dash
1 teaspoon savory seasoning of your choice.
2 to 3 bay leaves

This is one of my favorite soup recipes. It is high in fiber and protein.

Cover the split peas with 4 to 5 cups of water and allow to cook for 15 minutes on medium heat. Add the rest of the ingredients. Simmer until tender and creamy, stirring often. Last, add ½ tablespoon olive oil (optional). Taste and add extra spice if needed. Serve hot.

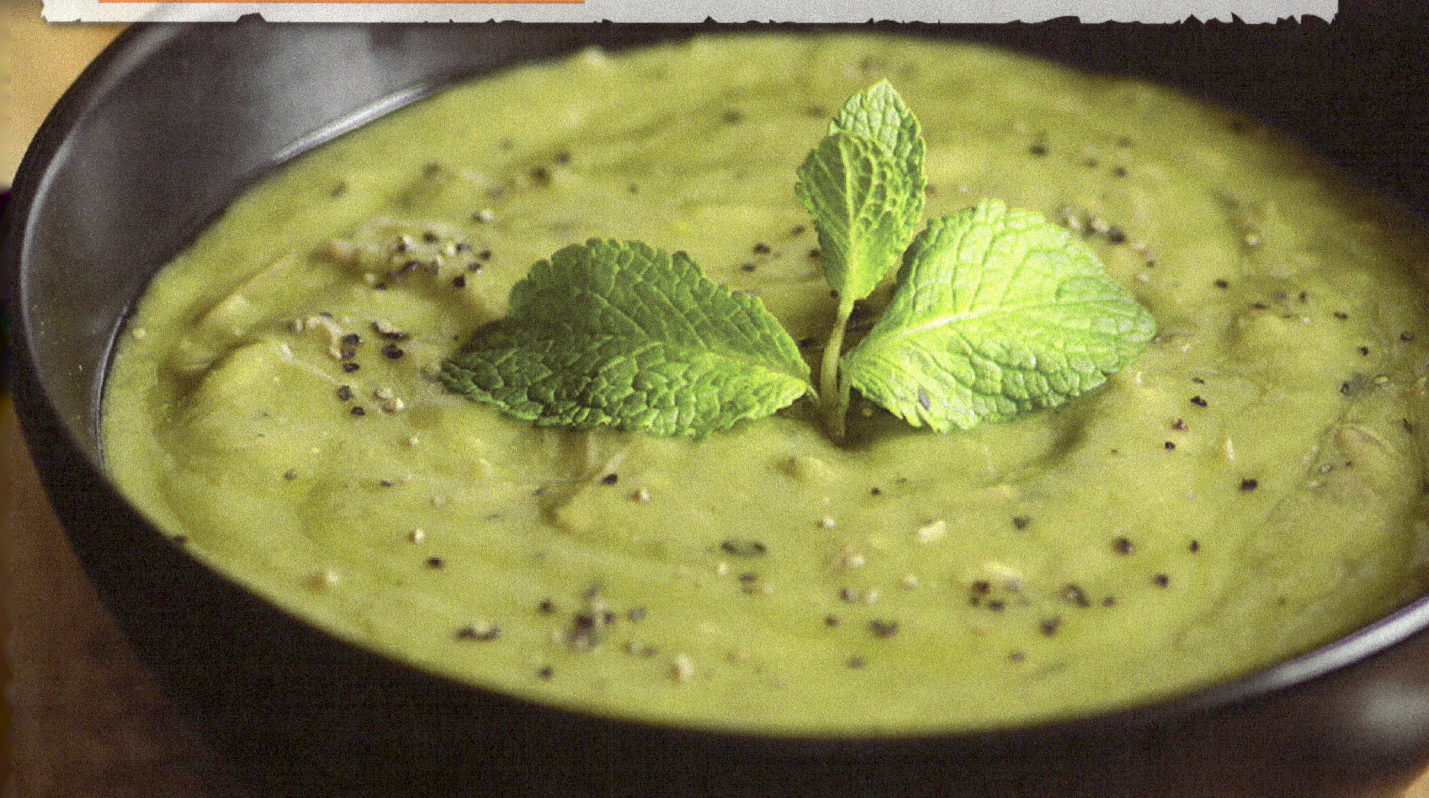

Italian Minestrone Soup

10 cups pure water, boiling
1 large onion, sliced
4 medium carrots, sliced
2 cups cabbage or fennel, chopped
2 large celery stalks, sliced or diced
1 (10 ounce) package frozen cut green beans
½ cup elbow noodles
1 (15-ounce) can kidney beans
3 garlic cloves, mashed and minced
1 (10-ounce) package frozen peas
1 (15-ounce) can kidney beans or chickpeas
1 (28-ounce) can Italian tomatoes, cut
1 bay leaf
4 sprigs of parsley
4 sprigs of sweet basil
2 teaspoons of salt

Vegetable soup is a great way to consume the recommended daily servings (5 to 6) of vegetables in one meal.

Bring water to boil. Add all ingredients except noodles. Simmer for 30 minutes, and then add noodles. Continue to simmer for 15 minutes, stirring occasionally until noodles are tender. Sprinkle vegan parmesan cheese over before serving, if desired.

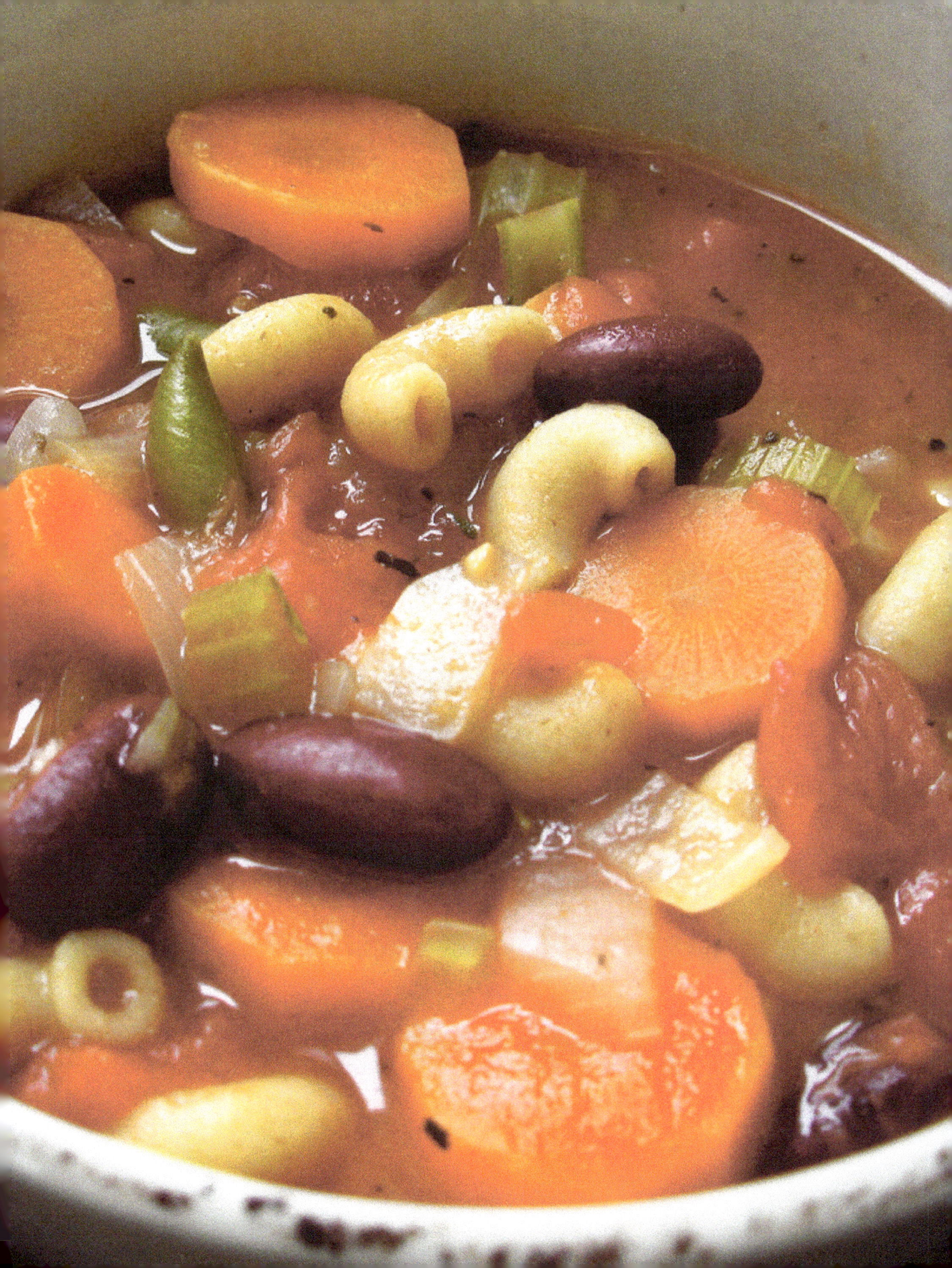

Lentil Soup with Vegetables

2 cups lentils
1 ½ cups onion, chopped
2 cup carrots, cubed
2 large potatoes, cubed
8 cups water
½ cup celery, chopped
2 tablespoons savory seasoning
4 garlic cloves, minced
1 bay leaf
2 teaspoon Italian herbs or Mrs. Dash
1 teaspoon thyme

This is a great dish to serve on a cold winter day. You can add other vegetables if desired. Serve with whole wheat bread.

In a large pot, combine the lentils and water and allow to cook for about 60 minutes until lentils are tender. Then add the vegetables and all the other ingredients. Allow to cook for another 30 minutes, stirring occasionally. Serve hot.

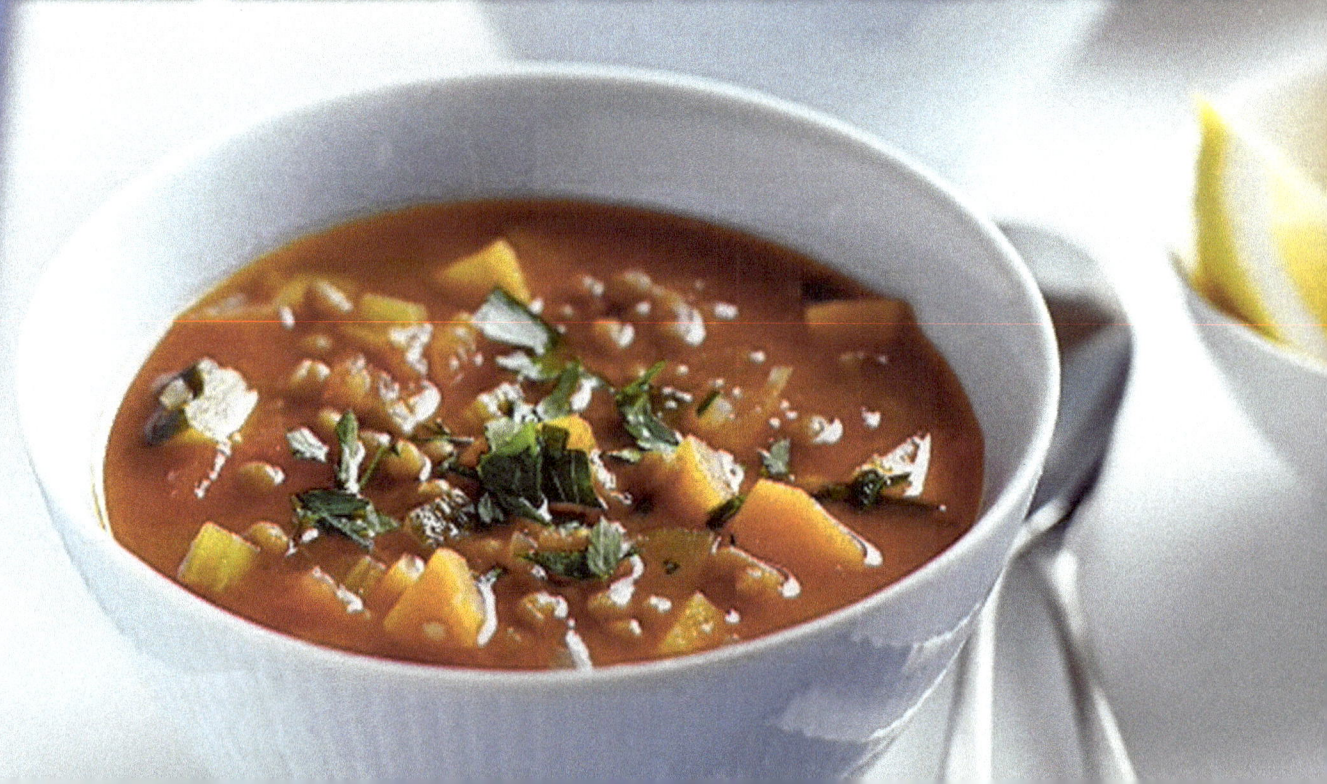

Indian Lentil Soup

1 cup dry red lentils
5 cups of water
1 garlic clove, crushed
1 tablespoon olive oil
1 cup onion, chopped
½ cup celery, thinly sliced
1 cup carrot, finely diced
15-ounce can chunky tomatoes
1 bay leaf
⅛ teaspoon chili powder
1 ½ teaspoons salt
½ cup fresh parsley, chopped

Combine lentils, water, garlic, oil, onion, celery, and carrots in a soup pot and bring to a boil. Reduce heat; cover and let simmer for 1 hour. Add the tomatoes, bay leaf, chili powder, and salt and let simmer a few more minutes. Just before serving, remove the bay leaf and add parsley.

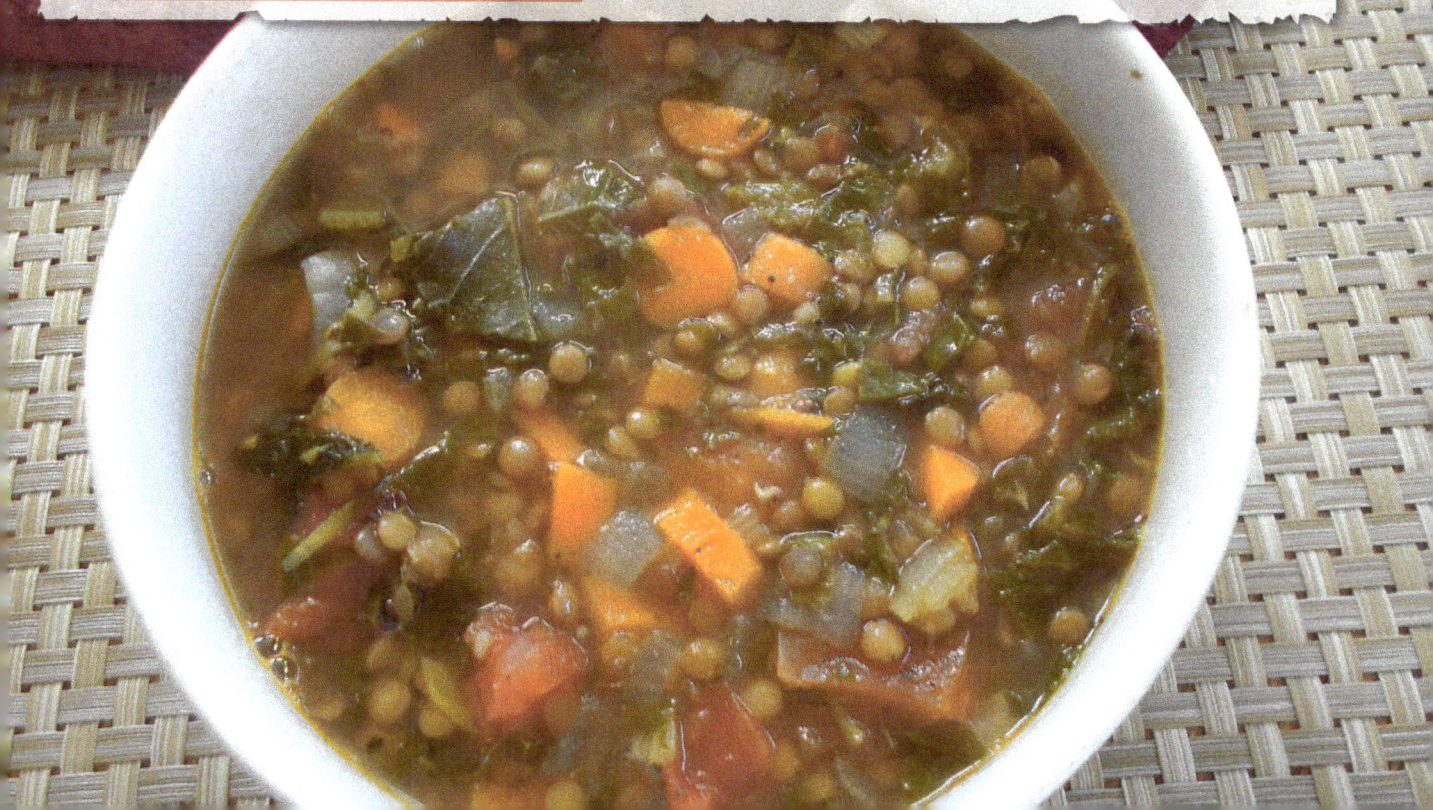

Jamaican Kidney Bean Soup

10 cups of water (better to use water from the cooked beans)
2 cups carrots, sliced
2 cups potatoes, cubed
1 cup coconut milk
4 cups red kidney beans, freshly cooked
3 garlic cloves, mashed and minced
1 cup onion, chopped
4 green onions, chopped
1 teaspoon Mrs. Dash seasoning
5 tablespoons McKay's chicken-style seasoning
4–6 sprigs fresh thyme
1 cup whole wheat elbow noodles

This dish is commonly served in the typical Jamaican home or restaurant. The elbow noodles are used to replace spinners. You can add a small slice of scotch bonnet pepper to give it the authentic Jamaican flavor.

In a large pot, place water, carrots, potatoes, and coconut milk and allow to cook for 30 minutes. Then add all the other ingredients and allow to cook an additional 20 minutes on low-to-medium heat.

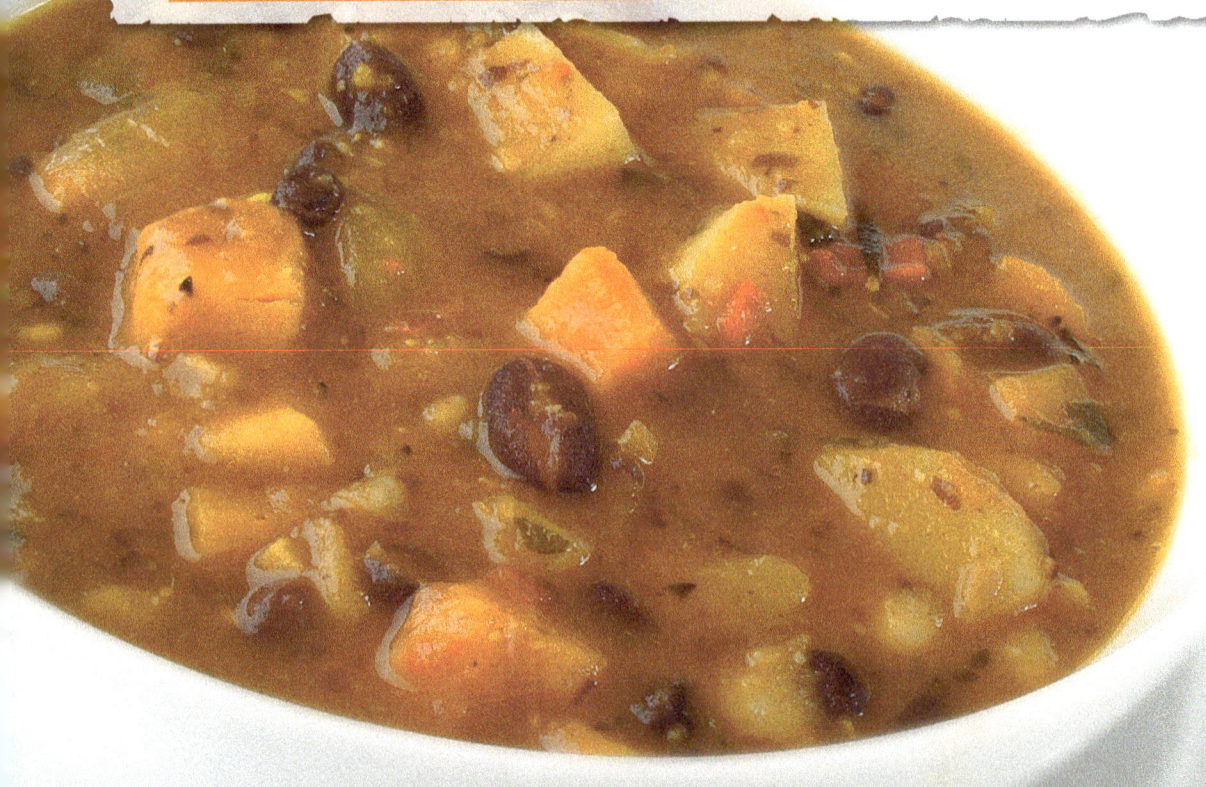

Spinach Kale Soup

½ pound yellow yam or 2 large potatoes or yucca
12 okras, cut in 1-inch cubes
8–10 cups water or vegetable stock
2 (10-ounce) packages spinach, frozen
2 cups kale, chopped
2 garlic cloves, mashed and minced
½ cup coconut milk
2 green onions, chopped
1 teaspoon Mrs. Dash seasoning
2 tablespoons beef-like seasoning
2 tablespoons Bragg's Amino Acids or soy sauce
4 sprigs of fresh thyme
Salt to taste

This dish is tasty, packed with antioxidants, and very filling. Serve hot.

Peel yellow yam, yucca, or potato and cut in 1-inch cubes and set aside. Wash okras, cut in 1-inch cubes, and set aside. In a large pot, add the water or vegetable stock and then add spinach and kale. Cook for 10 to 15 minutes. Take out the spinach and kale and blend in a food processor or blender and then set aside. Now add the okras, yam, potato, or yucca and garlic to stock and allow to cook on medium heat for 30 minutes. Now add the spinach-kale mixture, with green onion, thyme, coconut milk, and spices and allow to simmer for 15 minutes. Serve hot.

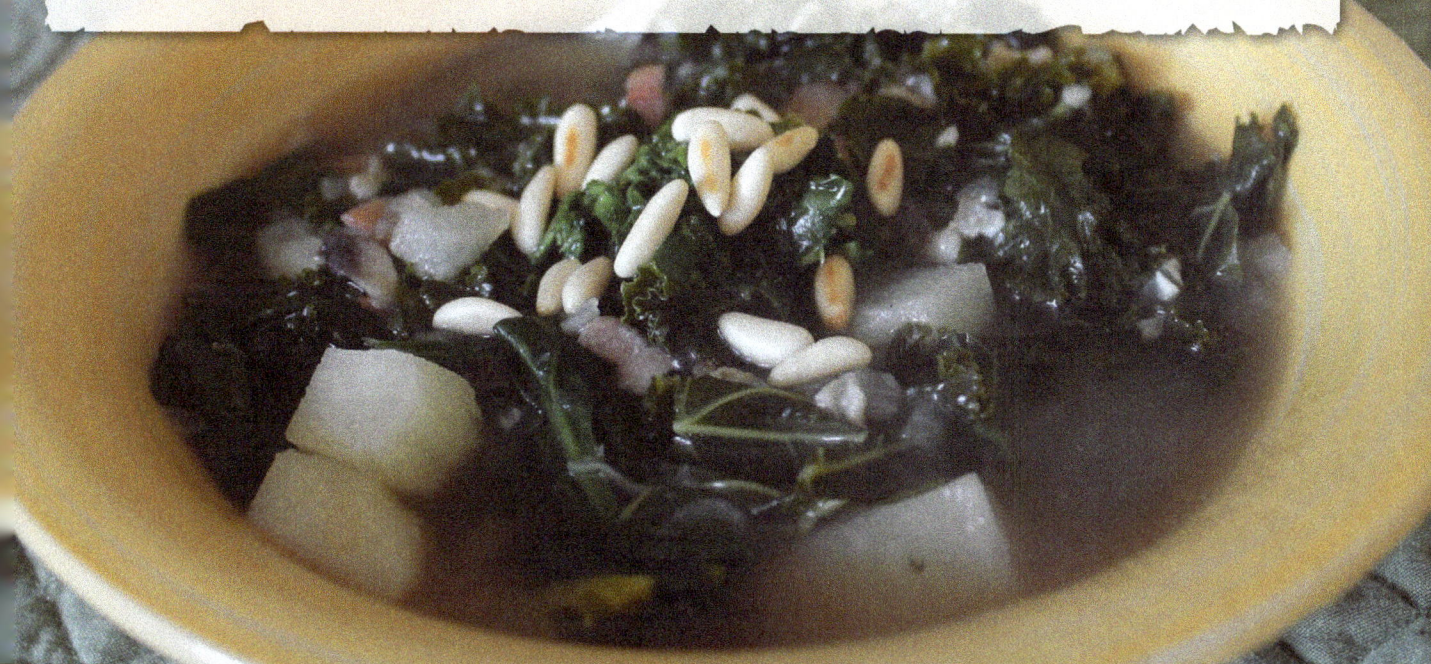

Cream of Pumpkin Soup

1 tablespoon olive oil
1 medium onion, chopped
2 cups soy milk
3 tablespoons whole-grain flour
1 teaspoon Mrs. Dash
2 cups (1 pound) boiled pureed pumpkin
Salt to taste

On low heat sauté in hot oil the onion for 2 minutes. Then add flour and Mrs. Dash. Add milk slowly and continue to stir until smooth and thickened. Combine pumpkin with mixture. Simmer for 5 minutes. Serve hot.

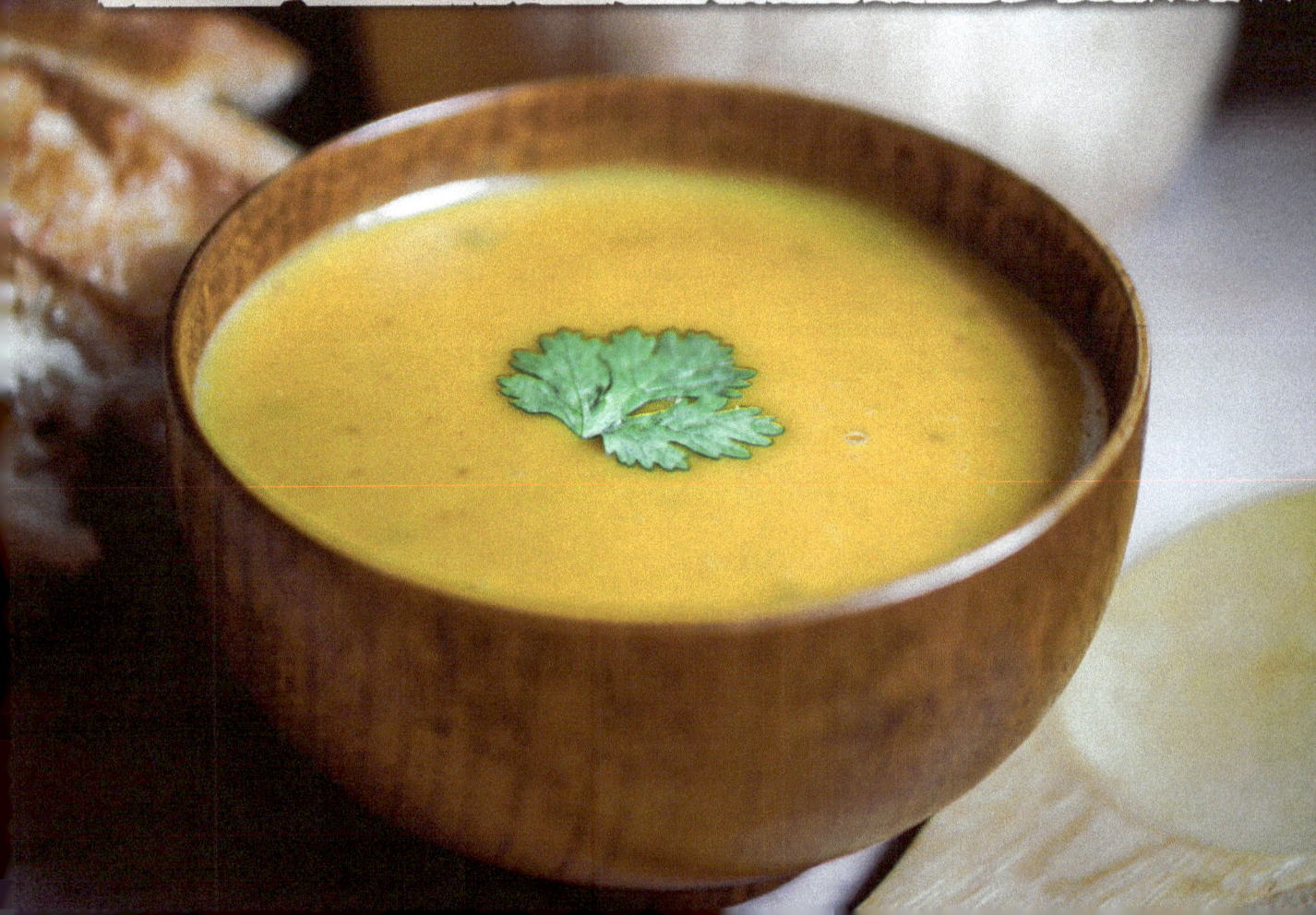

Lentil Stew

- 2 cups uncooked lentils
- 6 cups water
- 1 large onion, chopped
- 4 cloves garlic, mashed and diced
- 2 tablespoon thyme, fresh or dry
- 2 teaspoons Mrs. Dash (salt free)
- 2 teaspoon McKay's seasoning
- 2 tablespoons vegetable oil (optional)

This is a very simple but tasty dish. Serve over cooked brown rice, quinoa, or couscous or with potato, accompanied by a green salad.

Place lentils in large, deep pot. Add 6 cups water. Cook on medium heat for 90 minutes. Then add all the other ingredients. Allow to cook for another 30 minutes.

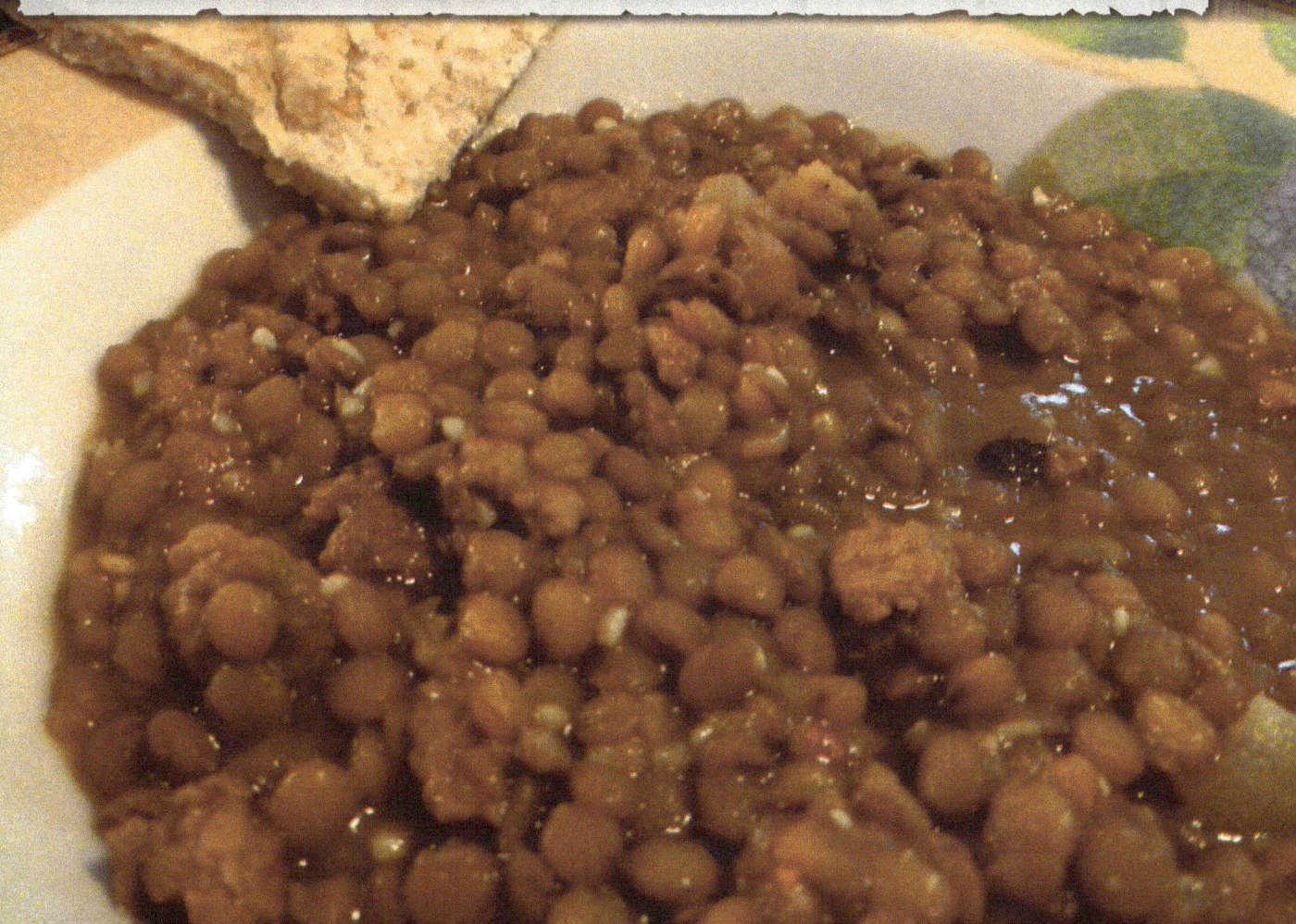

Easy Green Pea Soup

⅓ cup cashews or walnuts, raw
3 cups vegetable stock or water
1 (15-ounce) can peas
½ medium onion
1 tablespoon flour
Salt to taste

This soup is absolutely simple and easy to prepare. Serve as a side dish for lunch or dinner.

Blend nuts in vegetable stock until smooth. Then add other ingredients continue to blend until smooth. Heat mixture just enough until flour is cooked. Then serve hot.

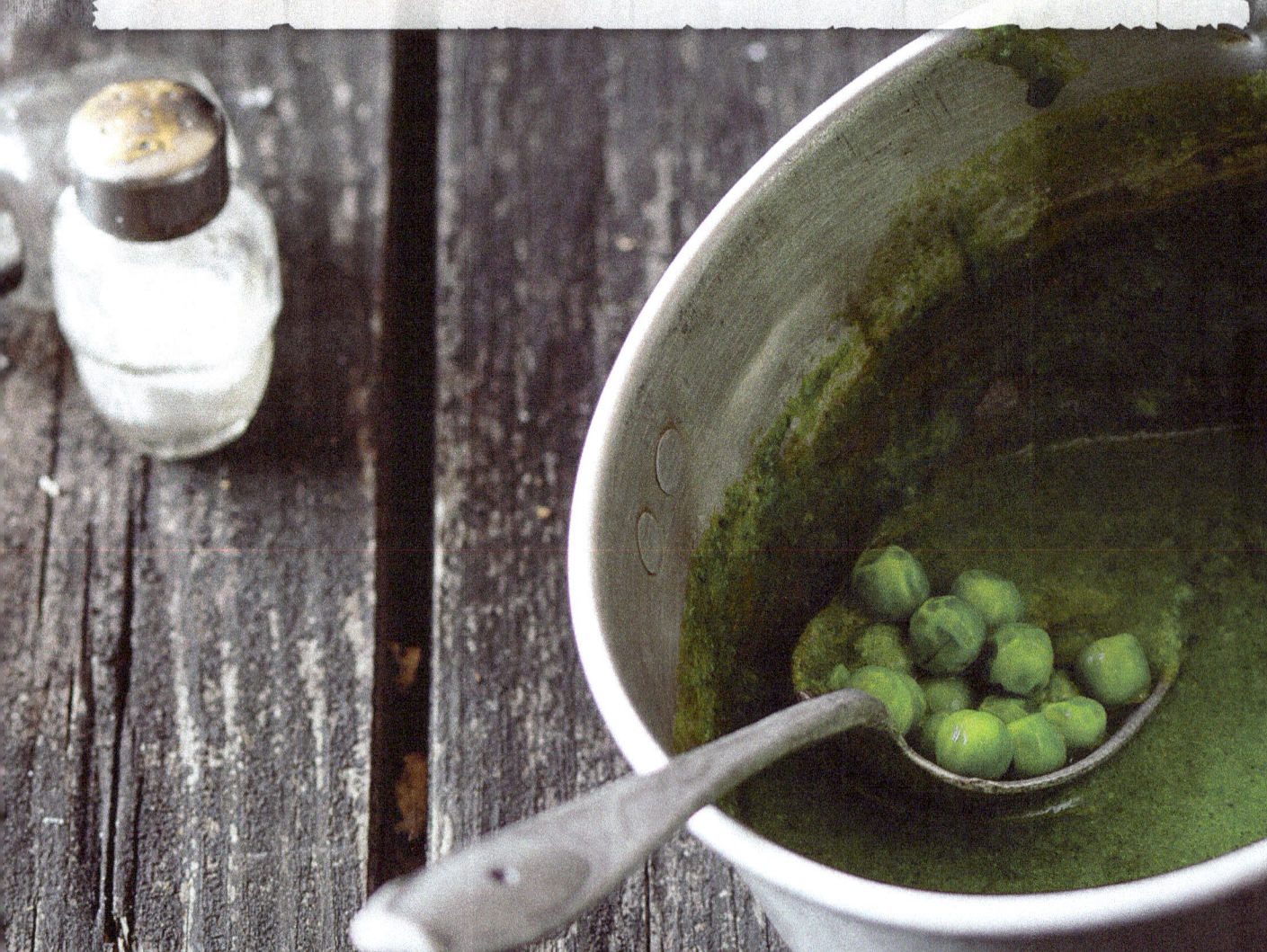

Summer Soup

- 2 cups water
- 1 pound tomatoes, ripe
- ½ medium cucumber
- ¼ medium onion
- 2 stalks celery
- ½ teaspoon salt
- ⅛ cup cashews, raw
- Pinch of cayenne pepper

Here is a cold soup you may relish on a hot summer day or evening. It is absolutely delicious and ideal for those who want to maintain a healthy weight and normal blood sugar.

Wash vegetables and then blend all ingredients and water in a high-speed blender. Chill in refrigerator before serving. Serves 4.

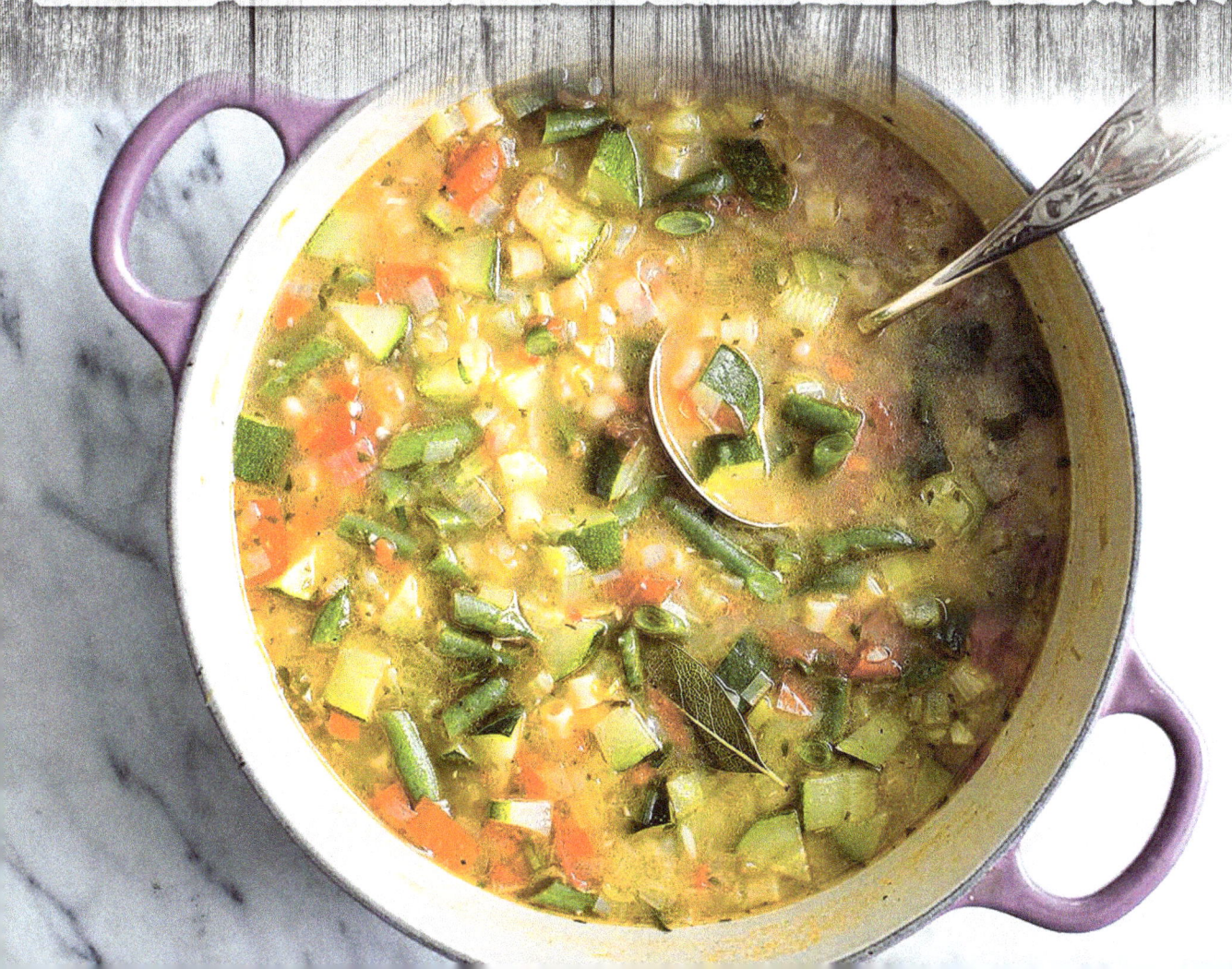

Cream of Broccoli Soup

2 scallion (green onions) stalks, washed and sliced
2 cloves garlic, minced
1 ½ cup vegetable stock
4 medium red potatoes, peeled and chopped
2 cups almond milk
2 medium stalks of broccoli, one chopped and one cut into small florets
½ teaspoon fresh thyme
1 teaspoon oregano
Freshly ground pepper to taste
Pinch of nutmeg

Sauté the leek and garlic in ⅓ cup of stock for 5 minutes. Add the remaining ingredients except the broccoli florets. Cover and cook over medium heat for 40 minutes or until potatoes are tender. Blend the mixture, in batches, in a blender or food processor until smooth and creamy. Return to the pan and keep warm. Meanwhile, place the broccoli florets in another saucepan with water to cover. Cover and cook over medium heat for 5 minutes. Drain. Add to the soup mixture. Season with freshly ground pepper to taste.

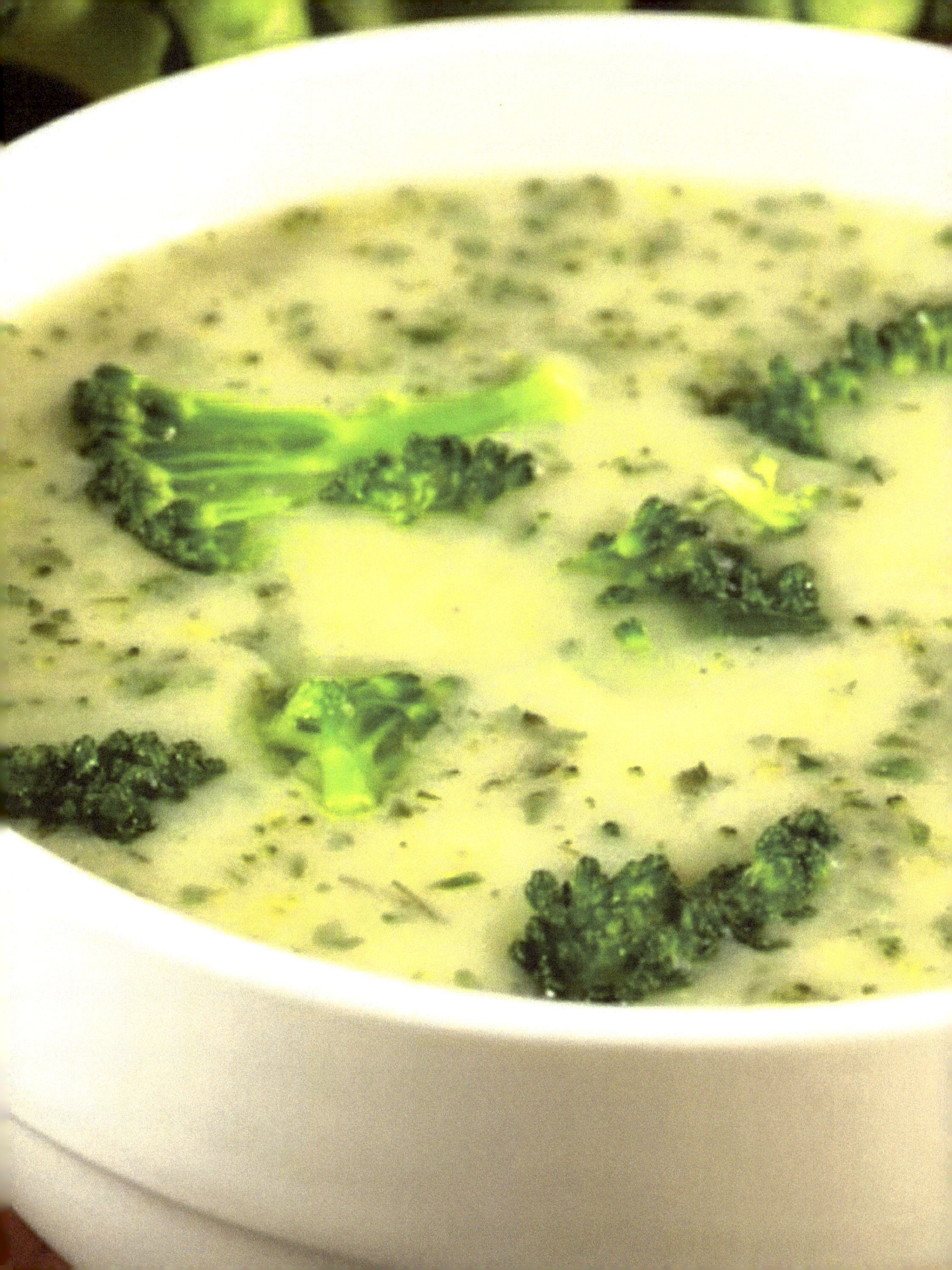

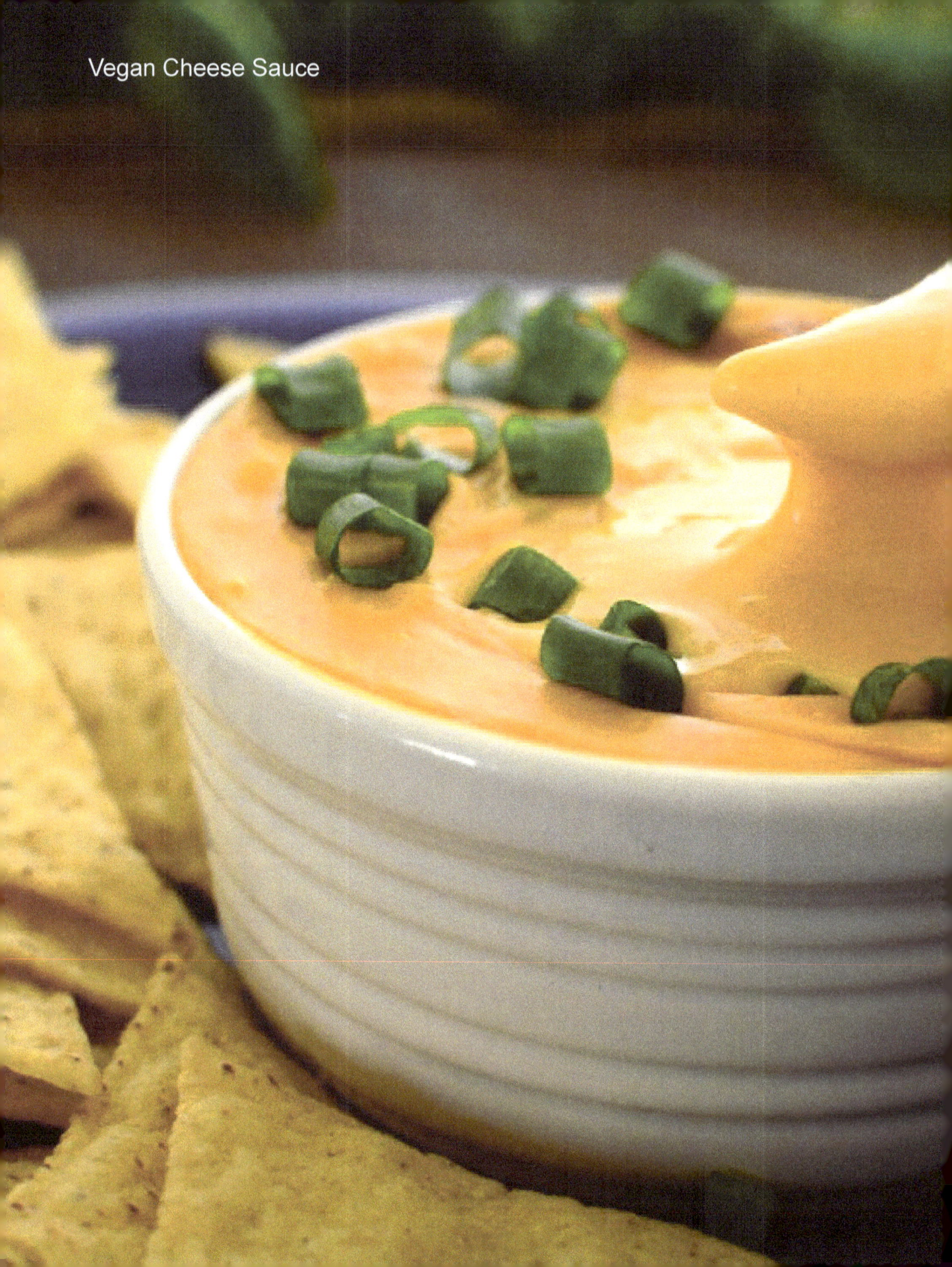
Vegan Cheese Sauce

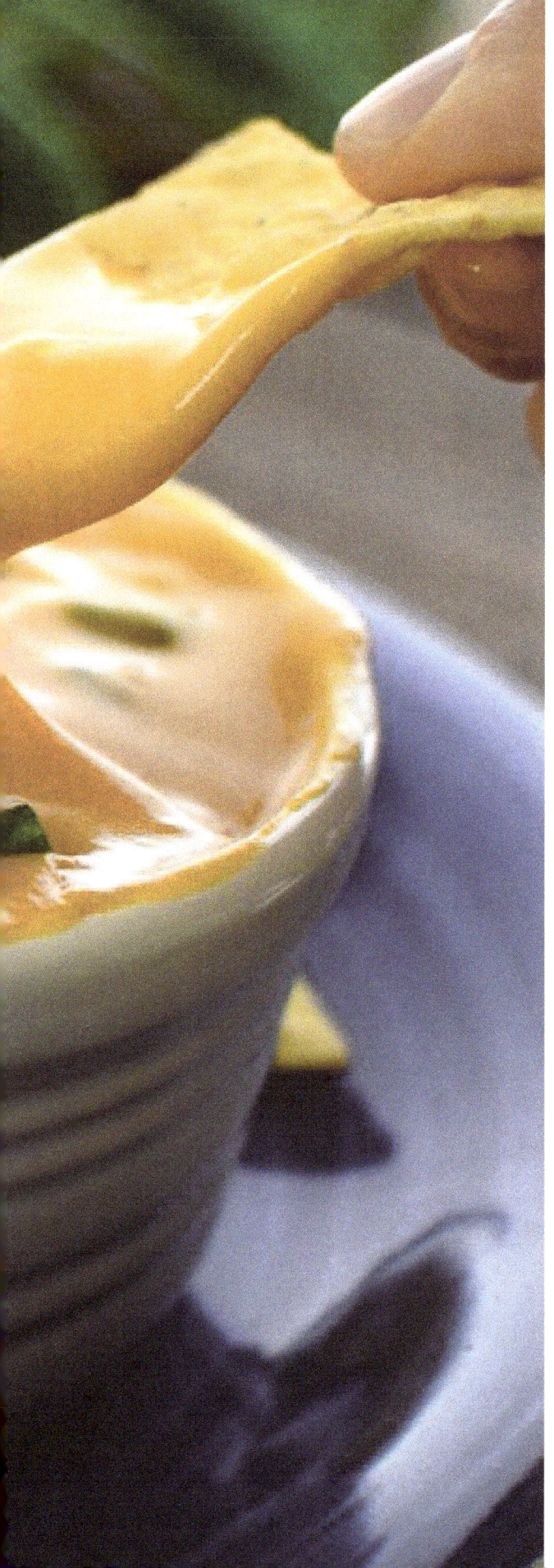

SAUCES, DIPS AND GRAVIES

"Meatball" Tomato Sauce

Alfredo Sauce

Lima Bean Cheese Sauce

Tofu Cheese Sauce

Vegan Cheese Sauce

Cashew Cheese Sauce

Hummus

Mango Avocado Salsa

Guacamole

Chickpea Spread or Dip

Mushroom Gravy

Country-Style Brown Gravy

"Meatball" Tomato Sauce

1 ½ cup tomato puree
½ cup onion, chopped
1 clove garlic, mashed and diced
2 teaspoon sweet paprika
1 ½ teaspoon thyme, dried
1 ½ cup water
2 tablespoons fresh basil, chopped
Salt to taste

Place 2 tablespoons of water in a nonstick pan on low-to-medium heat. Add onion and garlic. Sauté for 2 to 3 minutes and add the other ingredients. Continue to sauté for another 3 minutes. Then add meatballs. Enjoy with whole-grain spaghetti. (Refer to "Meatball" recipe on page 99.)

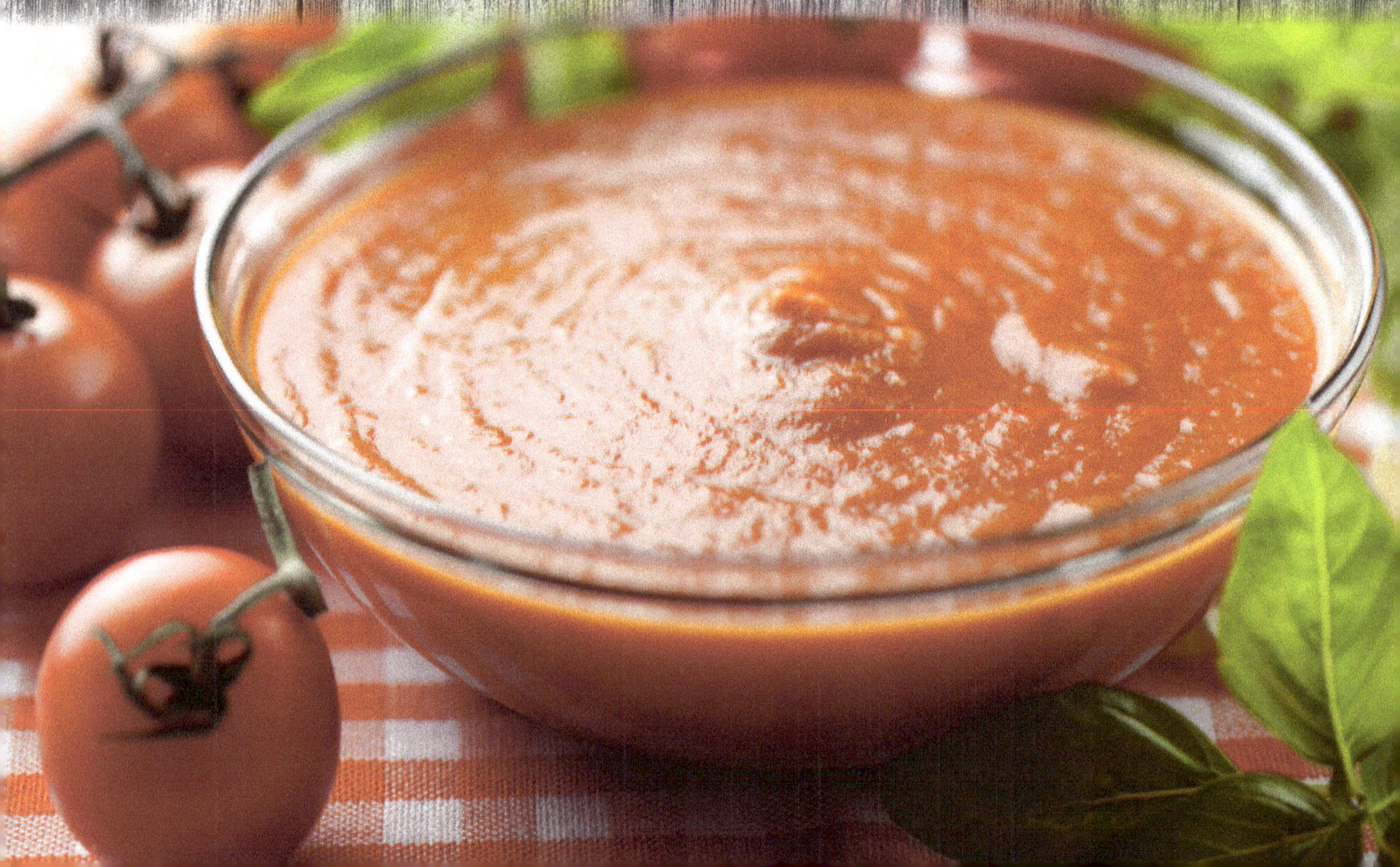

Alfredo Sauce

- ½ cup cashew nuts
- 1 ¾ cups water
- 1 tablespoon of cornstarch
- 1 teaspoon garlic powder
- 1 teaspoon onion powder
- 1 tablespoon chicken-like seasoning
- ½ teaspoon oregano

This is a great nondairy option. Feel free to add other herbs that you like.

Place all ingredients into a blender. Blend until smooth. Place in a medium-sized pot. Simmer on low heat, and stir continuously until thickened and smooth. Add salt to taste. Pour over pasta or enjoy with baked potato.

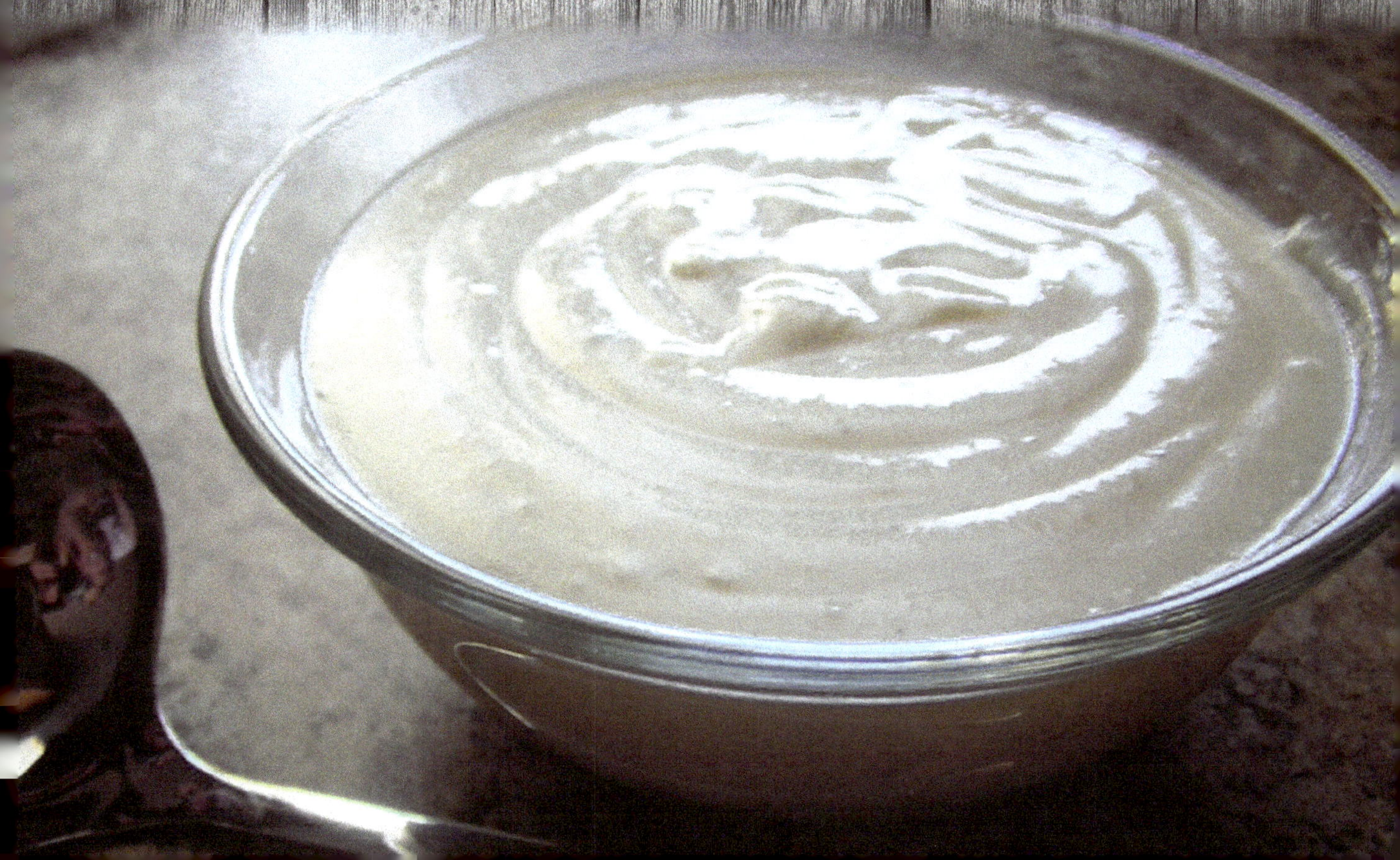

Lima Bean Cheese Sauce

15 ounces lima beans (cooked)
¾ cup nutritional yeast flakes
¾ cup soy milk (plain)
2 teaspoons onion powder
2 teaspoon of garlic powder
½ teaspoon paprika
½ teaspoon turmeric
1 teaspoon salt (or to taste)
1 small onion, chopped
1 medium red bell pepper
1 tablespoon vegetable oil

This is a great cheese sauce for those who might have a nut allergy. It has a good amount of fiber and protein.

Place all the ingredients except the onion and bell pepper in blender and blend until smooth. Sauté onion and bell pepper in oil on low heat for 2 to 3 minutes. Then add to pot and simmer on low heat for 7 to 10 minutes.

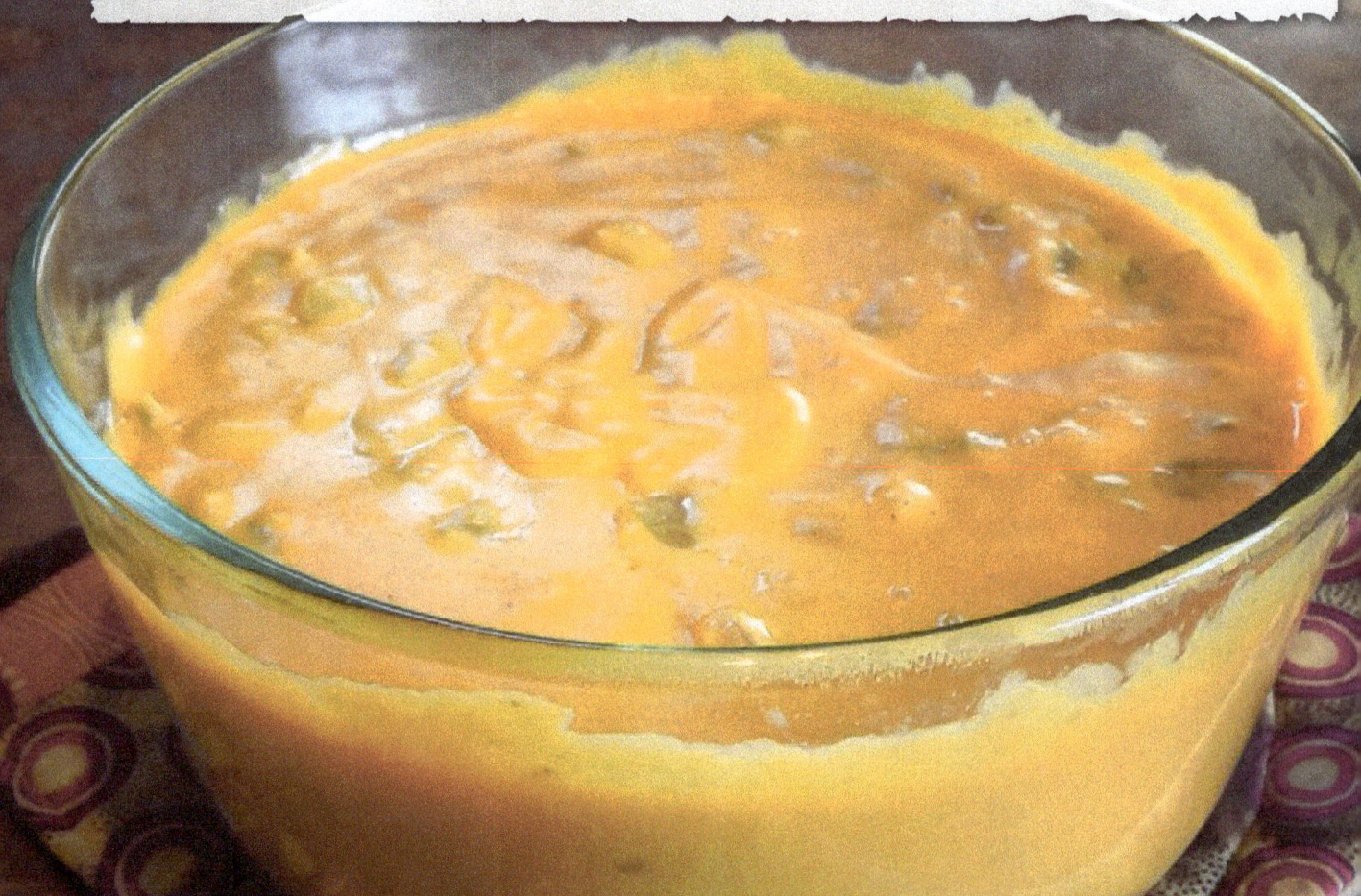

Tofu Cheese Sauce

- ½ cup of raw cashew
- 1 pack firm tofu
- ¾ cup nutritional yeast flakes
- 3 cups of water
- 1 large red bell pepper
- 2 tablespoon Bragg's Amino Acids
- 1 teaspoon turmeric
- 2 cloves garlic, mashed
- 1 large onion, chopped
- 1 tablespoon savory seasoning
- 1 ½ teaspoon salt
- 2 tablespoon cornstarch

This sauce can be used as a dip for raw vegetables but is also excellent for macaroni and cheese.

Blend cashew nuts with water. Then add the remaining ingredients and blend until smooth. Simmer on low heat for 7 to 10 minutes. Stir continuously until thickened.

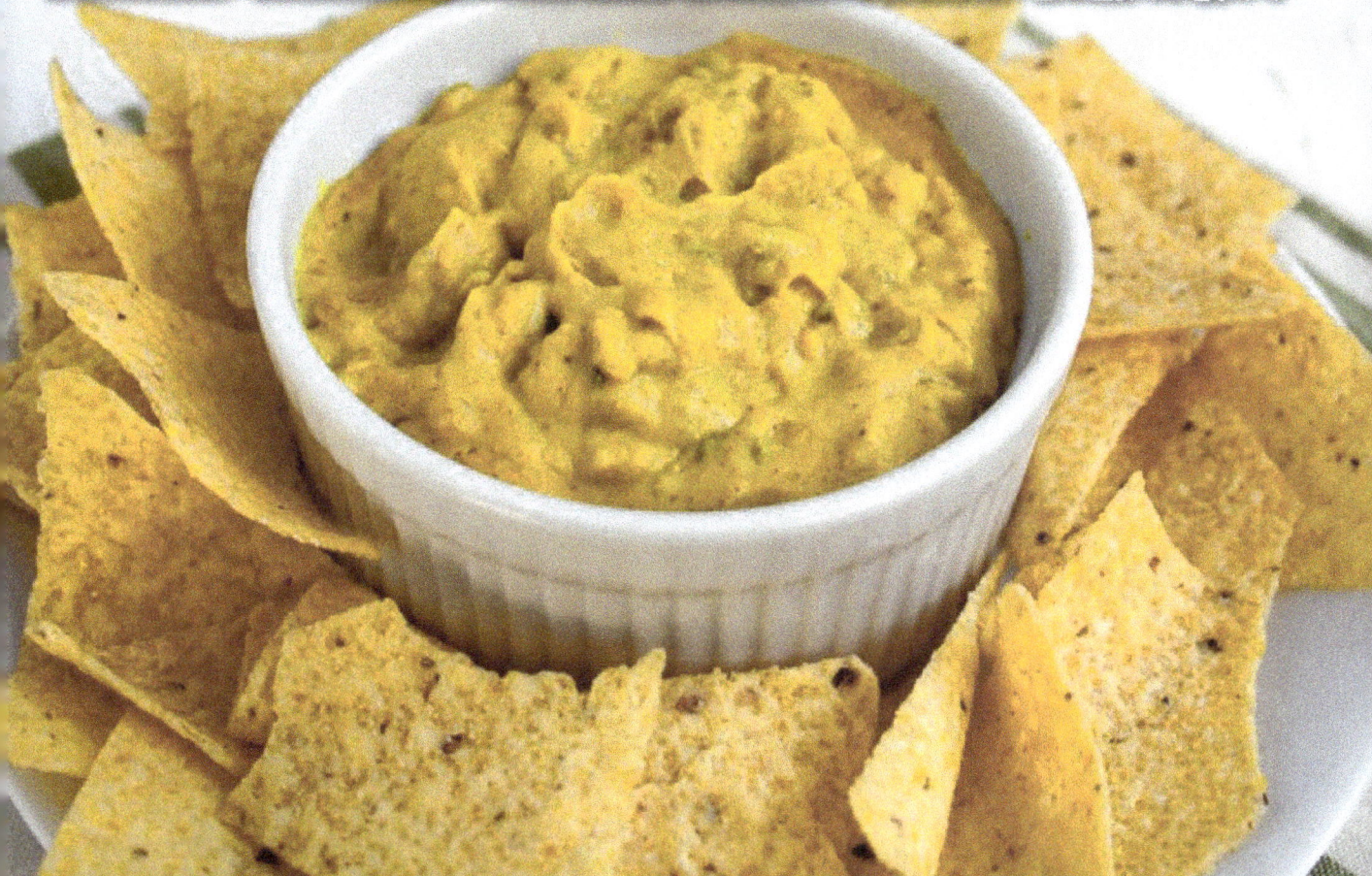

Vegan Cheese Sauce

- ¾ cup diced cooked carrot
- 1 ½ cups diced cooked potatoes
- ½ cup nutritional yeast flakes
- ½ teaspoon paprika
- 1 teaspoon garlic powder
- 2 teaspoon onion powder
- 1 cup water
- 1 small onion, cooked
- 1 teaspoon salt

This sauce can be served over pasta or poured over broccoli.

Blend all ingredients until smooth, then serve over broccoli or pasta.

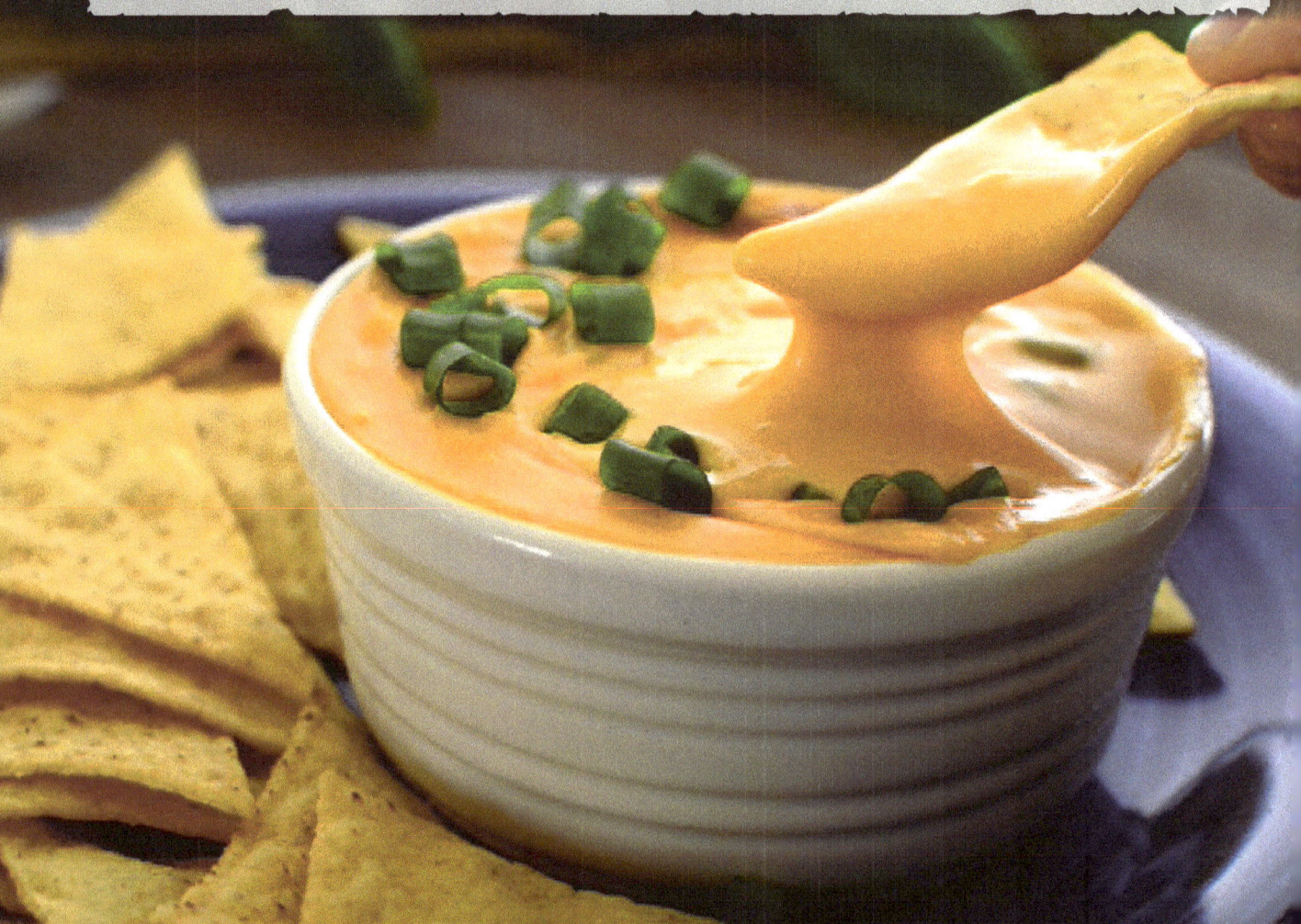

Cashew Cheese Sauce

- 2 cups water
- ½ cup clean, raw cashews
- 2-ounce jar pimientos, sliced or diced
- 3 tablespoons food yeast flakes
- 2 tablespoons cornstarch
- 2 tablespoons fresh lemon juice
- 1 ½ teaspoon salt
- 1 teaspoon onion flakes or powder
- 1 teaspoon garlic powder

This delicious cheese sauce is cholesterol free and is full of good, healthy fats. This can be used as a spread or for macaroni and cheese. It is also great with steamed broccoli.

Blend cashews in about ½ cup of water until very smooth. Add remaining water and other ingredients and continue blending until smooth. Simmer in a heavy saucepan until thickened, stirring constantly (5 to 6 min). Yields 2 ½ cups or 10 servings.

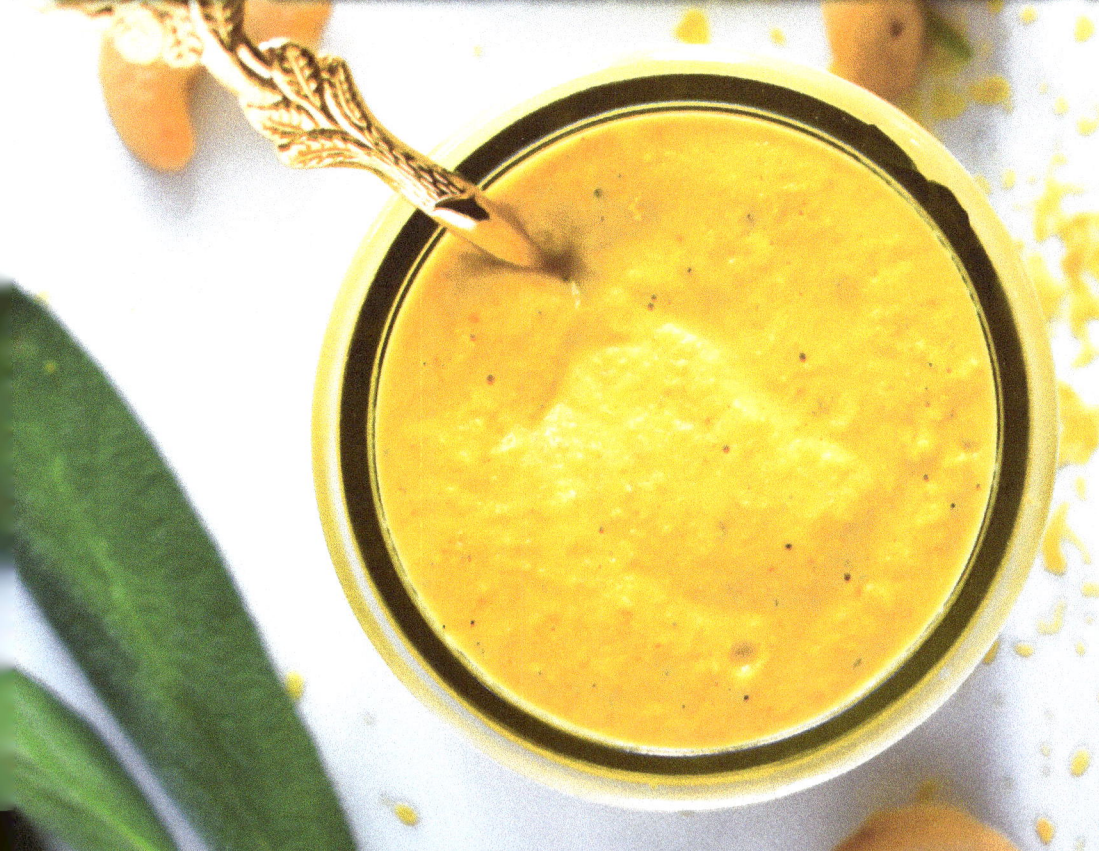

Hummus

- ¼ cup onion, chopped
- 2 cloves garlic, mashed and then minced
- 2 cups garbanzo beans, cooked
- ¼ cup lemon juice
- ⅓ cup tahini
- ½ cup water
- ½ teaspoon salt
- 1 tablespoon cumin
- ½ cup roasted bell pepper

Use as a dip for vegetables, pita, or multigrain chips. You may add vegetables, such as celery or bell pepper. This is a great party dish. Everyone enjoys hummus!

On low heat sauté onion and garlic, using a small amount of water. Then combine all ingredients in a food processor or high-speed blender and blend until smooth. Add water as needed. Taste and add more seasonings if desired.

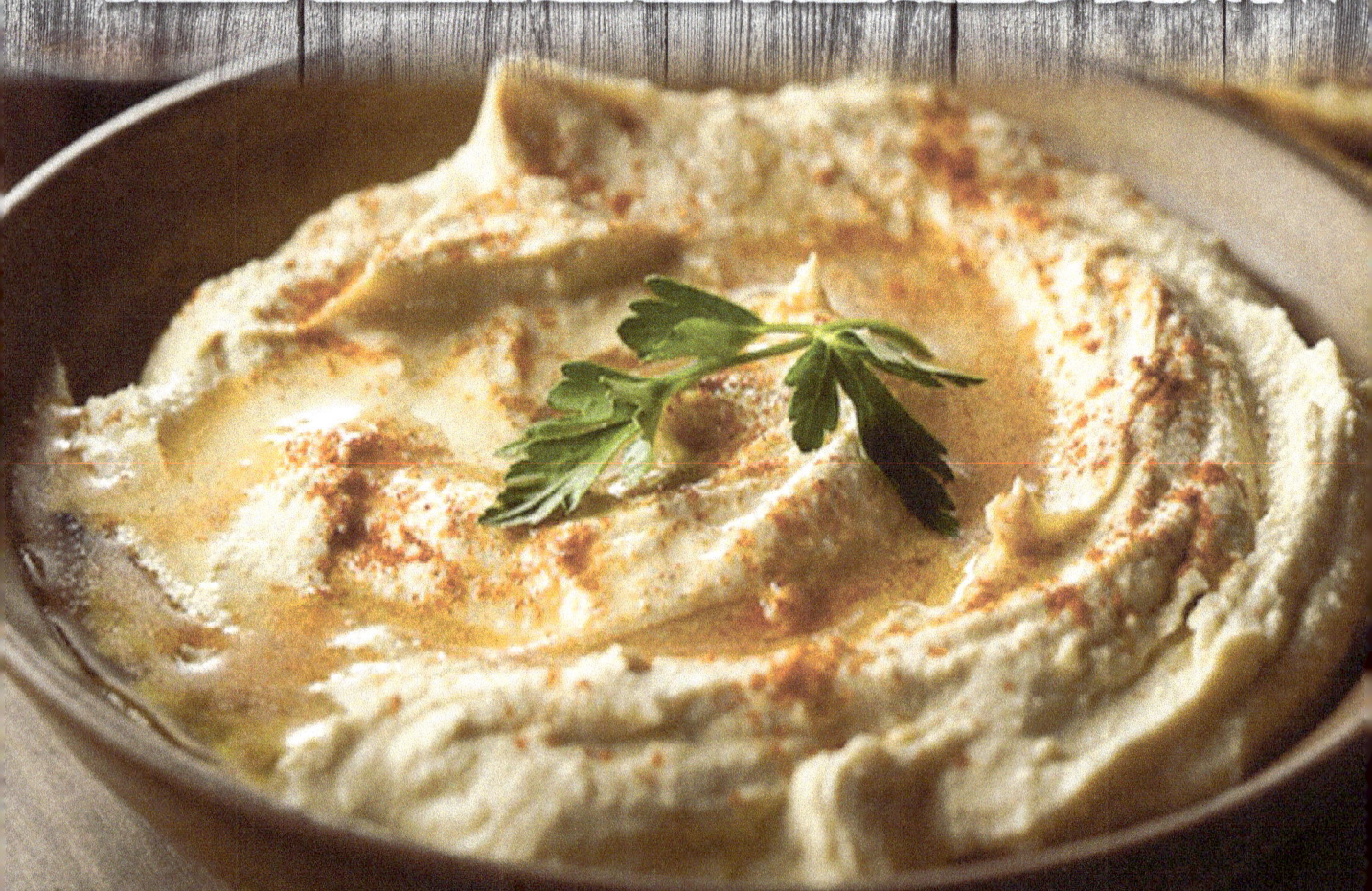

Mango Avocado Salsa

1 mango, peeled, seeded, and diced
1 avocado peeled, pitted, and diced
4 medium tomatoes, diced
1 jalapeño pepper, seeded and diced
½ cup chopped fresh cilantro
3 cloves garlic, minced
1 teaspoon salt
2 tablespoons fresh lime juice
¼ cup chopped red onion

Delicious salsa, best served with healthy tortilla chips or as a side dish for Mexican cuisine.

In a medium-sized bowl, combine the mango, avocado, tomatoes, jalapeño, cilantro, and garlic. Stir in the salt, lime juice, and red onion. Allow to stand in refrigerator for 30 minutes before serving.

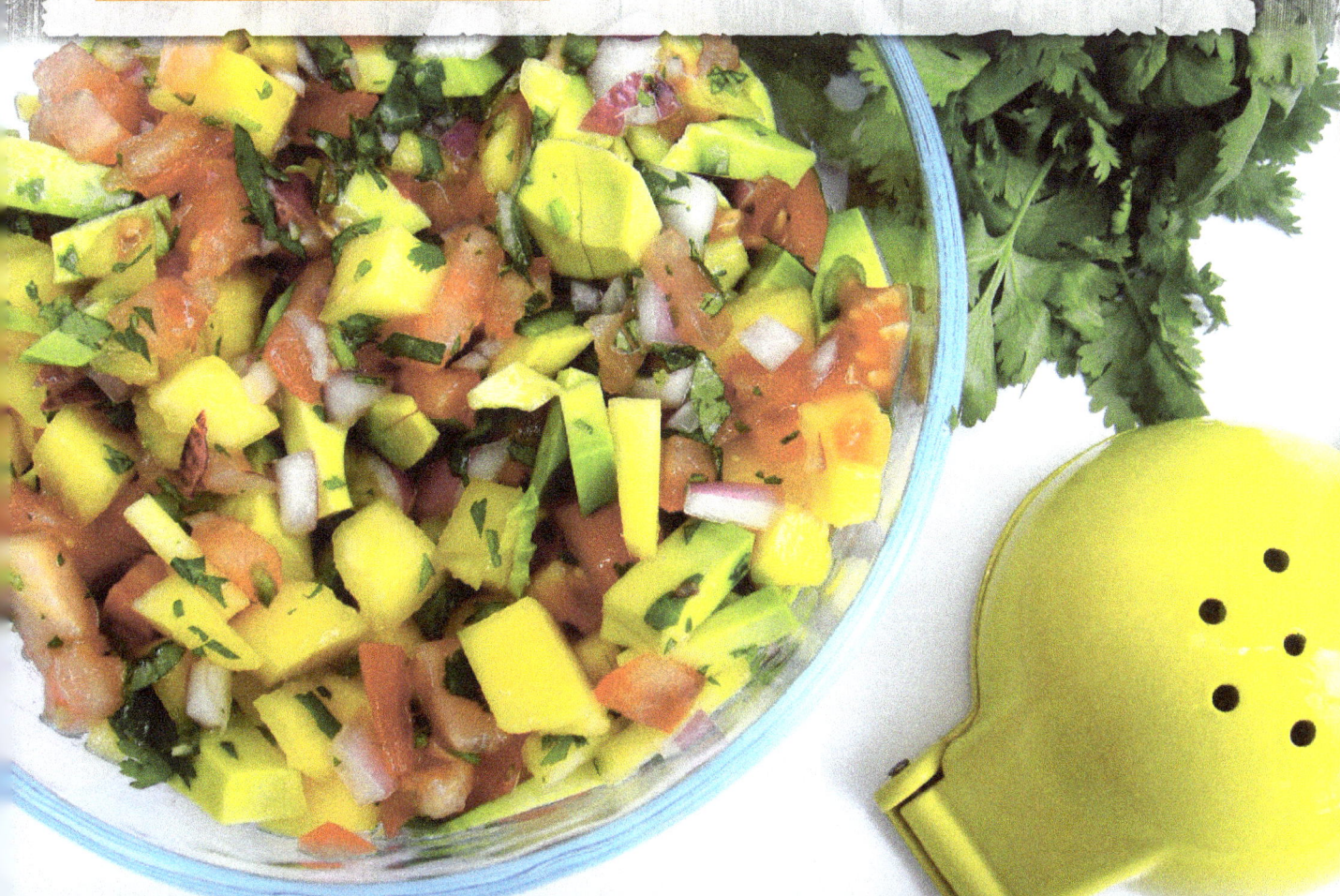

Guacamole

- 1 large avocado
- 2 tablespoons lemon juice
- 2 tablespoons onion, chopped
- ½ teaspoon salt

Please watch your portion size. Avocado has good fats, but this dish is high in calories.

Remove the skin and pit, cut avocado into small pieces, and mash with a fork. Add the remaining ingredients and mix well. Guacamole tends to become brown when exposed to air. To prevent this, store with the pit. Serve with Mexican dishes like tacos, nachos, burritos, or rice and beans.

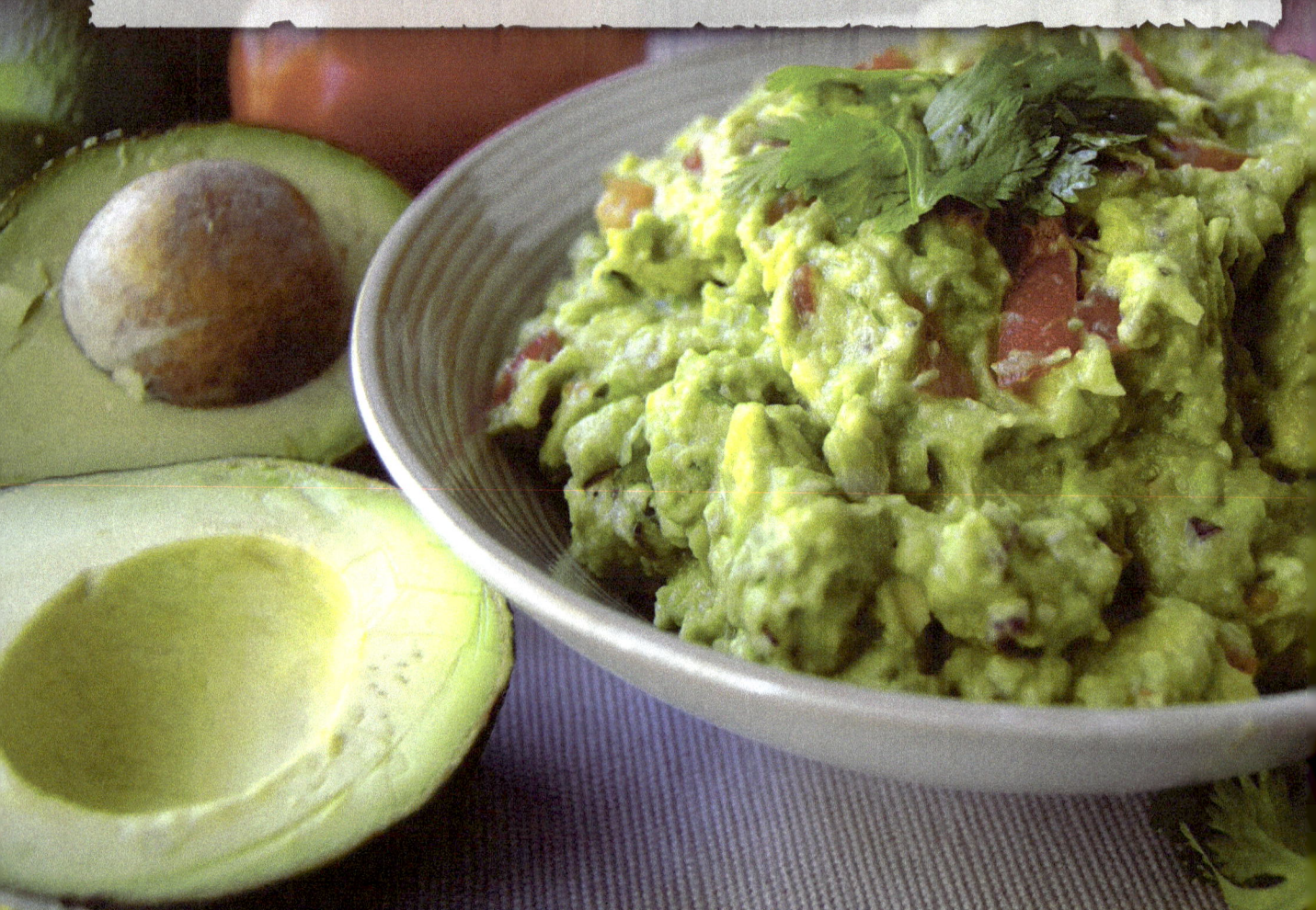

Chickpea Spread or Dip

¼ cup water
1–3 teaspoon ground cumin (to taste)
2 tablespoons lemon juice
1–2 garlic cloves
Water-packed chickpeas, drained and rinsed
1 small sweet onion
Chili powder to taste (optional)

This is better made the day before you plan to serve it and refrigerated. Use as a sandwich spread or as a dip for pita bread.

Combine the ingredients in a blender and process until smooth.

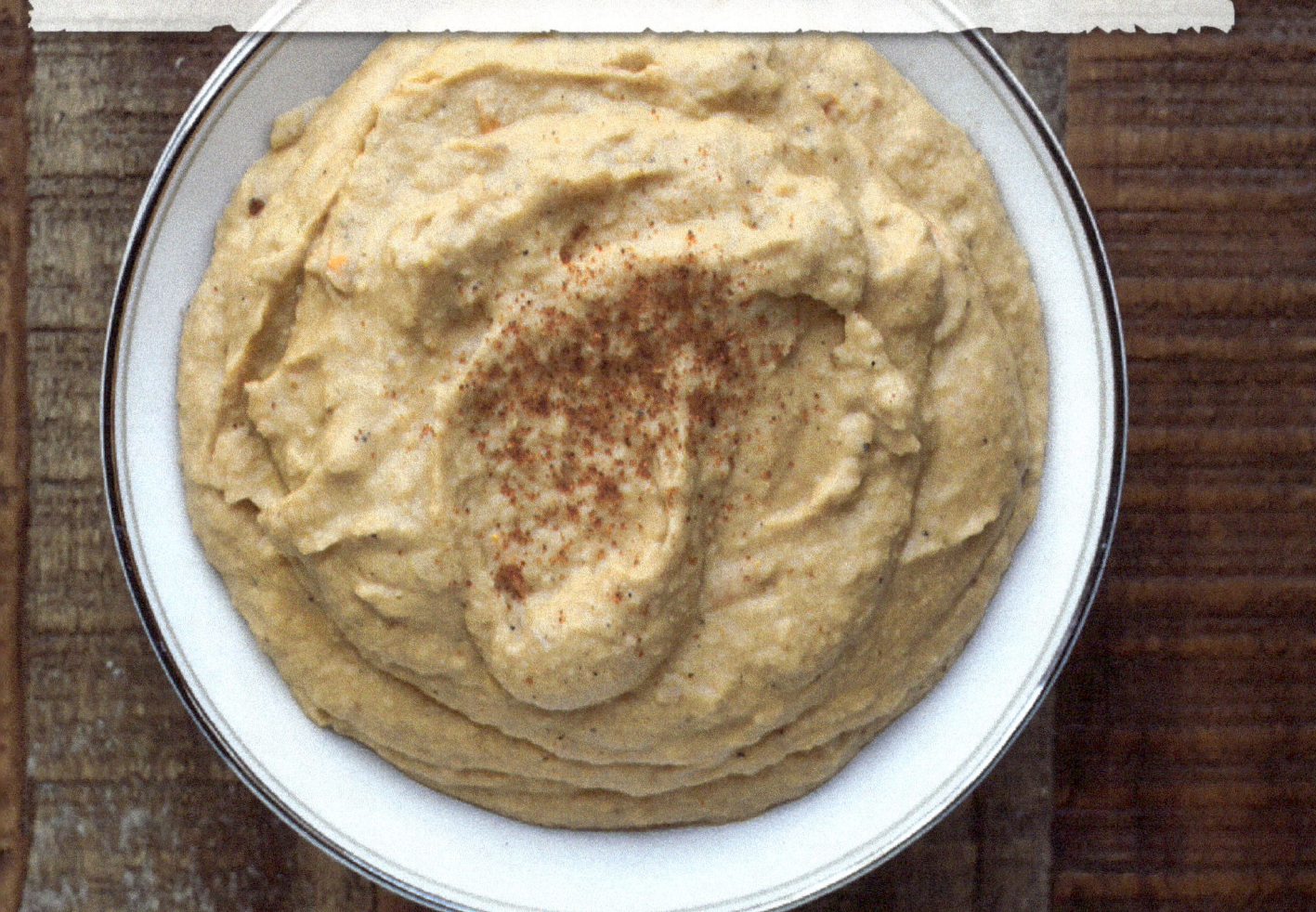

Mushroom Gravy

½ cup onions, chopped
2 cloves garlic, mashed then minced
2 cups mushrooms, sliced
3 cups soy milk
1 tablespoon Bragg's Amino Acids or soy sauce
3 tablespoons whole wheat flour
1 teaspoon basil or sage
1 ½ teaspoons chicken-style or savory seasoning
3 sprigs thyme

Great low-fat gravy that can be served over meatballs.

Sauté garlic, onions, and mushrooms in a medium-sized pot, using a small amount of water. Then add the remaining ingredients. Whisk flour in slowly to prevent clumping. Simmer for another 5 to 7 minutes until thickened.

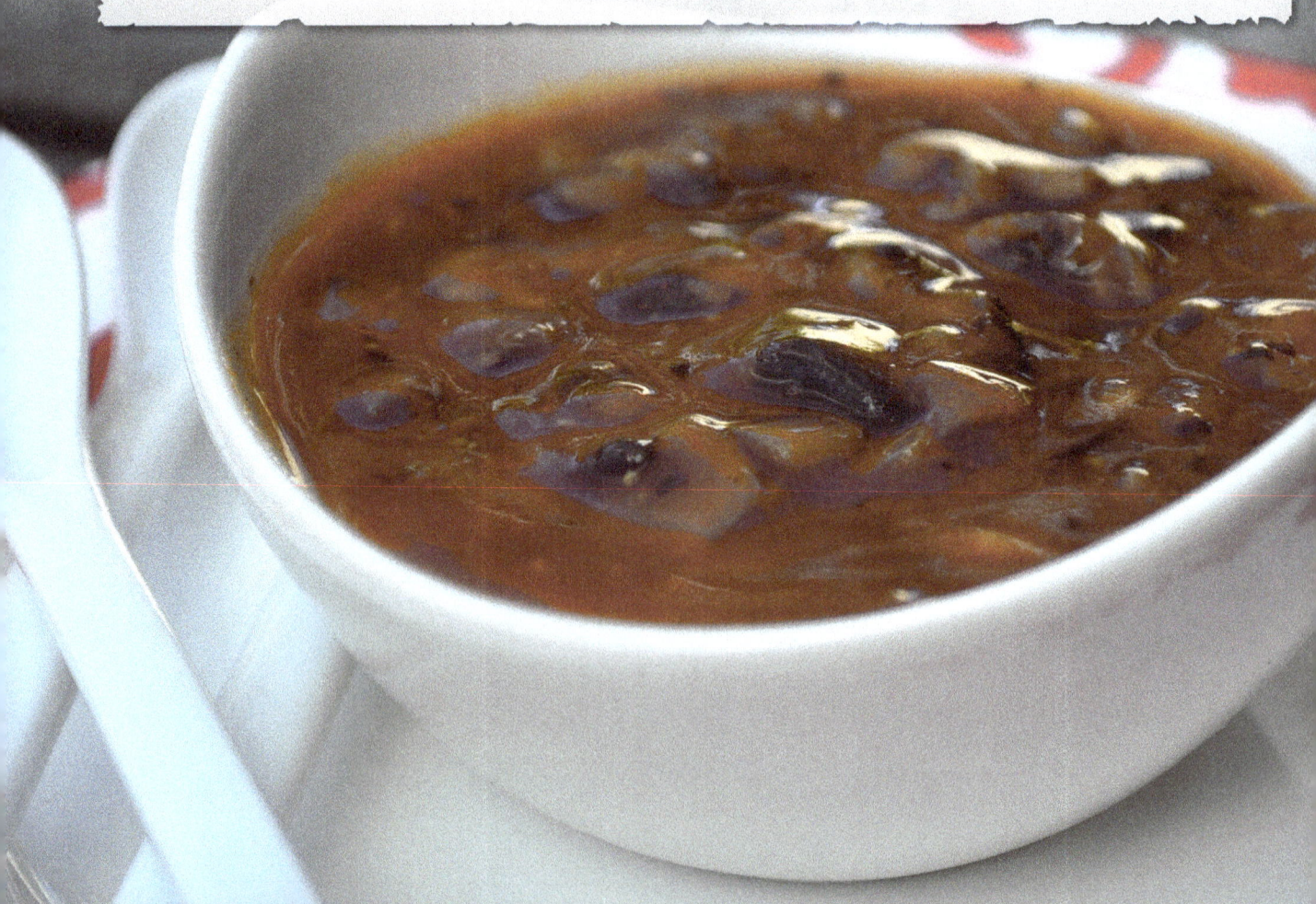

Country-Style Brown Gravy

- 2 cups warm water
- 3 cloves garlic, mashed then minced
- ⅛ cup cashews, rinsed
- ½ teaspoon garlic powder
- 1 tablespoon onion powder
- ½ teaspoon Italian herbs
- 2 tablespoon cornstarch
- 3 sprigs fresh thyme
- ½ tomato, chopped
- 3 tablespoons soy sauce
- 1 tablespoon parsley

This gravy is simple and easy to make. You can enjoy it over lentil patties, meatloaf, or meatballs.

Place ½ cup warm water and the other ingredients except the parsley in a blender or food processor and blend until smooth and creamy. When creamy, add 1 ½ cups more warm water and blend. Pour into a saucepan and cook over low-to-medium heat, stirring constantly, until thick (about 5 minutes).

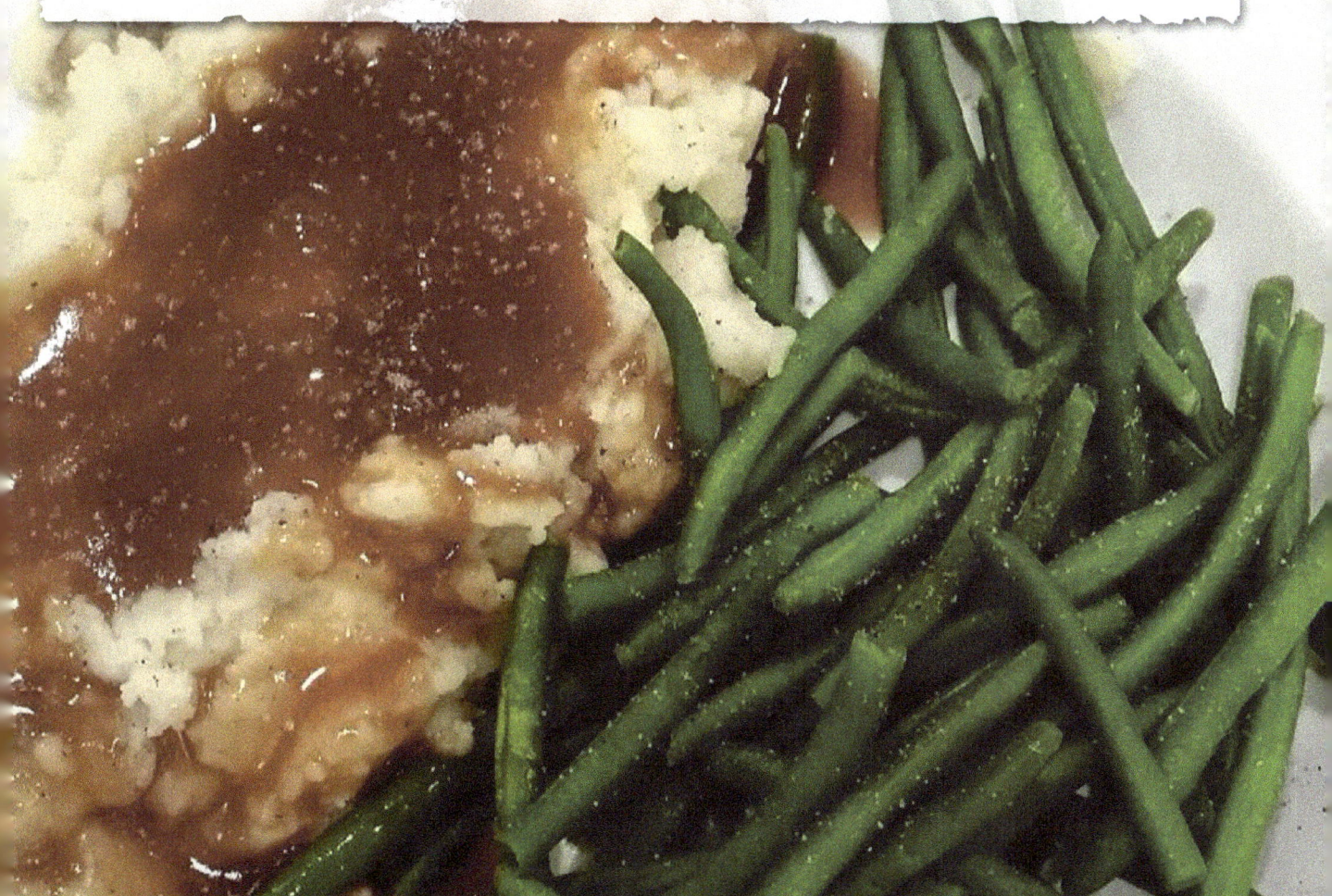

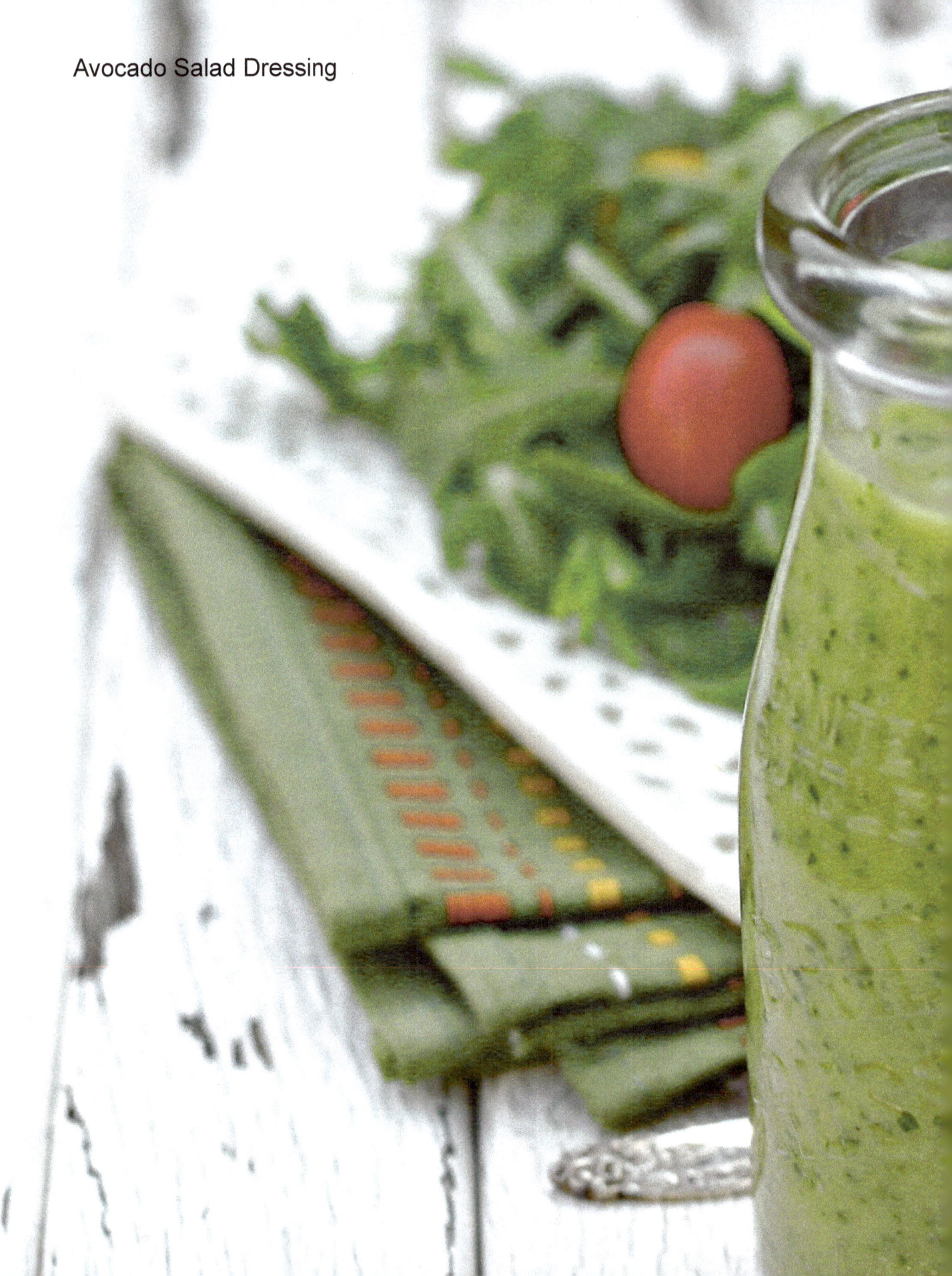

Avocado Salad Dressing

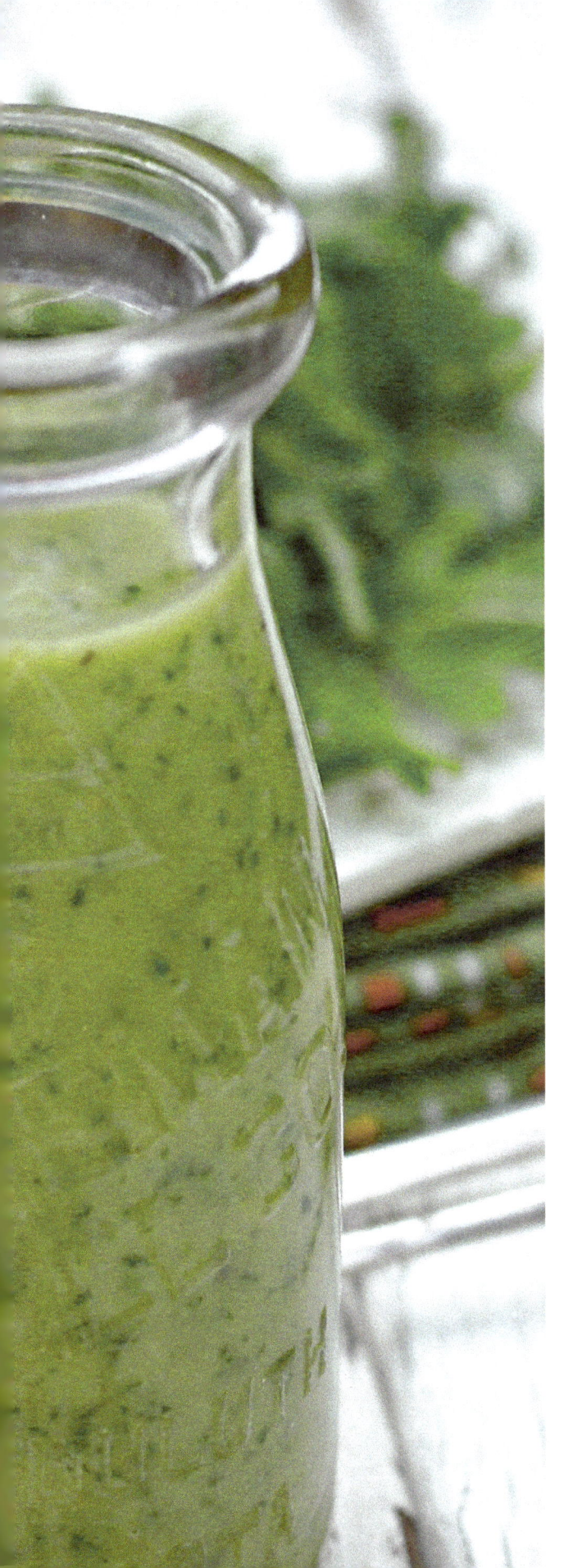

SALAD DRESSINGS

Cucumber Salad Dressing

Avocado Salad Dressing

Caesar Salad Dressing

Strawberry Salad Dressing

Orange Ginger Salad Dressing

Cucumber Salad Dressing

- 3 small cucumbers
- 2 tablespoons fresh lemon juice
- 1 small green onion
- 3 tablespoons tahini
- ½ teaspoon salt or to taste
- 2 gloves garlic
- 1 tablespoon Italian herbs

Easy to make, this delicious dressing goes well on green vegetables.

Place all ingredients in a blender and blend until smooth.

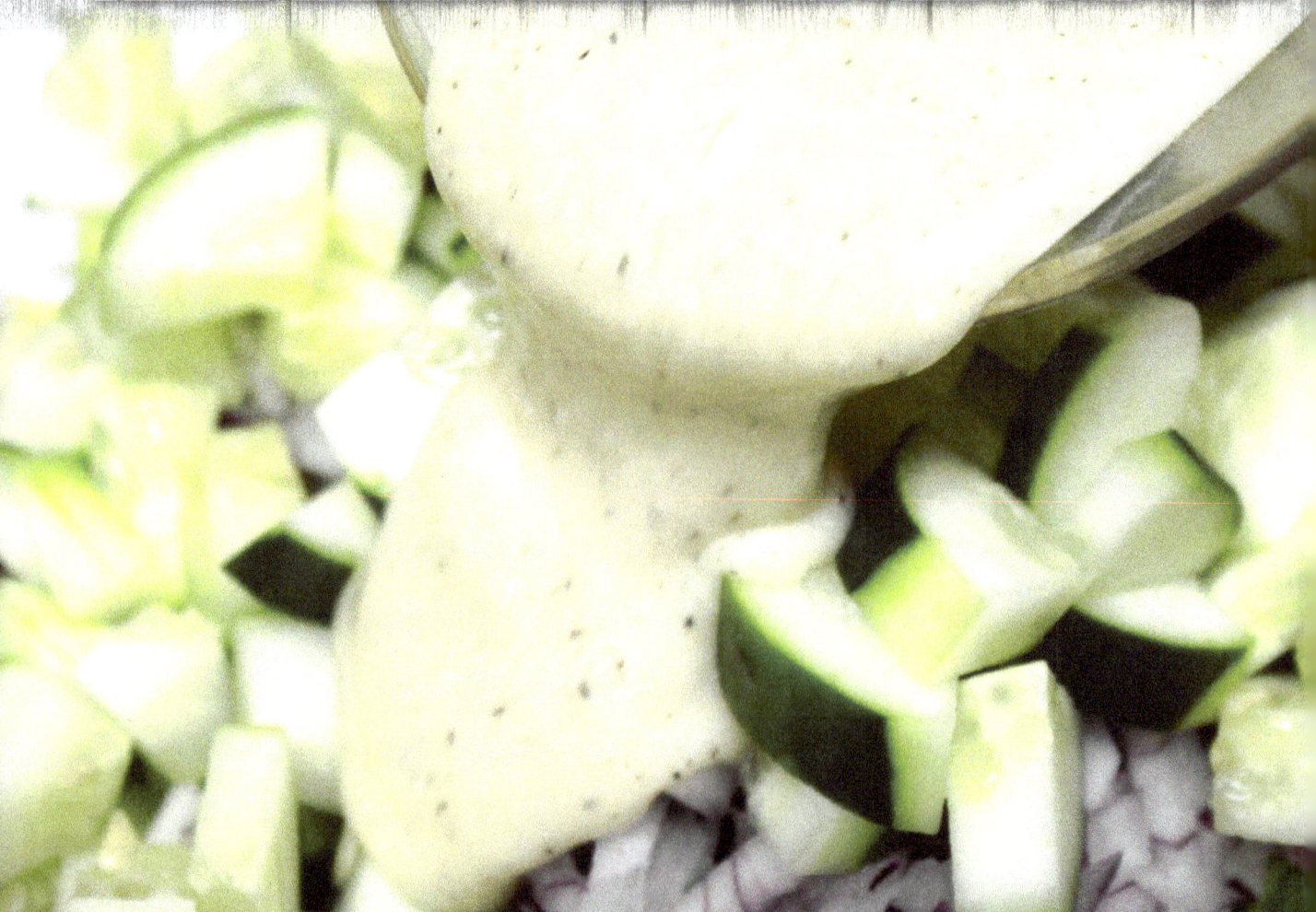

Avocado Salad Dressing

2 medium ripe avocados
3 tablespoons lemon juice
½ teaspoon sea salt, to taste
Pinch of dill, crushed
½ medium onion
½ cup cilantro, finely chopped
¼ cup water

Avocados are used in making this favorite tasty salad dressing.

Remove skin and seed from the avocado. Then cut it into pieces and place in blender with all the other ingredients. Blend until smooth. Delicious on salad greens.

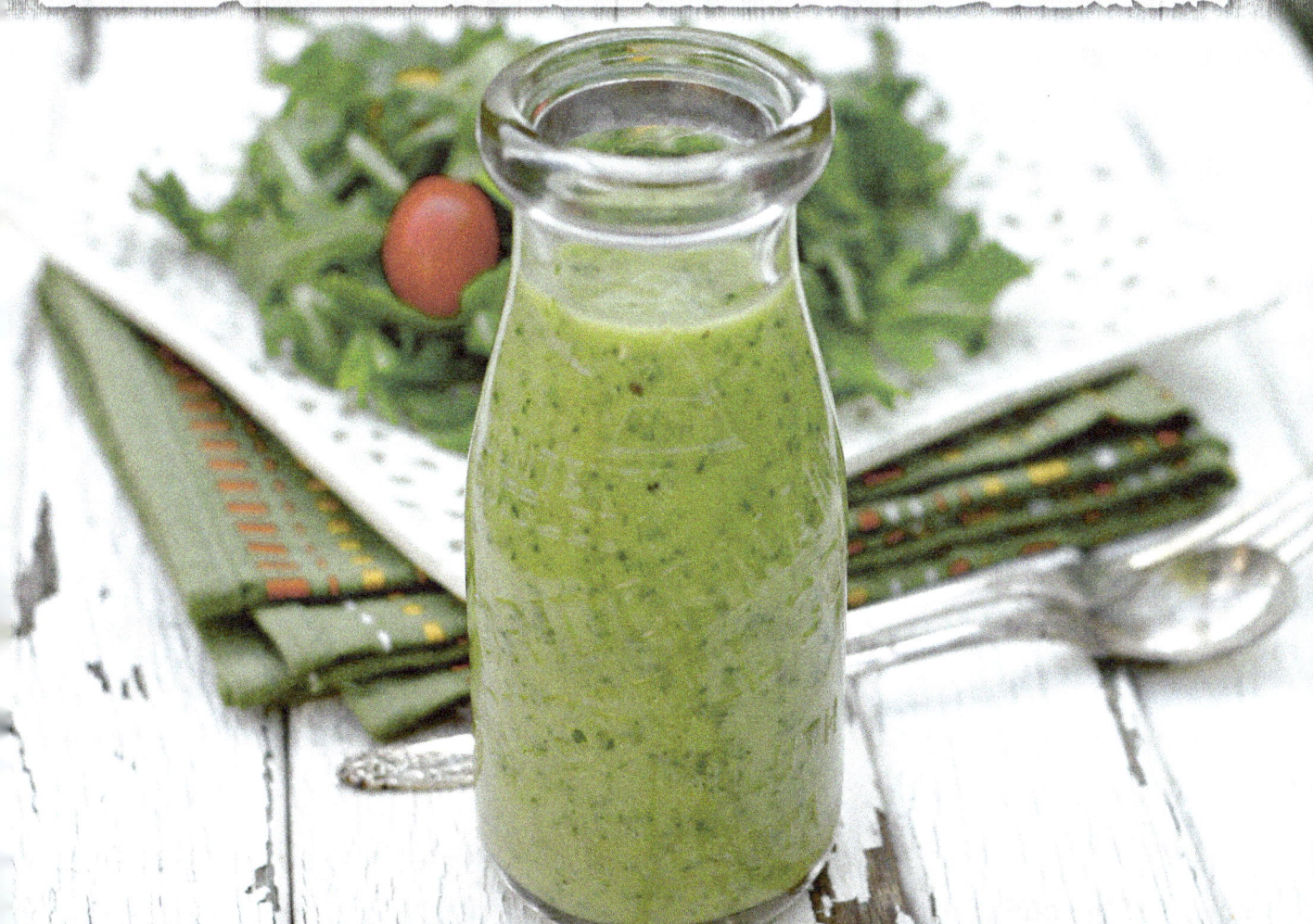

Caesar Salad Dressing

⅓ cup cashew nuts
1 tablespoon tahini
½ cup nut milk, unsweetened
3 teaspoons garlic powder
2 tablespoons lemon juice
2 teaspoons Mrs. Dash, Italian herbs
½ teaspoon salt to taste

This creamy dressing is very delicious. You can add a pinch of dill if desired. This dressing goes well with any green or steamed vegetables. Stores well in the refrigerator.

In a high-speed blender, blend cashews and milk until smooth. Then add the other ingredients until smooth.

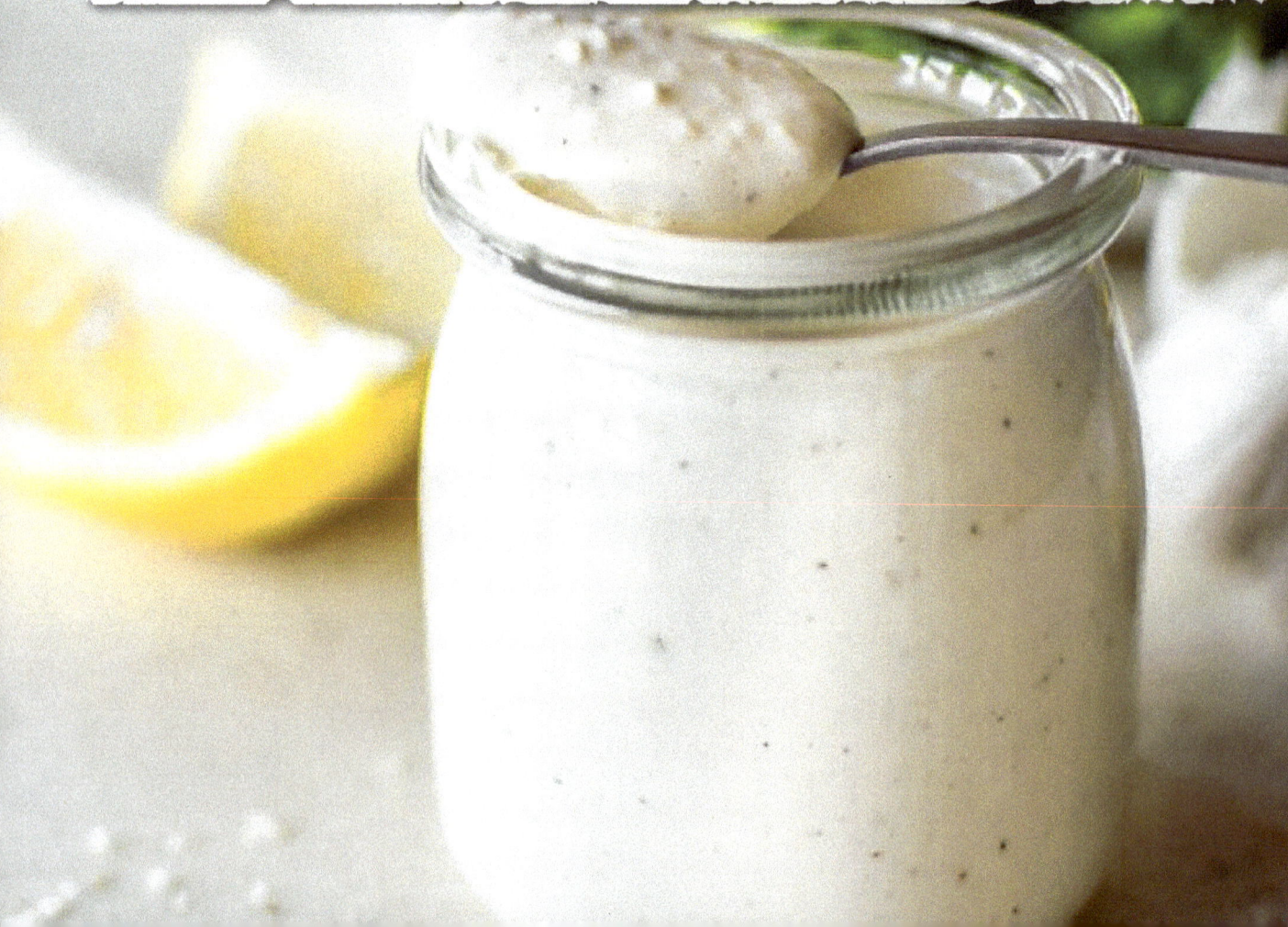

Strawberry Dressing

1 cup fresh strawberries, chopped

⅓ cup dried cranberries

⅓ cup walnuts

½ cup white grape juice

3 tablespoons lemon juice

This dressing goes well with fresh vegetables or salad. It is also delicious on waffles and pancakes and stores well in the refrigerator.

In a high-speed blender, blend walnuts and white grape juice until smooth. Then add the other ingredients until smooth.

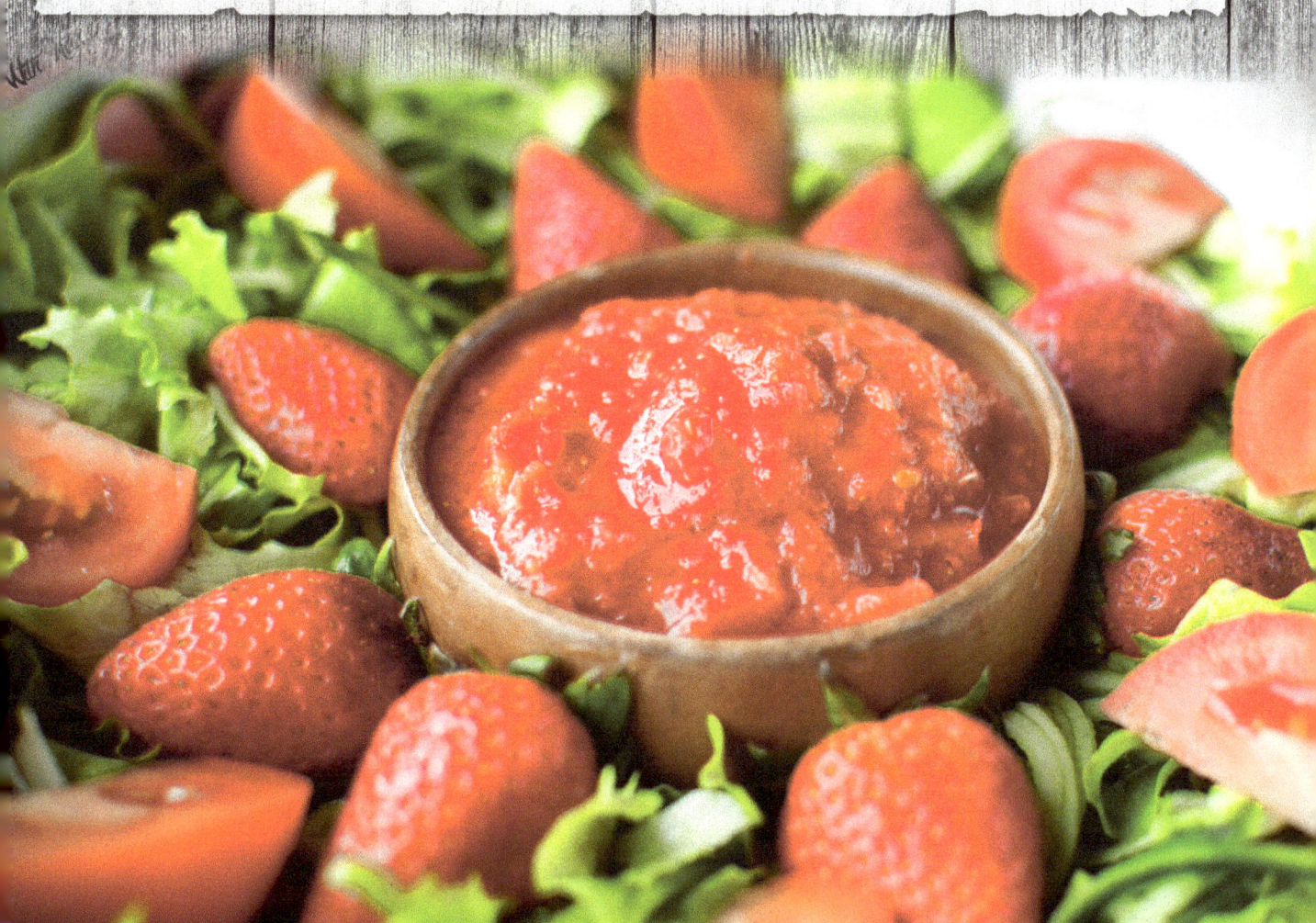

Orange Ginger Dressing

- 2 small oranges
- 1 teaspoon fresh ginger, grated
- 1 tablespoon lemon
- 2 tablespoons soy sauce
- ½ cup water
- 2 tablespoons tahini

This dressing goes well with fresh vegetables. It can also be used in preparing stir-fry tofu. Best when used freshly made.

In a high-speed blender, blend all of the ingredients until smooth.

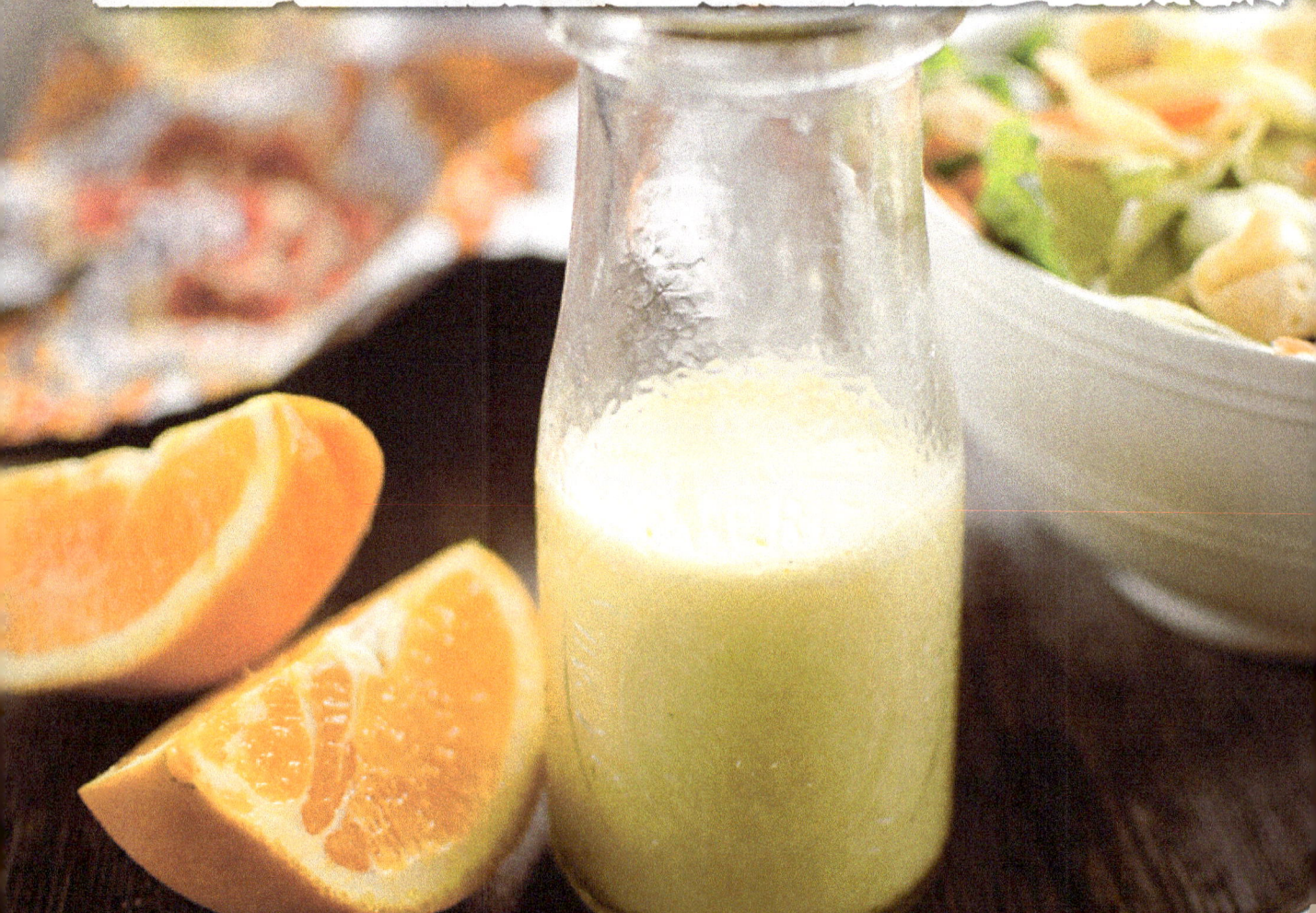

DESSERTS

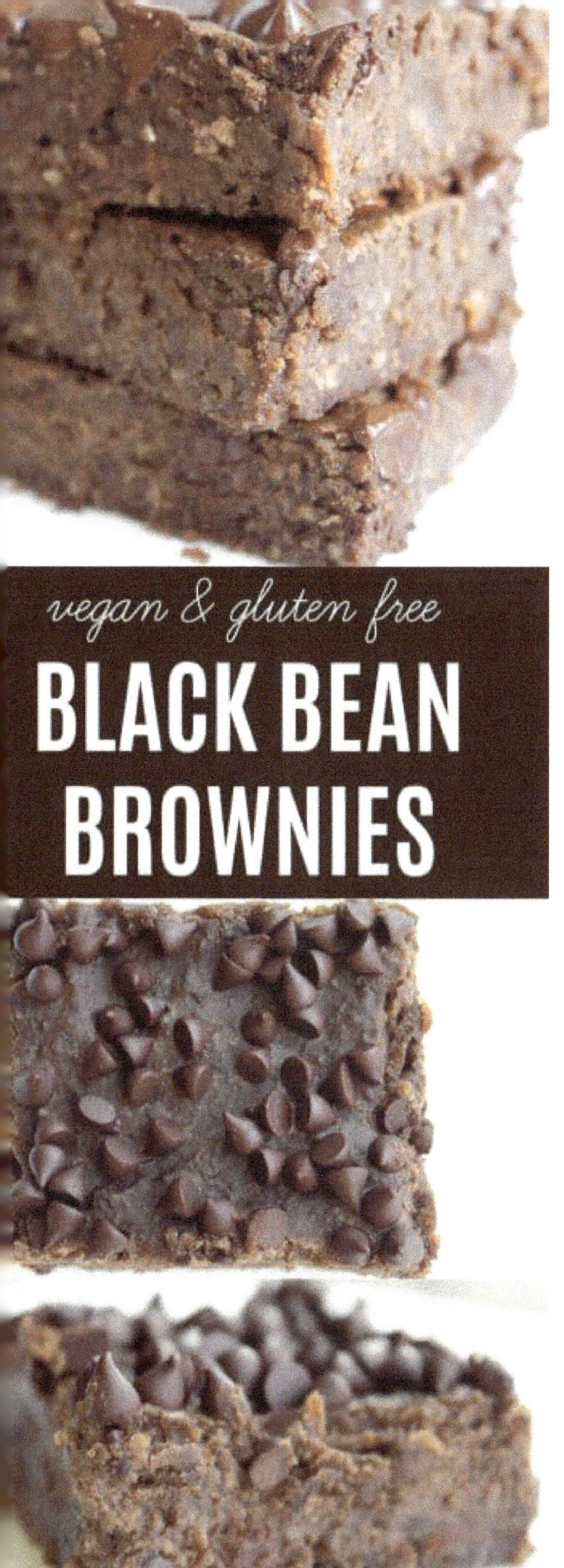

Vegan Gluten-Free Black Bean Brownies

Banana Peanut Butter Ice Cream

Banana Coconut Ice Cream

Papaya Banana Ice Cream

Strawberry Banana Sorbet

Carrot Cake

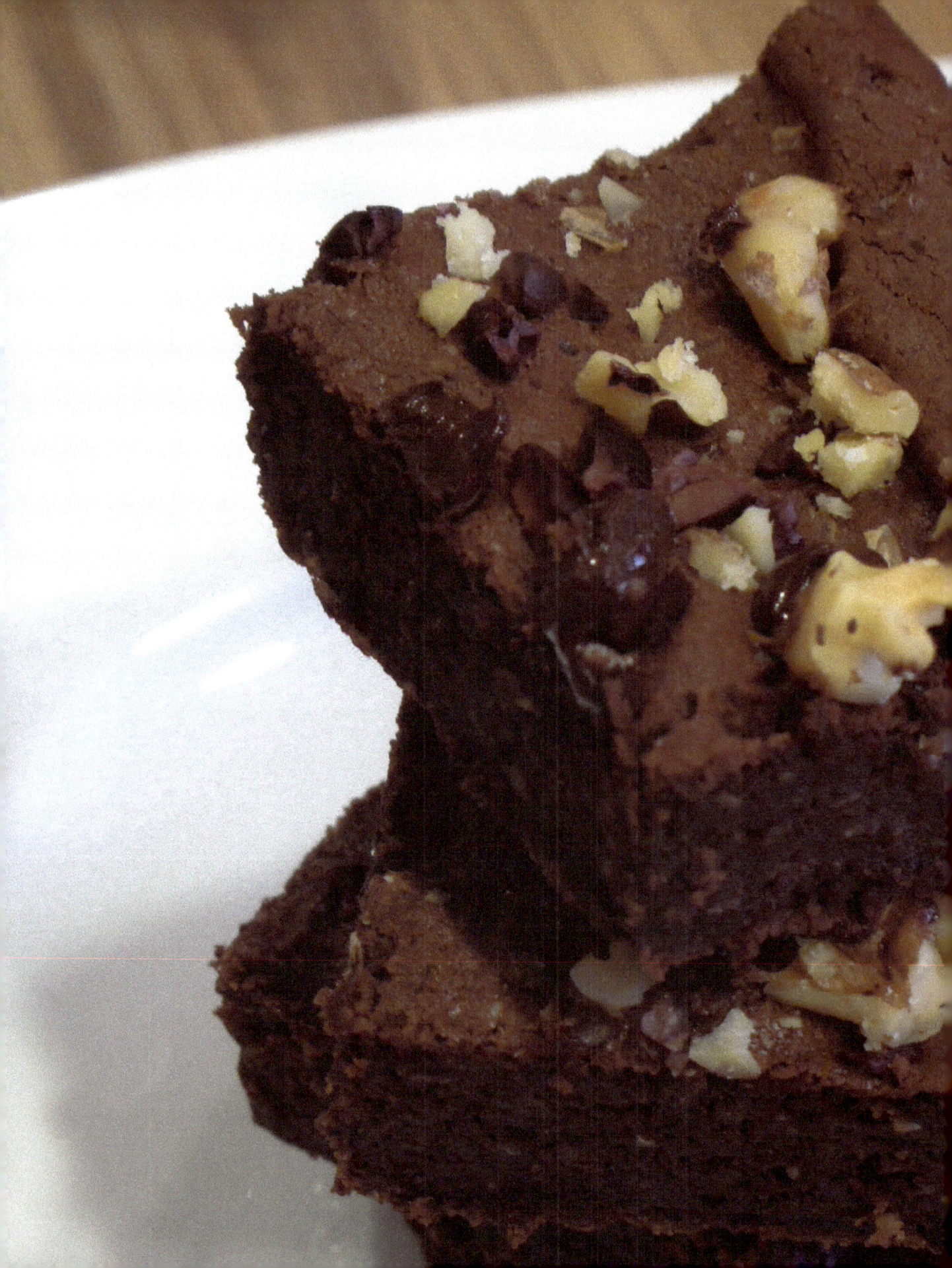

Vegan Gluten-Free Black Bean Brownies

2 ½ tablespoons flaxseed meal (and 6 tablespoons water)

1 (15-ounce) can black beans, rinsed and drained

3 tablespoons tahini

¾ cup carob powder

¼ teaspoon sea salt

1 teaspoon pure vanilla extract

½ cup agave

1 ½ teaspoon baking power

¼ cup crushed walnuts or pecans

Easy and delicious recipe. Please watch your portion, and don't overdo it.

Preheat oven to 350 degrees Fahrenheit. Lightly grease a 12-slot standard-size muffin pan. Prepare flax eggs by combining flaxseed and water in the bowl of the food processor; pulse a couple of times and then let it rest for a few minutes. Add the remaining ingredients (except walnuts) and pulse for about 3 minutes until smooth. If the batter is too thick, add a tablespoon or two of water and pulse again. Evenly distribute the batter into the muffin tin and smooth the top with spoon. Sprinkle with crushed walnuts. Bake for 20 to 26 minutes or until the tops are dry and the edges start to pull apart. Remove from the oven and let cool for 30 minutes before removing from pan. Store in an airtight container for a few days. Refrigerate to keep longer.

Banana Peanut Butter Ice Cream

- 3 frozen, ripe bananas, cut in pieces
- 2 tablespoons peanut butter
- ¼ cup almond milk

This ice cream is fat-free and delicious.

With blender on ice cream or frozen-dessert mode, blend all of the ingredients together until smooth; if needed, add a small amount of almond milk.

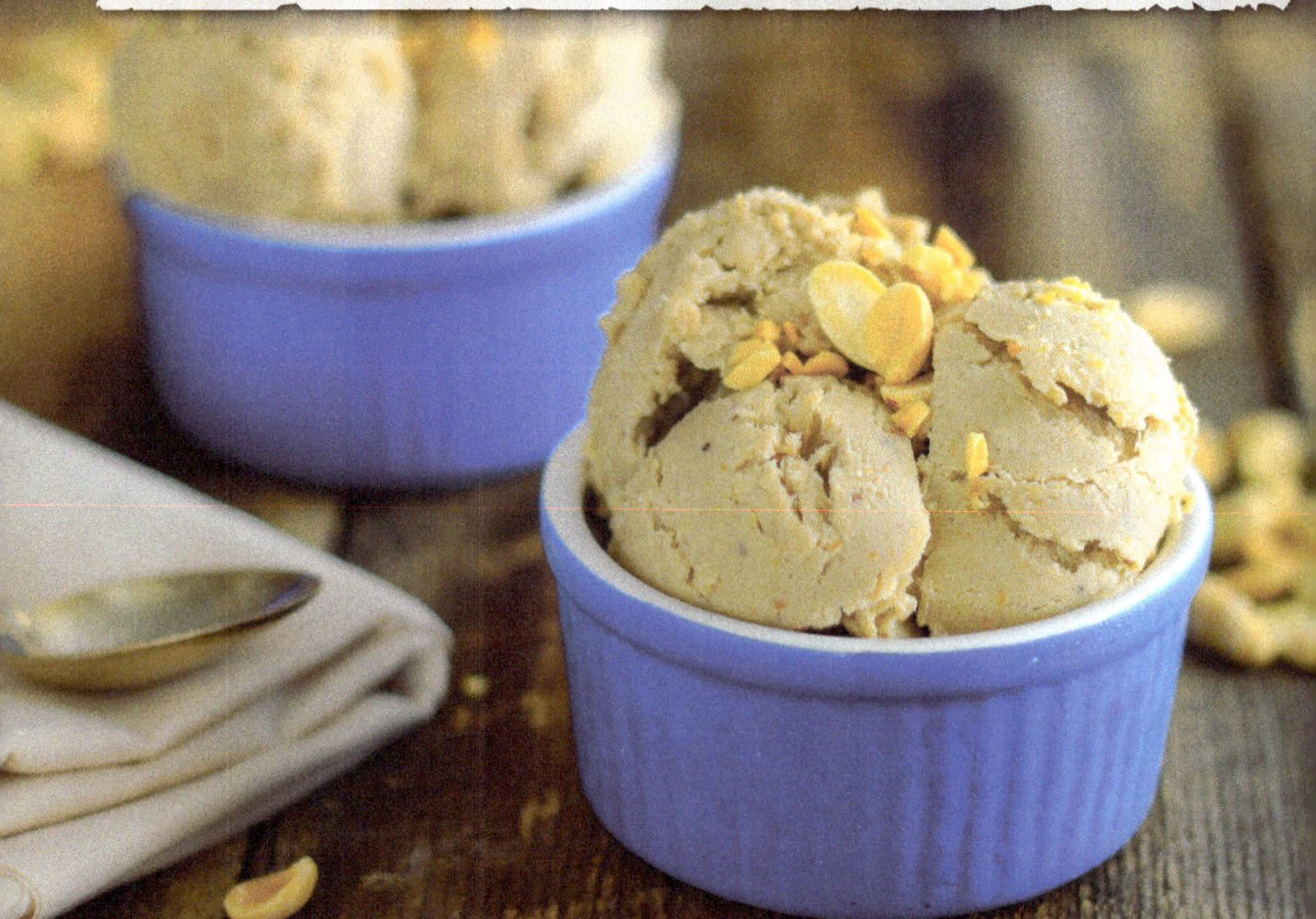

Banana Coconut Ice Cream

6 frozen, ripe bananas, cut in pieces

½ (15-ounce) can coconut cream

You can add a pinch of nutmeg or cinnamon if desired. Remember to be cautious with desserts. Do not overeat. Stores well in freezer.

With high-speed blender in ice cream mode, blend bananas and coconut cream until smooth.

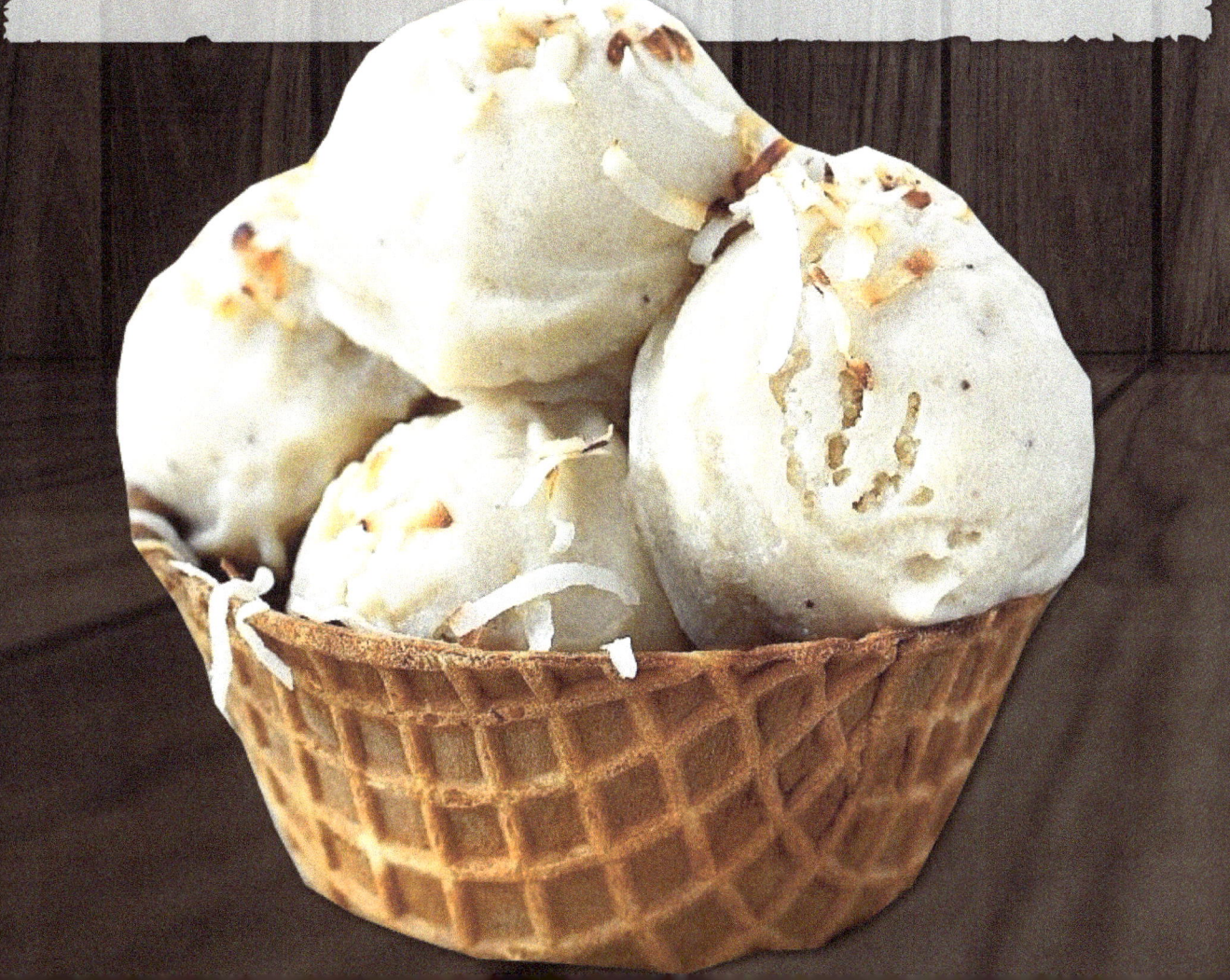

Papaya Banana Ice Cream

4 cups frozen, ripe bananas, cut in pieces

3 cups frozen, ripe papayas, cut in pieces

½ cup almond milk

3 tablespoons nondairy milk powder

This is one of my favorite desserts. It is delicious and stores well in the freezer.

With a high-speed blender on ice cream or frozen-dessert mode, blend all of the ingredients until smooth.

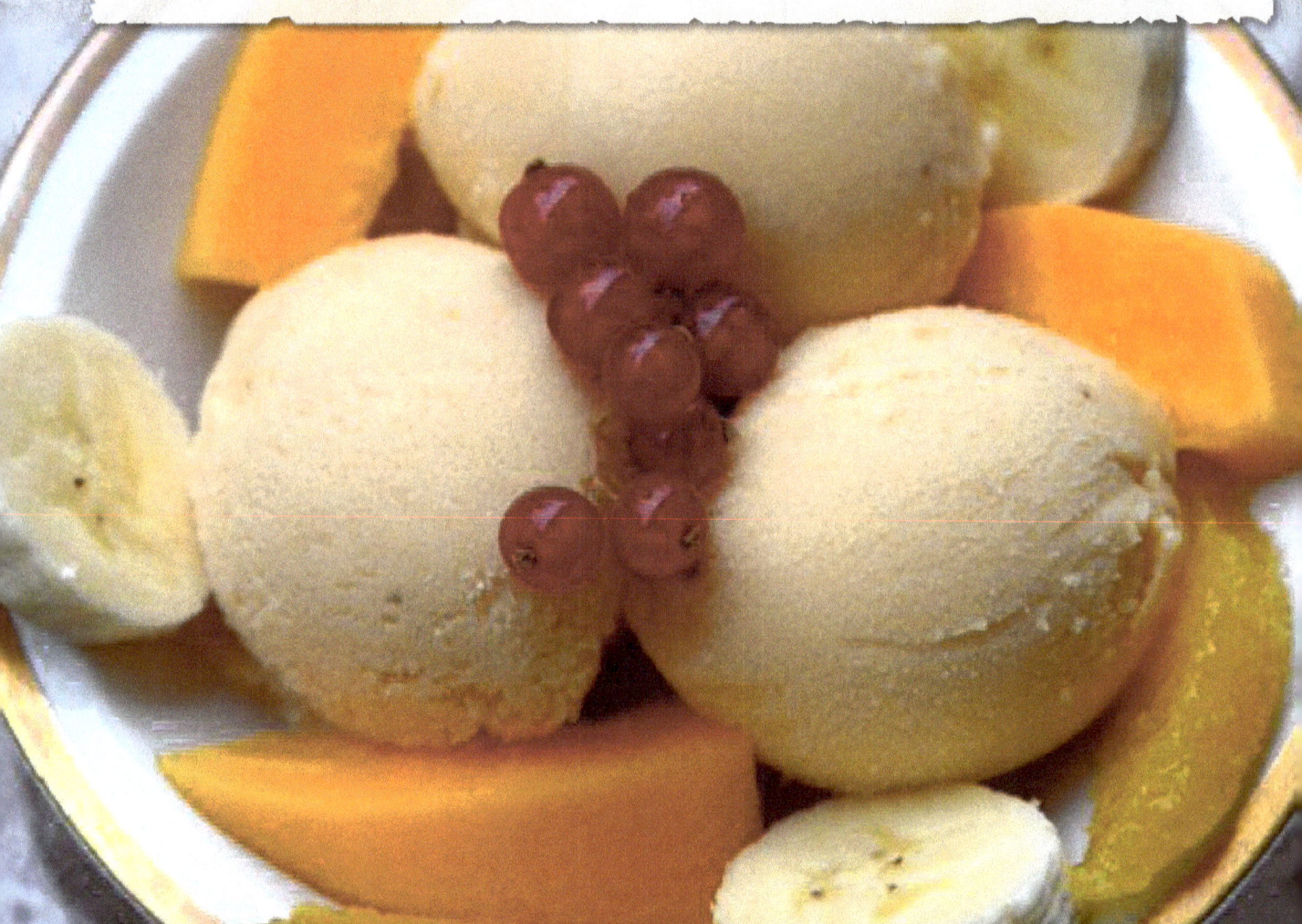

Strawberry Banana Sorbet

3 cups frozen strawberry, cut in pieces

2 cups frozen bananas, cut in pieces

½ cup fruit juice

This simple frozen fruit dessert is great for any age. You can use any type of frozen fruit.

With a high-speed blender on ice cream or frozen-dessert mode, blend all of the ingredients until smooth.

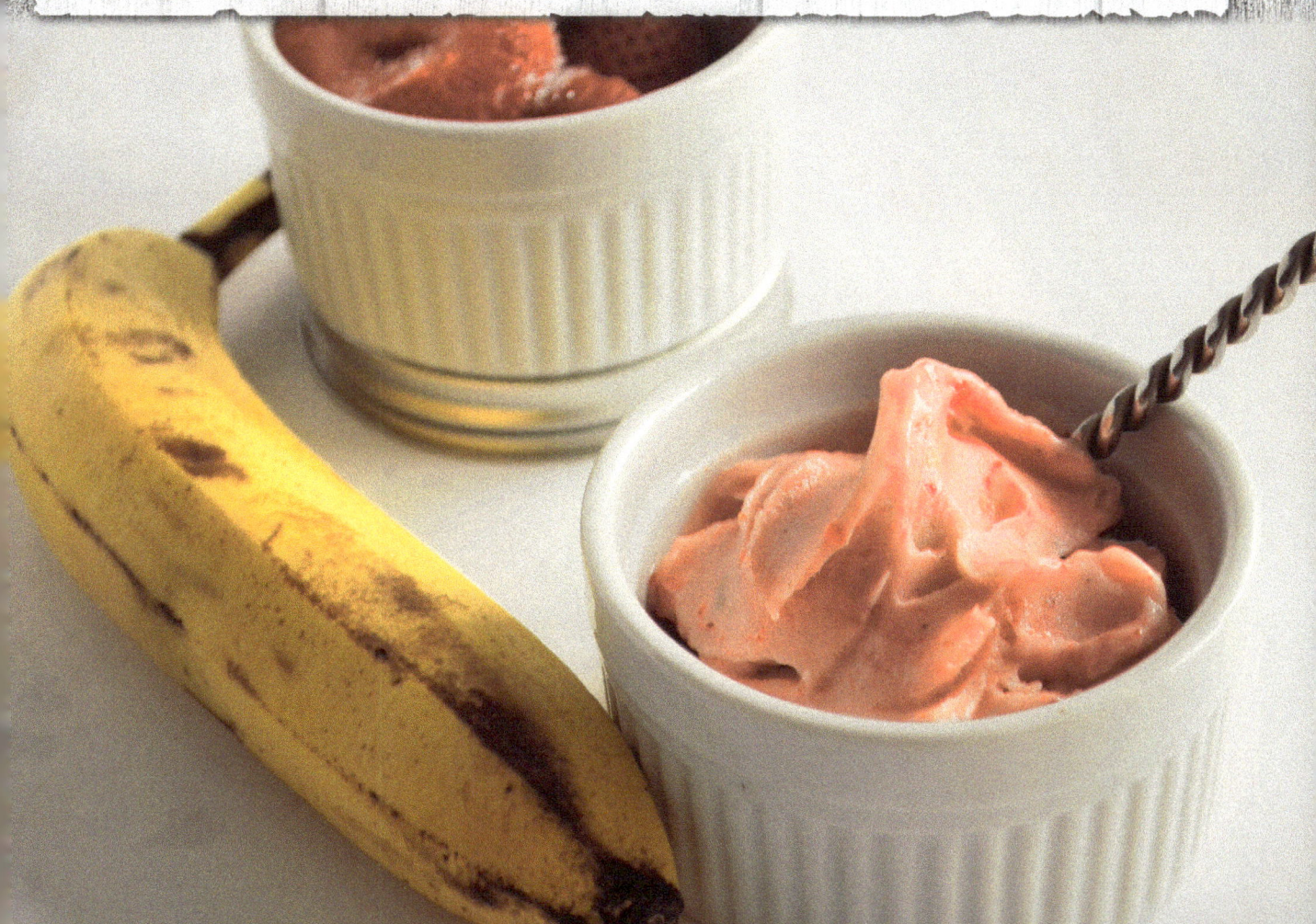

Berry Sorbet

2 cups frozen strawberries, cut in pieces

1 cup frozen blueberries

1 cup frozen blackberries

1 cup frozen cherries

½ cup white grape juice

This is a great dessert to enjoy on a hot summer day. These fruits are loaded with vitamins, minerals, and antioxidants.

With a high-speed blender on frozen-dessert mode, blend all of the ingredients until smooth.

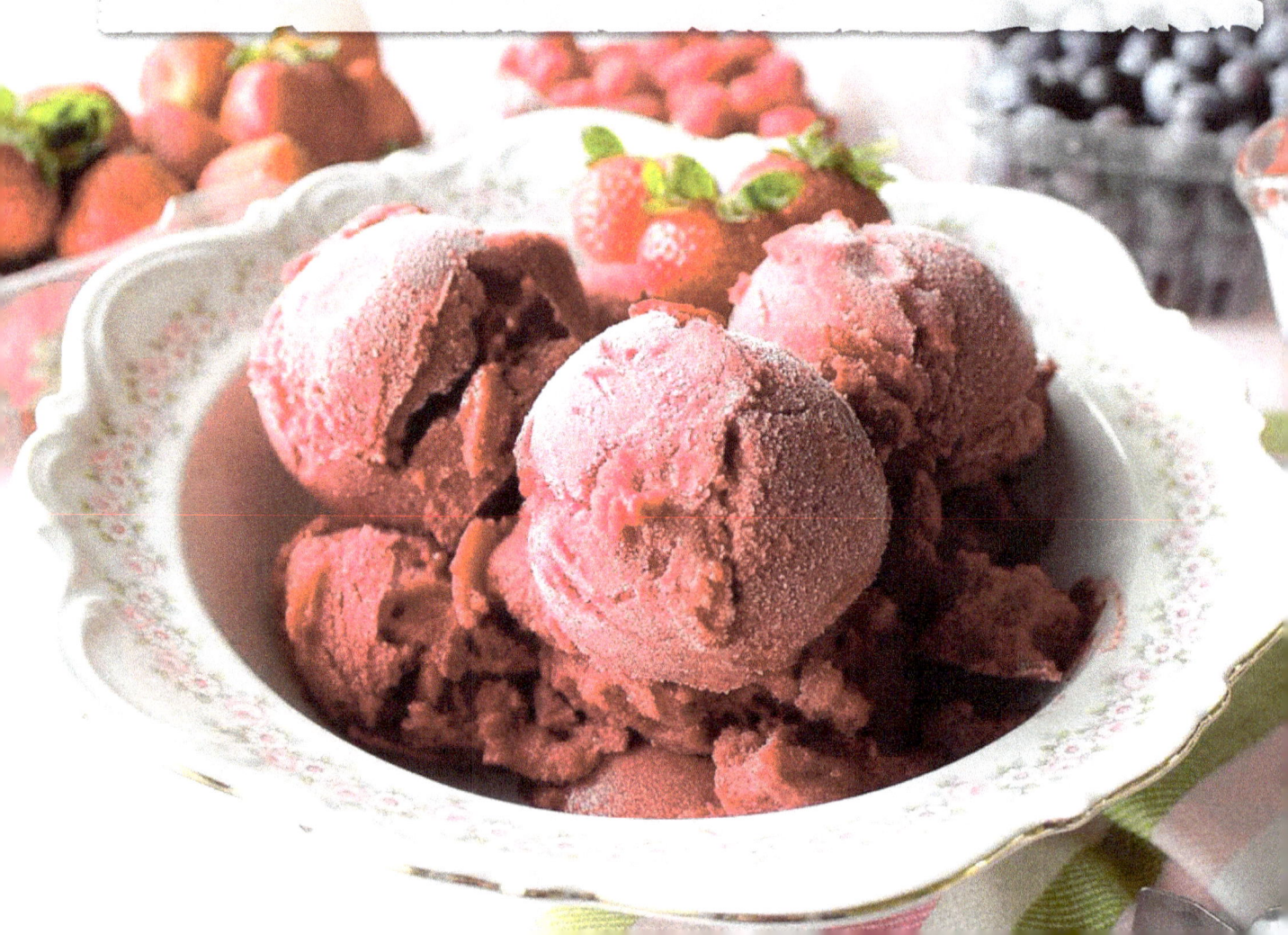

Carrot Cake

1 cup whole wheat flour
1 cup unbleached flour
4 teaspoons baking powder
1 teaspoon baking soda
½ teaspoon salt
8 oz. dates (pitted) or ½ cup maple syrup
¾ cup apple (grated)
2 cups coconut cream
⅓ cup lemon juice (freshly squeezed)
½ cup orange juice (freshly squeezed)
½ cup raisins
2 cups carrots, grated
1 teaspoon vanilla
¼ teaspoon clove
1 teaspoon cinnamon
½ teaspoon nutmeg

Place dates in blender add milk and blend until smooth, then pour in a medium sized bowl. Add orange juice, vanilla, mix thoroughly. Add flour, and other dry ingredients and spices to the liquid ingredients, mix well, then add in the grated carrots, apples, and continue to mix. Now incorporate the lemon and orange juice and continue to mix. Pour mixture in a greased cake baking pan, pre-heat oven at 350 degrees Fahrenheit and bake for 67 minutes.

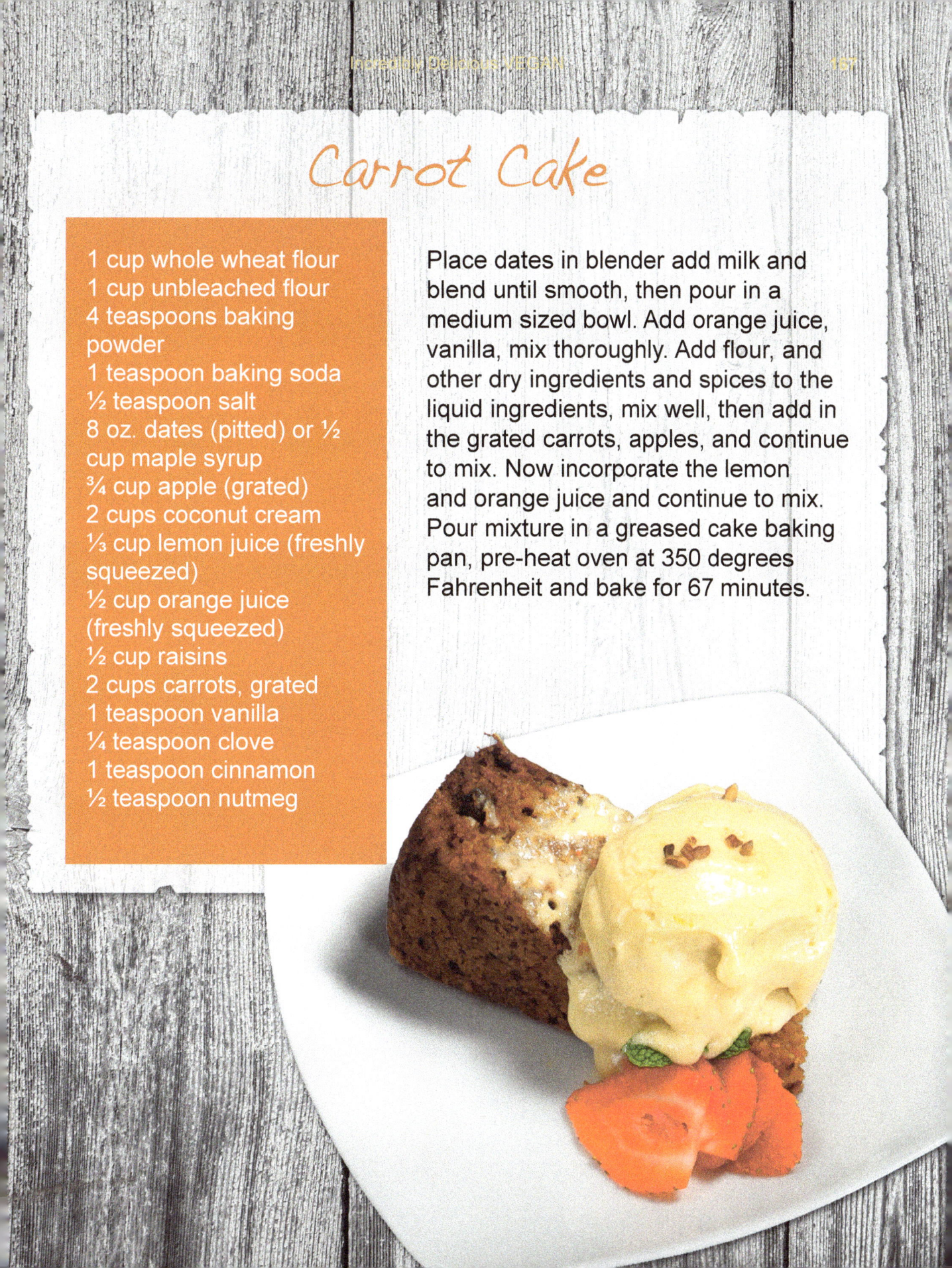

ENDNOTES

1 BBC. (n.d.). BBC - History - Historic Figures: James Lind (1716-1794). Retrieved from http://www.bbc.co.uk/history/historic_figures/lind_james.shtml.

2 Christiaan Eijkman, Beriberi and Vitamin B1. Nobelprize.org. Nobel Media AB 2014. Web. 22 Mar 2016. Retrieved from http://www.nobelprize.org/educational/medicine/vitamin_b1/eijkman.html

3 Sir Frederick Gowland Hopkins. (2016). In Encyclopedia Britannica. Retrieved from http://www.britannica.com/biography/Frederick-Gowland-Hopkins.

4 Centers for Disease Control and Prevention. (2015, March 31). IMMPaCt: Micronutrient Facts | DNPAO | CDC. Retrieved from http://www.cdc.gov/immpact/micronutrients.

5 Kim, S., & Radecki, J. (n.d.). Nutrients. Retrieved from http://www.diet.com/g/nutrients. 6 Ibid.

7 Harvard Health Publications. (n.d.). Vitamins & Minerals: Are You Getting What You Need? Retrieved from http://www.helpguide.org/harvard/vitamins-and-minerals.html.

8 Butler, N. (2015, November 6). Nutritional Deficiencies (Malnutrition). Retrieved from http://www.healthline.com/health/malnutrition.

9 Kim, S., & Radecki, J. (n.d.). Nutrients. Retrieved from http://www.diet.com/g/nutrients

10 World Health Organization (n.d.). Micronutrient deficiencies. Retrieved from http://www.who.int/nutrition/topics/ida.

11 Butler, N. (2015, November 6). Nutritional Deficiencies (Malnutrition). Retrieved from http://www.healthline.com/health/malnutrition.

12 Please see https://www.ncbi.nlm.nih.gov/pubmed/19103324).

13 See https://www.ncbi.nlm.nih.gov/pubmed/20112497.

14 See Journal of American Dietetic Association, 2009.

15 Pomplano-Roger, George D. Encyclopedia of Foods and Their Healing Powers. 2001, Madrid, Spain, Editorial Safeliz, Vol 2 (pages 56, 88, 119-120, 286-287, 288-289).

16 See https://www.ncbi.nlm.nih.gov/pubmed/12452674.

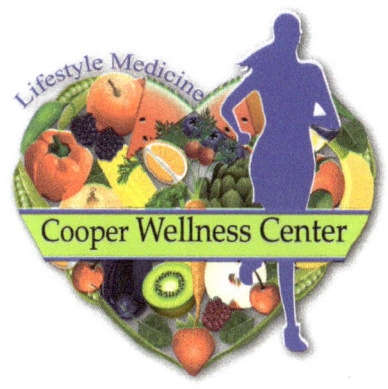

COOPER WELLNESS AND DISEASE PREVENTION CENTER

At the Wellness Center, we focus on patients with diabetes, hypertension, obesity and other chronic diseases who want to decrease medications or reverse diseases through lifestyle modifications.

956.627.3106
3604 N. McColl Rd.
McAllen, TX 78501
CooperWellnessCenter.com

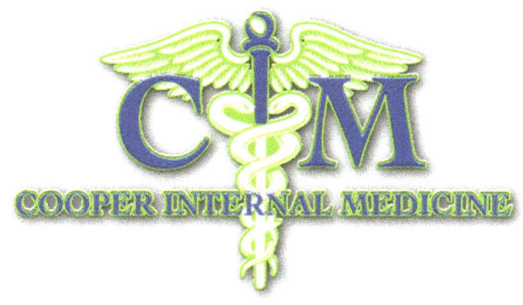

COOPER INTERNAL MEDICINE

956.686.8802	**956.287.9797**
801 E. Nolana, Ste. 12	5411 W. Monte Cristo Rd.
McAllen, TX 78504	Edinburg, TX 78541

CooperInternalMedicine.com

www.ingramcontent.com/pod-product-compliance
Lightning Source LLC
Chambersburg PA
CBHW061125070526
44584CB00033B/4227